DOPE HUNTERS

The Influence of Scientists on the Global Fight against Doping in Sport, 1967-1992

Jörg Krieger

DOPE HUNTERS

The Influence of Scientists on the Global Fight against Doping in Sport, 1967-1992

Jörg Krieger

COMMON GROUND PUBLISHING 2016

First published in 2016 in Champaign, Illinois, USA
by Common Ground Publishing LLC
as part of Sport and Society book series

Library of Congress Cataloging-in-Publication Data

Names: Krieger, Jörg.
Title: Dope hunters : the influence of scientists on the global fight against
  doping in sport, 1967-1992 / Jörg Krieger.
Description: Champaign, Illinois : Common Ground Publishing, 2015. | Includes
  bibliographical references and index. | Description based on print version
  record and CIP data provided by publisher; resource not viewed.
Identifiers: LCCN 2015045088 (print) | LCCN 2015042653 (ebook) | ISBN
  9781612298344 (pbk) | ISBN 9781612298351 (pdf) | ISBN 9781612298344 (pbk :
  alk. paper) | ISBN 9781612298351 (pdf : alk. paper)
Subjects: LCSH: Doping in sports--History. | Athletes--Drug use--History.
Classification: LCC RC1230 (print) | LCC RC1230 .K75 2015 (ebook) | DDC
  362.29/088796--dc23
LC record available at http://lccn.loc.gov/2015045088

Cover image credit: Manfred Donike in his anti-doping laboratory in Cologne. The Institute of Biochemistry, German Sport University Cologne and the Family of Manfred Donike have provided the cover image

From the Institute for Sport History
of the German Sport University Cologne
Head: Univ.-Prof. Dr. Stephan Wassong

Approved dissertation with the title:

**The Contribution of Anti-Doping Laboratory Experts
to the International Olympic Committee´s Fight Against Doping, 1967-1992**

Submitted by Jörg Krieger from Ochsenhausen

in fulfilment of the requirements for the academic degree of

Doktor der Sportwissenschaft

Cologne, 2015.

First Referee:	Univ.-Prof. Dr. Stephan Wassong Institute for Sport History German Sport University Cologne
Second Referee:	Prof. Thomas Hunt, J.D., Ph.D. Department of Kinesiology and Health Education University of Texas at Austin
Chairman of the Examination Board:	Univ.-Prof. Dr. med. Wilhelm Bloch Institute of Cardiology and Sports Medicine German Sport University Cologne
Day of the Oral Exam:	10 July 2015

Table of Contents

LIST OF ABBREVIATIONS

Note: For all abbreviations, the original title is given in the respective language of the country once introduced in the main text. For all other indications, the English title is used.

AMA	American Medical Association
BAWLA	British Amateur Weightlifters Association
BDR	German Cycling Federation (Federal Republic of Germany)
BISp	German Institute for Sports Science (Federal Republic of Germany)
BOA	British Amateur Athletic Association
CDDS	Committee for the Development of Sport (Council of Europe)
CIS	Commonwealth of Independent States
CNOSF	French National Olympic Committee
CoE	Council of Europe
COJO	Organising Committee of the 1976 Montreal Olympic Games
CuLDA	Carl and Liselott Diem-Archive
DLV	German Athletics Association (Federal Republic of Germany)
DOSB	German Olympic Sports Confederation (reunified Germany)
DSHS	German Sport University Cologne (Federal Republic of Germany)
EHSM	Swiss Federal Institute of Sports Magglingen
EPO	Erythropoietin
FEI	International Federation for Equestrian Sports
FIFA	International Football Federation
FIMS	International Federation of Sports Medicine
FINA	International Swimming Federation
FIVB	International Volleyball Association
FMSI	Italian Sport Medicine Federation
FRG	Federal Republic of Germany
GC	Gas Chromatography
GC-MS	Gas Chromatography and Mass Spectrometry
GDR	German Democratic Republic
GLP	Good Laboratory Practice Guide
hCG	Human Chorionic Gonatropin
hGH	Human Growth Hormone
IAAF	International Amateur Athletics Federation
IAF	International Athletic Foundation
IAODC	International Olympic Anti-Doping Committee
IAOMO	International Association of Olympic Medical Officers

ACKNOWLEDGEMENTS

Finishing this book was only possible through tremendous support of many people.

I want to thank my supervisor Stephan Wassong, head of the Institute of Sport History and director of the Olympic Studies Centre of the German Sport University Cologne, in the first place. He has prompted me to conduct this research project, and has become my mentor and friend. He has been motivating, encouraging, and enlightening with his proven expertise in Sport History and Olympic Studies. His patience, flexibility, caring, and faith in me were key to finalising this project. For his long-term support, I am entirely grateful.

My gratitude is extended to Thomas Hunt for his help. He has continuously encouraged me with his motivating words and advised me with his expertise. My thanks goes also to Keith Gilbert for his fantastic support. Without him and Ian Nelk from Common Ground Publishing this work would never have gotten off the ground. I also want to thank Marcel Reinold for sharing his historical sources with me. They contained valuable information that helped me to structure my work. At the International Olympic Committee Library and Archives, it was Sabine Christe, who has supported me continuously. Other people that have to be mentioned are Norbert Müller, Paul Dimeo, Ian Ritchie, Hans Geyer, Jordi Segura, Don H. Catlin, Peter Hemmersbach, Arne Ljungqvist, Derek Casey and Elvira Ramini. Their academic advice and input were greatly appreciated.

I would also like to thank my current and former colleagues at the Institute of Sport History. This accounts especially for Caroline Meier and Ansgar Molzberger, who always had a sympathetic ear for my questions and concerns. But I also want to express my gratitude to Claudia Grote, Kuno Schuch and Ralf Sühl. The student assistants Kersten Hilgers, Sina Schäper, Rory Flindall, Robin Austermann and Nils Mielke were always prepared to help me. Special thanks goes to Hedi Richter, who has shown great understanding for my project and supported me throughout. It is a pleasure to work with you all.

My proofreaders, Liam Kelly, who has also been a great friend and motivator throughout the entire process, and Jennifer Barber, have also contributed a great deal to the improvement of the final version.

I do not want to miss out in thanking my friends for showing much understanding for this lengthy task. They were always there for me when I needed some distraction, especially throughout Karneval. They have encouraged me to pursue my goals and I can consider myself blessed to have such wonderful friends in my life.

My family also played a major role during the time of writing. My parents Sonja and Frank, and their partners Peter and Regina, have supported me throughout the four years of compiling this work. They have taught me about hard work and independence, whilst encouraging me to pursue my dreams. This also applies for my brother Stefan. Finally, the backing through my grandparents Hella and Albert Grad, and Friedhelm and Marlene Krieger, was a key factor during the time of the research project. They were always concerned with my progress and how stressed I might be, whilst showing great interest in my work.

Last, but by no means least, I want to thank my wife Eunkyung. She had to live with the brunt of my stress and had to do without me for a great deal of the time since we are married. However, her love, care, and belief in me were a treasure. I could not have finished this project without her by my side. There are no words that can express my appreciation for all the things she has done for me. It means the world to me that I can share my dreams with her.

CHAPTER 1

Introduction

The history of doping and anti-doping in sport is immense and many researchers with extremely distinctive backgrounds have dedicated parts of their academic life investigating the history of the usage of performance-enhancing drugs.[1] In recent years, research on the matter has increased, caused mainly by the enhanced public attention to the doping problem. This goes as far as that the International Olympic Committee (IOC), representatively its former president Jacques Rogge[2], has labelled the usage of doping one of the most essential and perennial threats for the entire Olympic Movement,[3] and has encouraged and promoted academics to investigate into the issue.[4] Many such projects are of a historical nature in order to obtain a better understanding for the roots of doping and anti-doping.

Researchers dealing with the early usage of performance-enhancing substances have established the most basic foundation for any research on doping

---

[1] Those researchers will be named in this chapter and short overviews on the contents of their contributions will be given in order to draw a picture of the state of research and acknowledge their valuable work.

[2] Chevalier Dr. Jacques Rogge (born 1942) served as the eighth IOC president from 2001 until 2013. A medical doctor with a degree in sports medicine and competitor at the 1968, 1972 and 1976 Olympic Games in the yachting events, he became an IOC member in 1991. Before his presidency, he worked on several IOC commissions, amongst them the IOC Medical Commission from 1992 onwards (see Appendix 3). He was vice-chairman of the IOC Medical Commission from 1994 until 1999. INTERNATIONAL OLYMPIC COMMITTEE, *Biographies of the Members of the International Olympic Committee* (Lausanne: International Olympic Committee, 2009), 90.

[3] Jacques ROGGE, "Foreword," *Olympic Review* 47 (2003), 7.

[4] For example in the period from 2009 to 2011, the IOC Postgraduate Research Grant awarded two grants to research projects dealing with historical research on doping and anti-doping within the Olympic Movement. Kathryn HENNE, "The Origins of the International Olympic Committee Medical Commission and its Technocratic Regime: An Historiographic Investigation of Anti-Doping Regulation and Enforcement in International Sport," *Final Report to the IOC 2009 Postgraduate Research Grant Programme*, submitted December 31, 2009. Marcel REINOLD, "Arguing against doping: a discourse analytical study on Olympic anti-doping between the 1960s and the late 1980s," *Final Report to the IOC 2011 Postgraduate Research Grant Programme*, submitted May 7, 2012.

in sport. They have revealed that athletes have used substances to boost their performances ever since the beginning of any athletic competitions. Doping is therefore not only a phenomenon of modern sport. The word "doping" originates from the South African word "dope," which was used to describe a primitive alcoholic drink that caused a stimulating effect on their natives during ceremonial dances.[5] Wolfgang DECKER, one of the most renowned researchers on the Ancient Olympic Games, claims that methods such as oracles, oneiromancy and magic can be considered as "doping replacements".[6] However, he advances the opinion that these methods have to be distinguished from contemporary doping because the effects were beyond the training and athletic grounds. Thereby, DECKER argues similarly to Egon MARÓTI, who suggests that there was no conscious doping in the careers of Ancient Olympic athletes.[7] The usage of substances to improve performance at the end of the nineteenth century was often a consequence of the interest in the substance itself instead of its actual effect on performance in sport. Paul DIMEO outlines this in his excellent account on the history of drugs use in sport between 1876 and 1976.[8] In England, doping had made its way into the dictionary as early as 1869.[9] John M. HOBERMAN describes how mixtures of opium and narcotics were used to improve the performance of racehorses, but how they were also applied to decrease the performance of an opponent's animal in order to influence betting results.[10] He also claims that the behaviour of medical doctors, such as Dr. Philippe Tissié, to recommend performance-enhancing substances in order to finish the long cycling races at the end of the nineteenth century, is an important reason for doping in sport. Additionally, HOBERMAN considers the wider stimulant use of athletes from the 1920s onwards and suggests that German scientists were at the forefront of sports medicine in the interwar period from 1920 to 1940.[11] This could be seen as an explanation for the appearance of a first German doping definition related to

---

[5] Robert VOY and Kirk D. DEETER, *Drugs, Sports and Politics* (Champaign, Ill: Leisure Press, 1991), 5.

[6] Wolfgang DECKER, *Sport in der griechischen Antike* (Hildesheim: Arete Verlag, 2012), 126ff.

[7] Egon MARÓTI, "Gab es Doping im Altgriechischen Sportleben?" *Acta Classica universitatis scientiarum Debreceniensis* 40/41 (2004/2005), 71.

[8] Paul DIMEO, *A History of Drug Use in Sport 1876-1976* (London: Routledge, 2007), 19f.

[9] Ludwig PROKOP, "Zur Geschichte des Dopings und seiner Bekämpfung," *Sportarzt und Sportmedizin* 21, no. 6 (1970), 126.

[10] John M. HOBERMAN, *Mortal Engines: the Science of Performance and the Dehumanization of Sport* (New York, NY: The Free Press, 1992).

[11] Ibid., 314f.

sport, found in the German encyclopaedia *Beckmanns Sport Lexikon*, published in
1933, which describes doping as the "use of stimulating (performance enhancing)
agents, which shall push the athlete beyond his/her normal limits of
performance".[12] Ludwig PROKOP[13], later amongst the first members of the IOC
Medical Commission, has conducted some of the earliest research on the history
of drug *use* in sport and the early doping incidents such as the swimmers, who
took wide-ranging (supposedly) performance-enhancing substances during the
Amsterdam channel races.[14] The first doping case on the Olympic level occurred
during the marathon race at the 1904 St. Louis Olympic Games, in which the
American Thomas Hicks suffered from the effects of consuming strychnine and
almost died.[15] However, whilst these incidents all took place at the end of the
nineteenth and the beginning of the twentieth century respectively, it is often
forgotten that doping in horseracing was already quite advanced by this time.[16] As
early as 1666, a decree was put into place in Great Britain, which aimed to stop
the usage of performance-enhancing substances in horseracing.[17] John GLEAVES
outlines the first doping concerns by the race-horsing associations in America and
Europe at the end of the nineteenth century and illustrates that these concerns
were triggered by a sense of fair play, in order to create a level playing field for

---

[12] Rudhard K. MÜLLER, "History of Doping and Doping Controls," in: *Doping in Sports*,
ed. Detlef THIEME and Peter HEMMERSBACH (Berlin: Springer, 2010), 15.

[13] Professor Dr. Ludwig Prokop (born 1920) was one of the most influential medical
experts on the IOC Medical Commission in its early years and supported the argument that
testing was needed in order to control the usage of performance-enhancing substances. He
was also president of the International Federation of Sports Medicine (Fédération
Internationale de Médicine Sportive, FIMS) from 1976 until 1980. Ludwig Prokop was
also a successful athlete as he was a former Austrian Champion in swimming, fencing and
modern pentathlon. "Olympic Order," *Olympic Review* 214 (1985), 472.

[14] Ludwig PROKOP, "The struggle against doping and its history," *Journal of Sports
Medicine and Medical Fitness* 10 (1970), 46.

[15] Terry TODD, "A History of the Use of Anabolic Steroids in Sport," in: *Sports and
Exercise Science: Essays in the History of Sports Medicine*, eds. Jack W. BERRYMAN and
Roberta J. PARK (Urbana: University of Illinois Press, 1992), 323.

[16] Jürgen COURT and Wildor HOLLMANN, "Doping," in: *Lexikon der Ethik im Sport*, ed.
Ommo GRUPE and Dietmar MIETH (Schorndorf: Hofmann Verlag, 2001), 98.

[17] E.G.C. CLARKE and M. MOSS, "A Brief History of Dope Detection in Racehorses,"
British Journal of Sports Medicine 10, no. 3 (1976), 100. It has been attempted to list all
first names of the authors of academic publications. However, it was not possible to obtain
all of them, since it is uncommon to list the first names in publications in the natural
sciences and the medical sciences.

the betting public.[18] Neither the athletes nor the public felt the sense of explicit cheating.[19]

Building on the research conducted on the history of performance-enhancing substances in sport, academics have looked into the origins of the first rules and regulations against what sport organisations labelled "doping." It is evident that in the increasingly common use of the word doping in the 1920s and 1930s, one can also find the origins of anti-doping. The Council of the International Amateur Athletics Federation (IAAF)[20] approved the first doping definition by a sport organisation in 1928:

> Doping is the use of any stimulant not normally employed to increase the power of action in athletic competition above the average. Any person knowingly acting or assisting as explained above shall be excluded from any place where the rules are in force or, if he is a competitor, be suspended for a time or otherwise from further participation in amateur athletics under the jurisdiction of his Federation.[21]

Erkki VETTENNIEMI links the introduction of the definition to rumours that distance runners such as Otto Peltzer (Germany), and Paavo Nurmi (Finland), had taken stimulants in order to enhance their performance.[22] The IAAF definition

---

[18] John GLEAVES, "Enhancing the Odds: Horse Racing, Gambling and the First Anti-Doping Movement in Sport, 1889-1911," *Sport in History* 32, no. 1 (2012), 26-52.

[19] Michael KRÜGER, "Doping in Cycling – Comments from the Theory of Civilization Point of View to a Long History," *Sport and Society* 3 (2006), 349. In his article, KRÜGER gives an excellent overview of the history of doping in cycling arguing that sport federations in general and the UCI in particular undertook enormous efforts in order to solve the problem of doping. Against the public opinion, this is specifically the case in cycling although in recent years most doping cases have come from within the sport.

[20] It was only in 2001 that the IAAF Congress unanimously decided to rename its federation in International Association of Athletics Federations.

[21] Minutes, "9th Congress of the IAAF in Amsterdam, July 27 and August 6-7", 1928, archive collection "IAAF Congresses," IAAF Archive, Monaco, 55.

[22] Erkki VETTENNIEMI, "Runners, Rumours, and Reaps of Representations: An Inquiry into Drug Use by Athletes in the 1920s," *Journal of Sport History* 37, no. 3 (2010), 427. In this very interesting study, VETTENNIEMI argues that there is a possibility that the German distance runner Otto Peltzer was faced with drug allegations in 1927, shortly before the IAAF began to discuss rules to forbid the usage of performance-enhancing drugs. Interestingly though, in his homeland Germany, Otto Peltzer has not been brought in relation with doping but is rather remembered as a sporting hero.

only referred to amateur competitions and to the exclusion of athletes who used stimulating substances to enhance their performances during amateur meetings. Doping contradicted the ideal of the amateur that was connected to the health and character education of sport at the time.[23] This educational purpose was not fulfilled if an athlete was a professional.[24] The IOC also advocated the amateur status of athletic competitors at the time and did so until the 1980s. Likewise, Frenchman Baron Pierre De Coubertin, founder of the modern Olympic Movement, was a backer of strict compliance with the amateur rules at the Olympic Games.[25] However, in contrast to the IAAF, the IOC did not react to the early doping developments in the 1920s, in particular in cycling, athletics and football. Ruud STOKVIS reports that Paul Rousseau, member of the French National Olympic Committee (Comité National Olympique et Sportif Français, CNOSF), made the first mention of doping in the Olympic context in a report in 1933.[26] In this report, he referred to drug use at the 1932 Los Angeles Olympic Games, arguing that it was in strong contrast to the ideals of amateur sport. But it was only during the IOC Session in Warsaw in June 1937 that doping made its first appearance on the agenda of the IOC, when the British IOC member Lord

---

[23] John HOLT, *Sport and the British. A Modern History* (Oxford: Oxford University Press, 1989), 74ff.

[24] John GLEAVES, "A Critique of Contemporary Sanctions for Anti-Doping Violations: Changing Directions," in: *Doping and Anti-Doping Policy in Sport: Ethical, Legal and Social Perspectives, eds.* Mike MCNAMEE and Verner MØLLER (New York, NY: Routledge, 2011), 237.

[25] Hart CANTELON, "Amateurism, High-Performance Sport, and the Olympics," in *Global Olympics. Historical and Sociological Studies of the Modern Games*, eds. Kevin YOUNG and Kevin B. WAMSLEY (Bingley: JAI Press, 2007), 86.

[26] Ruud STOKVIS, "Moral Entrepreneurship and Doping Cultures in Sport," (ASSR Working Paper 03/04: 6); http://dare.uva.nl/document/2264 [accessed June 16, 2013].

David Burghley[27] raised the issue[28] According to the minutes of the IOC, he informed the IOC members about the effects of doping, whereupon a Commission was founded to have a closer look at the problem and to present its result on the following IOC Session in Cairo in 1938.[29] The members of the Commission were Avery Brundage[30] (USA), Karl Ritter von Halt[31] (Germany),

---

[27] Lord David Burghley (1905-1981) had joined the IOC in 1933, after successful participation at the Olympic Games in 1924, 1928 and 1932. He won the gold medal in the 400m event at the 1928 Olympic Games in Amsterdam and devoted his sport political activities on the IOC (from 1933 until 1976), the IAAF (from 1947 until 1976) and as president of the British Amateur Athletic Association (BOA) (from 1936 until 1976) to the protection of the amateur rules. "The Biographies of all IOC members, No. 162 David George Lord Burghley," *Journal of Olympic History* 19, no. 2 (2011), 51. He also proved to have sport political ambitions within the IOC. At the 47th IOC Session in Helsinki in 1952, he competed for the IOC presidency against Avery Brundage but lost as he only obtained 17 votes in contrast to Avery Brundage´s 30 votes. After the voting, he was proposed by the Canadian IOC member Sydney Dawes for the position of vice-president of the IOC. However, David Burghley also lost the election for vice-president, this time against the former French fencer Armand Massard by 25 votes to 23. Minutes, "47th Session of the IOC in Helsinki, July 16-27, 1947", archive collection "IOC Sessions 1894-2009," IOC Archive, Lausanne, 4ff.

[28] Minutes, "37th Session of the IOC in Warsaw, June 7-11, 1937", archive collection "IOC Sessions 1894-2009," IOC Archive, Lausanne, 2.

[29] Minutes, "37th Session of the IOC in Warsaw, June 7-11, 1937," 2. During the four days of the Session, organisational issues raised by the National Olympic Committees (NOCs) and the International Federations (IFs), the controversial Worker´s Olympics and the status of the Olympic amateurs were discussed. Pierre de Coubertin, who died only a few months later on September 2, 1937, criticised these kinds of agenda as he was of the opinion that they would not contribute to the development of the Olympic Games and its educational purpose. He had already made this point during the 21st IOC Session in Prague in 1925 when he argued that the IOC would only deal with technical matters and not address the educational importance of the Olympic Movement anymore. On the basis of this, Pierre de Coubertin resigned from the position of the IOC president. Pierre De COUBERTIN, "Speech Given at the Opening of the Olympic Congress at the City Hall of Prague," in: *Olympism. Selected Writings*, ed. Norbert MÜLLER (Lausanne: International Olympic Committee, 1925/2000), 555.

[30] Avery Brundage (1887-1975) was participant in the decathlon event at the 1912 Stockholm Olympic Games. He was president of the Amercian Amateur Athletic Union and became an IOC member in 1936. Already one year later, he was voted onto the IOC Executive Board and became vice-president in 1945. In 1952, Avery Brundage became IOC president and dedicated his presidency (until 1972) to the fight against professionalism and the commercialisation of the Olympic Games. "The Biographies of all IOC members, No. 172 Avery Brundage," *Journal of Olympic History* 19, no. 3 (2011), 57ff.

Alberto Bonacossa[32] (Italy), Sigfrid Edström[33] (Sweden) and David Burghley himself.[34] Although it is not clear how intensive the Commission looked into the problem, a report was presented in Cairo and the IOC decided to publish the following statement regarding the doping problem:

> L'usage des drogues ou des stimulants artificiel [sic] de toutes sortes est des plus condamnables, et toute personne qui reçoit ou offre du doping, sous quelque forme que ce soit, ne devrait pas être admise aux meetings d'amateurs ou aux Jeux Olympiques.
>
> [The use of drugs or artificial stimulants of any kind must be condemned most strongly, and everyone who accepts or offers dope, no matter in what form, should not be allowed to participate in amateur meetings or in the Olympic Games].[35]

---

[31] Karl Ferdinand Ritter von Halt (1891-1964) was a German decathlon champion that had participated at the 1912 Stockholm Olympic Games. From 1931 until 1945, he was the president of the German National Athletics Federation. He was an IOC Executive Board member from 1937 until 1946 and again from 1958 until 1963. "The Biographies of all IOC members, No. 149 Karl Ferdinand Ritter von Halt," *Journal of Olympic History* 19, no. 2 (2011), 45.

[32] Count Alberto Bonacossa (1883-1953), a former Italian champion in tennis and figure skating, was a member of the Organising Committee for the 1924 European Ice Hockey Championships in Milan. In 1932, he became the owner of the Italian sports newspaper *Gazetta dello Sport*. "The Biographies of all IOC members, No. 133 Comte Alberto Bonacossa," *Journal of Olympic History* 19, no. 1 (2011), 65.

[33] Johannes Sigfrid Edström (1870-1864), a business man, was founder of the Swedish National Sports Federation in 1903, and served as its president from 1903 until 1913. He was the vice-president of the Organising Committee of the 1912 Stockholm Olympic Games. He initiated the foundation of the IAAF in 1912, and was the IF's president until 1946, when became IOC president. "The Biographies of all IOC members, No. 99 Johannes Sigfrid Edström," *Journal of Olympic History* 18, no. 3 (2010), 43.

[34] Minutes, 37th Session of the IOC in Warsaw, June 7-11, 1937, archive collection "IOC Sessions 1894-2009," IOC Archive, Lausanne, 8.

[35] Minutes, 38th Session of the IOC in Cairo, March 13-18, 1938, archive collection "IOC Sessions 1894-2009," IOC Archive, Lausanne, 20. The author of this book has already dealt more extensively with this issue previously and published the results in a joint paper in 2013. Jörg KRIEGER and Stephan WASSONG, "Die institutionelle Formierungsphase und das frühe Wirken der Medizinischen Kommission des Internationalen Olympischen Komitees," in *Doping. Kulturwissenschaftlich betrachtet*, eds. Eckhard MEINBERG and Swen KÖRNER (St. Augustin: Academia Verlag, 2013), 101-116.

John GLEAVES and Matthew LLEWELLYN illustrate convincingly that this definition was based on a handwritten note by Avery Brundage.[36] However, the IOC did not pursue the doping issue any further until 1960. Instead, the IOC concentrated on the rebuilding of the Olympic Movement after the Second World War and the continuously developing commercialisation of the Olympic Games.[37] It focused on the issues of legitimising the amateur paragraph, the prohibition of starting money and the participation of professionals in the Olympic competitions more extensively in this period.[38] Doping was a known problematic, but was not yet regarded as endangering the integrity of the IOC and the Olympic Movement. It has been argued that the 1960s marked the real beginning of the international doping fight,[39] even though GLEAVES and LLEWELLYN are entirely correct that rules banning doping existed before.[40] The most noteworthy and lengthy studies on more increased initiatives have been compiled by Thomas M. HUNT,[41] Barrie HOULIHAN,[42] Alison WRYNN,[43] and Rob BEAMISH and Ian RITCHIE,[44] all illustrating that the deaths of the cyclists Knud Jensen at the 1960 Rome Olympic

---

[36] John GLEAVES and Matthew LLEWELLYN, "Sport, Drugs and Amateurism: Tracing the Real Cultural Origins of Anti-Doping Rules in Sport," *The International Journal of the History of Sport* 31, no. 8 (2014), 849.

[37] Robert K. BARNEY, Stephen R. WENN and Scott G. MARTIN, *Selling the Five Rings* (Salt Lake City: University of Utah Press, 2002), 31ff.

[38] Stephan WASSONG, "'Clean Sport:' A Twofold Challenge in the Contemporary History of the Modern Olympic Games," in: *Pathways: Critiques and Discourse in Olympic Research. Ninth International Symposium for Olympic Research*, eds. Robert K. BARNEY, Michael K. HEINE, Kevin B. WAMSLEY and Gordon H. MACDONALD (London, Ontario: International Centre for Olympic Studies, 2008), 86.

[39] Marcel REINOLD, Christian BECKER and Stefan NIELSEN, "Die 1960er Jahre als Formationsphase von modernem Doping und Anti-Doping," *Sportwissenschaft* 42 (2012), 156.

[40] GLEAVES and LLEWELLYN, "Sport," 850.

[41] Thomas M. HUNT, *Drug Games: The International Olympic Committee and the Politics of Doping, 1960-2008* (Austin, TX: University of Texas Press, 2011).

[42] Barrie HOULIHAN, *Dying to Win: Doping in Sport and the Development of Anti-doping Policy* (Strasbourg: Council of Europe Publishing, 1999).

[43] Alison WRYNN, "The Human Factor: Science, Medicine and the International Olympic Committee, 1900–70," *Sport in Society: Cultures, Commerce, Media, Politics* 7, no. 2 (2004), 211-231.

[44] Rob BEAMISH and Ian RITCHIE, *Fastest, Highest, Strongest: A Critique of High-Performance Sport* (London: Routledge, 2007).

Games,[45] and Tom "Tommy" Simpson at the 1967 Tour de France caused the IOC to take doping seriously. The IOC was at the forefront of the international fight against doping from this point onwards. It first established a doping subcommittee in 1961 in cooperation with the International Federation of Sports Medicine (Fédération Internationale de Médicine du Sport, FIMS) and then founded the IOC Medical Commission in 1967. The most significant agent on the political level was Prince Alexandre De Mérode, who headed the IOC Medical Commission from 1967 until his death in 2002.[46] Barrie HOULIHAN, with a focus on the role of the Council of Europe (CoE),[47] concentrates more extensively on the establishment of anti-doping rules since the late 1960s and illustrates the different events and processes that led to the rules and regulations in place today.

It is at this point that a third area of research in the history of doping and anti-doping in sport, namely the history of technical developments, needs to be addressed. It is certainly not new to state that the IOC and the IAAF, along with other sport federations based their first concrete anti-doping initiatives on the testing of forbidden performance-enhancing substances. In fact, this is, despite additional preventive measures, still the case today. Researchers have looked into the development of technical equipment used for doping tests as well. Amongst the most notable are the summaries by Mario THEVIS,[48] Peter HEMMERSBACH[49]

---

[45] Verner MØLLER, "Knud Enemark Jensen's Death During the 1960 Rome Olympics: A Search for Truth?" *Sport in History* 25, no. 3 (2005), 452ff. The diagnosis of the attending doctor as well as the official report of the Danish Olympic Committee state that Knud Jensen's cause of death was a brain injury, caused by a fall from his bike. The fall was triggered by a heatstroke. Dissident from this report, the IOC ascribes Knud Jensen's death the ingestion of amphetamines. Point of reference for this is the examination of Ludwig Prokop. He claims that traces of amphetamines were found during Jensen's autopsy. However, his findings are disputable. Although the Danish team doctor admitted that he gave his athletes ronicol to expand their blood vessels, no amphetamine abuse could be proved. It is, however, suspicious that Ludwig Prokop's documentation is not accessible anymore.

[46] Paul DIMEO, Thomas M. HUNT and Matthew BOWERS, "Saint or Sinner?: A Reconsideration of the Career of Prince Alexandre de Merode, Chair of the International Olympic Committee's Medical Commission, 1967–2002," *The International Journal of the History of Sport* 28, no. 6 (2011), 925-940.

[47] HOULIHAN, *Dying*, 151ff.

[48] Mario THEVIS, *Mass Spectrometry in Sports Drug Testing* (New Jersey: Wiley, 2010). THEVIS gives an outline of the history of MS in general and in sport in particular in the first chapter of his book.

and Rudhard Klaus MÜLLER.[50] They reveal that the first scientific initiatives lie even further in the past than the first definitions of the IAAF and the IOC. These first efforts were made in equestrian sport and the Polish pharmacist Alfred Bukowski invented the first doping tests in 1910. Thus, he is regarded as the "pioneer of anti-doping research" from a technical perspective.[51] Alfred Bukowski developed a set of procedures for sample collection and his own analytical method to detect alkaloids in horse saliva. Concrete anti-doping initiatives have therefore their origin in the inaugural inventions of a pharmacist, who started to develop methods to detect substances with extrinsic properties in urine. It was a sports club – the Warsaw Jockey Club – which was dissatisfied with the problem of doping and requested for help.[52] Later in 1910, the Budapest Jockey Club and the Vienna Jockey Club also approached Alfred Bukowski to present his method, and then adopted his testing procedures.[53] Since Alfred Bukowski´s first attempts to detect performance-enhancing substances in bodily fluids, the testing methods have advanced considerably. In his excellent book on mass spectrometry (MS) in sports drug testing, THEVIS dedicates his entire first chapter to explain the developments concerning MS as detector of prohibited substances in gas chromatography (GC). He stresses that initial efforts were individual initiatives without cooperation between different institutions.[54] Only a few different methods and procedures were developed between 1930 and 1960 that were solely used for the testing of drugs in sports which is understandable considering the lack of interest in the matter by sports organisations. First applications with paper chromatography were later replaced by thin-layer

---

[49] Peter HEMMERSBACH, "History of Mass Spectrometry at the Olympic Games," *Journal of Mass Spectrometry* 43 (2008), 839-853. HEMMERSBACH is solely looking at the usage of mass spectrometry at the Olympic Summer and Winter Games. His research is based on personal correspondence with the heads of the respective laboratories and the Official Reports compiled by the respective Organising Committees.

[50] MÜLLER, "History," 1-18.

[51] Andrzej POKRYWKA, Damian GORCZYCA, Anna JAREK and Dorota KWIATKOWSKA, "In memory of Alfons Bukowski on the centenary of anti-doping research," *Drug Testing Analysis* 2, no. 11/12 (2010), 540.

[52] Ibid.

[53] However, THEVIS reports that Alfred Bukowski never disclosed any details about his method, which led to some of the Jockey Clubs turning to other scientists about the development of similar testing procedures. Professor Dr. Sigmund Fränkel from the University of Vienna got involved and his developed methods based on the Sats-Otto process were later published by the chief chemist for the Jockey Club of England. THEVIS, *Mass Spectrometry*, 4.

[54] Ibid., 10.

chromatography (TLC), used primarily for the detection of morphine-related narcotics, amphetamines and diuretics.[55] At the end of the 1950s, the possibility to separate compounds through GC was realised. This achievement can be attributed to several research teams, but it is notable that Arnold Beckett from the King's College London (KCL) led the subsequent development of GC.[56] In 1969, Manfred Donike successfully synthesised N-Methyl-N-trimethylsilyl-trifluoracetamid on which the doping controls at the 1972 Munich Olympic Games were based.[57] In his excellent overview on the historical development of MS at the Olympic Games, HEMMERSBACH focuses on these tests, claiming, "many elements of doping analysis that are still important requirements for an Olympic laboratory were already introduced in 1972."[58] This shows significant links between the laboratories and the scientific developments made over 50 years ago and the methods and laboratories used by the World Anti-Doping Agency (WADA) today.

Previously undertaken historical research has been essential as the first step to reveal the truth about the historical situation on doping and anti-doping in sport. However, it also reveals gaps in research. In particular, how individuals with a scientific background have cooperated, interacted and set up a network to support the global fight against doping, based on their scientific expertise, has been largely neglected so far. This neglect is despite that the former head of WADA and former IOC vice-president Richard W. POUND[59] considers their impact as immense.[60] DIMEO has noted the lack of research on this matter. He contends, "the role of scientists is the great omission in the current historiography

---

[55] THEVIS, *Mass Spectrometry,* 11.

[56] Arnold H. BECKETT and M. ROWLAND, "Determination and identification of amphetamine in urine," *Journal of Pharmacy and Pharmacology* 17, no. 1 (1965), 59-60.

[57] Manfred DONIKE, "N-Methyl-N-trimethylsilyl-trifluoracetamide, ein neues Silylierungsmittel aus der Reihe der silylierten Amide," *Journal of Chromatography* 42 (1969), 103-104.

[58] HEMMERSBACH, "History," 841.

[59] Richard W. Pound (born 1942) is a Canadian lawyer and former world-class swimmer, who competed at the 1960 Rome Olympic Games and finished in 6th place. Following his sporting career, he became president of the Canadian Olympic Committee in 1977, a position he held until 1982, and an IOC member in 1978. He was a member of the IOC Executive Board from 1983 until 1991 and from 1992 until 1996. In the periods between 1987 and 1991, and 1996 until 2000, he was vice-president of the IOC. In 1999, he became the first president of the newly founded WADA. INTERNATIONAL OLYMPIC COMMITTEE, *Biographies,* 86.

[60] Richard W. POUND, *Inside the Olympics. A Behind-The-Scene Look at the Politics. The Scandals, and the Glory of the Games* (Toronto: Wiley, 2004), 75.

of doping and anti-doping."[61]Notably, the studies and books compiled following the publication of DIMEO's book in 2007 did not focus on this issue either. Rather, they tend to analyse the history of anti-doping from the multi-layered sport political perspectives similar to previous research. For example, whereas such very informative research papers as the one by Marcel REINOLD et al., which have been written in the context of the publicly funded research project on doping in the Federal Republic of Germany (FRG),[62] do take into consideration important agents situated within science, they do not give an in-depth analysis of their influence on the international level. This leads the research group to conclude that the history of anti-doping has to become more differentiated by focusing on specific aspects of the national and international fight against doping.[63] Alanah KAZLAUSKAS and Kathryn CRAWFORD explore the community of scientists and the contribution of the annual meetings of experts in the field of doping analysis to the work in accredited doping laboratories. In one of their papers, KAZLAUSKAS, who is the wife of the head of the Sydney anti-doping

---

[61] DIMEO, *A History*, 104.

[62] REINOLD, BECKER and NIELSEN, "Die 1960er Jahre". The German Institut for Sports Science (BISp) and the German Olympic Sports Confederation (DOSB) have funded the research project "Doping in Germany from 1950 until today from a historio-sociological perspective in the context of ethical legitimation" in 2009. The aim of the study was to implicitly rework and systemize the doping phenomena in the FRG. Two project groups from the University of Münster and the Humboldt-University Berlin investigated the issue until 2013.

[63] Michael KRÜGER, Christian BECKER, Stefan NIELSEN and Marcel REINOLD, *Doping und Anti-Doping in der Bundesrepublik Deutschland 1850 bis 2007* (Hildesheim: Arete, 2014), 25. This is also true for the publications of another German research group based at the Humboldt University of Berlin since it concentrates on the national level and investigates the usage of drugs by athletes and medical doctors from the FRG. Giselher SPITZER, Erik EGGERS, Holger J. SCHNELL and Yasmin WISNIEWSKA, *Siegen um Jeden Preis. Doping in Deutschland: Geschichte, Recht, Ethik 1972-1990.* (Cologne: Verlag Die Werkstatt, 2013), 409ff. In their final chapter "Desiderata", the authors separate the research fields in which they see the need for further studies in two categories: 1) Substantial questions and further doping methods and substances 2) doping analysis. It is argued that these two areas could not have been researched into depth as the decision was made to focus firstly on the dealings with doping in the FRG until 1977 and secondly on the research study "Regeneration and testosterone (1986-1993)" by the German Federal Institute for Sports Science.

laboratory Professor Dr. Rymantas "Ray" Kazlauskas [64], and CRAWFORD, conclude that the "co-configuration of knowledge mobilisation," advance the everyday laboratory practice. [65] However, whilst looking at the knowledge exchanges of the scientists, the work does not take into account the historical perspective, and does not address the interexchange between the scientific level and sports organisations such as the IOC. Barrie HOULIHAN´s groundbreaking book *Dying to Win* on the history of anti-doping policy does contribute to aspects of the scientific impact. He touches upon the accreditation of the international anti-doping laboratories without detailing how the institutions and heads of anti-doping laboratories cooperated with each other. [66] This is also true for other articles by HOULIHAN, in which he attempts to examine the influence of a group of scientists and doctors on the global fight against doping. He maintains that they "lack a prominent forum (...), the additional resources, such as organisational capacity, money and, to an extent, legitimacy, necessary for an effective intervention in policy debates."[67] Consequently, he concludes that the anti-doping network has failed to incorporate the scientific expertise.

In view of the missing historical research on the role of science and scientists in international anti-doping activities, this book leaves the focus on the political dimension and centres its analysis on the key agents and institutions from within the scientific world. It explores the formative processes that led to networks of scientists working together to support global anti-doping efforts through their professional competencies in doping analysis. With this divergent approach, it adds another perspective to the history of anti-doping in sport and outlines that anti-doping strategies went through extremely distinctive phases in which the decision-making bodies had variously informed knowledge about the scientific

---

[64] Professor Dr. Rymantas "Ray" Kazlauskas (born 1946) had obtained a Ph.D. in organic chemistry from the University of Sydney in 1972. After working at the Department of Pharmacology at the University of Sydney from 1982 until 1986, he joined the Australian National Measurement Institute and became the director of its anti-doping laboratory in Sydney in 1988. He retired from this position at the end of 2011.

[65] Alanah KAZLAUSKAS and Kathryn CRAWFORD, "The Contribution of a Community Event to Expert Work: an Activity Theoretical Perspective," *Outlines. Crtitical Pracice Studies* 6, no. 2 (2004), 74.

[66] HOULIHAN, *Dying*, 147ff.

[67] Barrie HOULIHAN, "Anti-Doping Policy in Sport: The Politics of International Policy Co-ordination," *Public Administration* 2 (1999), 332. Also see: Barrie HOULIHAN, "Building an international regime to combat doping in sport," in *Sports and International Relations. An emerging relationship*, eds. Roger LEVERMORE and Adrian BUDD (New York, NY: Routledge, 2004), 68.

dimensions of anti-doping. Hence, this book explores from a historical perspective, the contribution of scientists to the global fight against doping. The processes in which those agents but also their institutions and organisations were involved within anti-doping are described, analysed and discussed. It is outlined, examined and argued how these experts cooperated with each other in order to establish a science-oriented anti-doping network. This book demonstrates how they were involved on the political level and how they have influenced decision-making processes, in particular by the IOC and the IAAF, through their expertise in the field of doping analysis in different periods. Thereby, it is important to consider that the pivotal figures were closely linked to the IOC Medical Commission and various related anti-doping bodies. Consequently, this book is also an enquiry into the IOC body, even though it differs extensively from previous undertaken research on the IOC Medical Commission, because it looks at the personnel alterations and emphasises individual efforts and accomplishments from the group of influential scientists.

It is necessary to characterise which distinctive scientific fields are explored. This is not only vital for the understanding of the undertaken approach in this book, but also to distinguish between different fields of expertise necessary to legitimate and to conduct an anti-doping policy based predominantly on doping testing. Furthermore, it also allows avoiding generalisations about different fields of scientific expertise and consequently attempts to circumvent drawing hasty conclusions. Past historical research on doping appears to have overlooked not only the role of science in anti-doping but that experts from the medical sciences, which predominantly deal with the health of the athletes, need to be distinguished from experts in doping analysis. This distinction is inevitable if one considers the influence of science on the fight against doping and the distinction is deemed essential in order to conduct an in-depth analysis into the topic. When taking the historical perspective into account, this becomes clearly apparent. Other research has shown that medical doctors experimented with athletes to investigate into the performance-enhancing effects of specific substances from the late nineteenth century onwards, and many had considered the usage of artificial drugs as dangerous for one´s health.[68] In fact, according to Ivan WADDINGTON, support to improve athletic performance has become an integral aspect of sport medicine

---

[68] HOBERMAN, *Mortal*, 126ff. Also see: Vanessa HEGGIE, "Volunteers for Science: Medicine, Health and the Modern Olympic Games," in Vivienne LO, *Perfect Bodies Sports Medicine and Immortality* (London: The British Museum, 2012), 97-109.

specialists' recent history.[69] In contrast to medicine's long-lasting involvement, experts dealing with the detection of substances in bodily fluids have been less involved in sport until doping controls had been established in the mid-1960s. Only then, they were needed to develop scientific techniques to detect performance-enhancing substances.

Besides the important distinction between sport medicine specialists and professionals working in doping analysis, sciences and scientific actors are not defined via clearly divided classifications of scientific disciplines in this book. Instead, it adopts Karin KNORR CETINA's concept to work with knowledge-related cultures.[70] KNORR CETINA claims that although science and expert systems are clear candidates to be put into different categories, "one needs to magnify the space of knowledge-in-action, rather than simply observe disciplines or specialities in organising structures."[71] In order to do so, she introduces the term "epistemic culture" and distinguishes between different settings of knowledge production. Her approach has the advantage that not only single fields of knowledge but complete contexts of expert work can be taken into consideration. KNORR CETINA thereby argues along the similar lines of Peter HAAS, who states that epistemic communities in policy also often come from a number of different disciplines and are "networks of knowledge-based communities with an authorative claim to policy-relevant knowledge within their domain of expertise."[72] In this way, communities attempt to support decision-makers and provide them with solutions and ideas whilst at the same time advancing their own expertise and their status.[73] Accordingly, this book tries to extend parts of HOULIHAN's investigations, in which he includes the group of scientists and doctors as stakeholder within his networks of anti-doping policy.[74] He reduces the

---

[69] Ivan WADDINGTON, "The Development of Sports Medicine," *Sociology of Sport Journal* 13 (1996), 186.

[70] Karin KNORR CETINA, *Epistemic Cultures: How the sciences make knowledge* (Cambridge, MA: Harvard University Press, 1999).

[71] Ibid., 3.

[72] Peter HAAS, "Epistemic communities," in: *International encyclopedia of political science*, eds. Bertrand BADIE, Dirk BERG-SCHLOSSER and Leonardo MORLINO (Thousand Oaks, CA: SAGE Publications, 2011), 787f.

[73] Alanah KAZLAUSKAS and Kathryn CRAWFORD in their study on the support of scientific experts to the fight against doping adopt the term "Communities of Practice". Alanah KAZLAUSKAS and Kathryn CRAWFORD, "Understanding International Scientific Expert Work," in *Recent Advances in Doping Analysis (11)*, ed. Wilhelm SCHÄNZER, Hans GEYER, Andrea GOTZMANN and Ute MARECK-ENGELKE (Cologne: Sportverlag Strauß, 2003), 253.

[74] HOULIHAN, "Anti-Doping Policy," 319 and 325..

involvement of this group in the period from the mid-1960s to the late 1980s to the early awareness of steroid use by the American Dr. John Ziegler,[75] and claims for the following period until today that "doctors, scientists and doping control officers" were marginalised within policy debates.[76] However, he does not specify the group nor does he outline their historical involvement or their role in the transformation of the Olympic doping fight. It is at this point that this publication ties in with, and attempts to investigate whether these arguments can be supported from a sport historical perspective through a more in-depth analysis.

Against the background of these theoretical considerations, the main experts under investigation are summarised under the term "anti-doping laboratory experts" and exclude sport medical specialists. This allows a conduction of more elaborate research on this particular knowledge culture of anti-doping laboratory experts rather than mixing up various scientific disciplines. The anti-doping laboratory experts are the centre of the investigation. This allows a discussion of their involvement on important anti-doping commissions and in decision-making processes. However, an attempt is made to examine their role from within, from the perspective of science. In this context, it is important to emphasise that the term "political" as used in this book refers to the decision-making level within sport.

The in-depth investigation into the inter-personal relationships of the anti-doping laboratory experts allows conclusions that go beyond the profile change of Olympic anti-doping. The focus on those dealing with doping analysis highlights power shifts within the inner circle of leading anti-doping laboratory experts. This is important, because it gives relevant information on how and why the controlling bodies made fundamental decisions, and hence steered the anti-doping

---

[75] John B. Ziegler played a crucial role in the early history of doping in sport. He was the team doctor of the American weightlifting team and accompanied them to the 1954 World Weightlifting Championships in Vienna. There, he was told by a Soviet doctor that the Soviet athletes were using the growth hormone testosterone in order to improve their performances. Apparently, he had not known about the effects of testosterone at the time. Bob GOLDMAN, Ronald KLATZ and Patricia J. BUSH, *Death in the Locker Room* (South Bend, IN: Icarus Press, 1984). However, DIMEO does not agree with this construction of the story and argues that the Americans had previously known about testosterone and its usage in the Second World War and were dissatisfied that American athletes were underperforming despite using the drug. DIMEO, *A History*, 72ff. In his book, DIMEO mainly draws on the historical research of John FAIR, which he published in 1993. John D. FAIR, "Isometrics or Steroids? Exploring New Frontiers of Strength in the Early 1960s," *Journal of Sport History* 20, no. 1 (1993): 1-24.

[76] HOULIHAN, "Anti-Doping Policy," 329.

efforts in a certain direction based on the knowledge and influence of anti-doping laboratory experts. Due to the numerous involved individuals and the multiplicity of institutions with little orthographical differences, particular attention is paid to granularity. Footnotes provide additional background information on people who reappear in various parts, as well as on all IOC members and IOC Medical Commission members.[77] Key figures – in particular the most relevant anti-doping laboratory experts – are introduced in the main text. In addition, to allow a clear understanding, all persons are labelled with their forename and surname.

Clearly, investigating in-depth into the history of the establishment of an anti-doping laboratory expert network to support global anti-doping efforts is impossible without briefly sketching the earlier developments in drug detection techniques, the early interest of sport medicine specialists in doping and the passive approach to combat doping by sport organisations. These three streams came together in the 1960s and therefore, the investigation of this book begins with the preparation phase for the doping controls at the 1968 Winter Olympic Games in Grenoble. From this point onwards, competencies in doping analysis became relevant for the IOC.[78] The processes of anti-doping laboratory experts' involvement are explored until the immediate aftermath of the 1992 Barcelona Olympic Games. This endpoint can be justified with the citation of three arguments. First, the book predominantly explores the individual-related contributions of anti-doping laboratory experts. In this context, the preliminary investigations revealed that Arnold Beckett and Manfred Donike were the key figures within this group. Significantly, the 1992 Barcelona Olympic Games were the last Summer Olympic Games at which both of them participated as members of the IOC Medical Commission. Second, the consulted archival material decreases considerably in the beginning of the 1990s, mainly due to legally fixed embargo regulations. Third, the inspection of a longer period would have resulted in significant issues in terms of feasibility.

The knowledge acquisition was affected by means of a hermeneutical analysis. Hermeneutics is the method or theory of the interpretation of texts.[79]

---

[77] In the majority of cases, the sources for the bibliographical data have been listed in the footnote. If this is not the case, the data stems from the archival sources.

[78] Jörg KRIEGER and Stephan WASSONG, "Munich 1972: Turning Point in the Olympic Doping Control System," in: *Problems, Possibilities, Promising Practices* (Proceedings of the 11th International Symposium for Olympic Research), eds. Janice FORSYTH and Michael HEINE (London, Ontario: University of Western Ontario, 2012).

[79] Judy PEARSALL, ed., *The new Oxford Dictionary of English* (Oxford: Clarendon Press, 1999), 858.

Martin HEIDEGGER's attempts to justify that the aim of epistemology is hermeneutical as it tries to distribute an interpretation of "Dasein [Being there],"[80] are essential for the understanding of a hermeneutic analysis. Accordingly, he claims that every interpretation is based on historically embedded ways of thinking which needs to be open for revision and enhancement.[81] In this way, it is emphasised that within Hermeneutics it is necessary to move from the whole to the specific and reverse. This systematic interpretation process, HEIDEGGER labels the hermeneutic circle.[82] Its basic assumption is that the original evidence of the truth is the starting point for the circle. Only if this is given, one is in a position to further expand the truth and therefore encourage the way of understanding and interpretation. Hans-Georg GADAMER established the understanding of a text on a historical pre-knowledge, which is changed through a re-evaluation and eventually leads to a modified comprehension.[83] He refers to this concept as "wirkungsgeschichtliches Bewusstsein [historically affected consciousness],"[84] and criticises historians who believe that their understanding is based on some kind of objectivity. He claims that one has to acknowledge the impact of historical pre-knowledge.[85] A hermeneutic analysis, as applied within this research, is therefore a constant interaction between the limits of past understandings and new insights. Consequently, the leading thought is that all explicit knowledge is based upon the pre-knowledge and can never been seen entirely as independent from it.[86] For this book, the pre-knowledge has been gained through the in-depth analysis of the literature available. Continuous reference to past research is made throughout. The regress onto the previously introduced literature enables the communication process with the pre-knowledge and is used to build new knowledge on its foundation. Additionally, the pre-knowledge is enhanced through the consultation of new sources and a new perspective. Therefore, the indention into the history of reception is achieved.[87] In accordance with GADAMER, understanding the truth within this research is thereby an intervention into the previous ways of transmission. Consequently, the hermeneutic circle is not only applied as a methodological tool but also even

[80] Martin HEIDEGGER, *Sein und Zeit* (16th ed.) (Tübingen: Max Niemeyer, 1986), 11.
[81] Ibid., 151.
[82] Ibid., 153.
[83] Hans-Georg GADAMER, *Truth and method* (2nd ed.) (New York, NY: The Crossroad Publishing Corporation, 1989), 300.
[84] Ibid., 274f.
[85] Karen JOISTEN, *Philosophische Hermeneutik* (Berlin: Akademie Verlag, 2009), 145.
[86] Matthias JUNG, *Hermeneutik zur Einführung* (Hamburg: Junius Verlag, 2001), 115.
[87] GADAMER, *Truth*, 274f.

more as "ein ontologisches Strukturmoment des Verstehens [an ontological structural element for understanding]."[88]

The documents that underwent the hermeneutical analysis and allowed addressing the above-stated research topic were written sources, acquired from various national and international archives. It was necessary to focus on sources in written form in order to base the undertaken research on an assured state of facts. It was possible to do this because the history of anti-doping is well documented in official protocols, reports and other written correspondences found in the conducted archives. The comparison of varying sources from different archives allowed a verification of the documents and enabled the researcher to examine facts and circumstances from multiple perspectives instead of conducting a one-dimensional and possibly preoccupied analysis. Three archives proved to be most useful. First, the IOC Library and Archives in Lausanne, at which the complete collections of the minutes of the IOC Sessions from 1894 to 2010, and the minutes of the IOC Executive Board from 1921 to 1975 are available, were viewed. Moreover, at the IOC archive, the researcher examined all the historical material on the IOC Medical Commission from 1967 until 1995. It was possible to obtain an exceptional authorisation for all the minutes and protocols of the IOC Medical Commission until 1995. It is the first time that these documents could be used to reveal historical processes in the IOC's fight against doping. Second, the IAAF Archive in Monaco made the minutes of the IAAF Council and the IAAF Congress available to the researcher. Documents on the IAAF Medical Committee such as minutes of meetings and various reports to the IAAF Congress could also be obtained. Third, the Carl and Liselott Diem-Archive (Carl und Liselott Diem-Archiv, CuLDA) at the DSHS was accessed to retrieve important information on the IAAF Council, the Cologne anti-doping laboratory and the role of Manfred Donike. In particular, the documents from the estate of the former director of the FRG's Institute for Sports Science

---

[88] Ibid., 277.

(Bundesinstitut für Sportwissenschaft, BISp), Professor Dr. August Kirsch[89], proved to be valuable in this regard. A detailed inventory for this archival collection exists.[90] Moreover, the German Federal Archives in Berlin-Lichterfelde and the KCL Archives & Special Collections in London provided valuable material.

Finally, material examined at the private archives of Professor Dr. Don H. Catlin[91] in Los Angeles, and Professor Dr. Jordi Segura[92] in Barcelona, was an extremely useful addition to the official archives. Both professors were contacted to try to gain information through oral interviews with contemporary witnesses, such as anti-doping laboratory experts and international anti-doping policy makers. Thereby, the research tried to consider Eckhard MEINBERG's argumentation that the possibilities and the practices of hermeneutical analysis go beyond the mere interpretation of texts.[93] According to MEINBERG, it is important that the indention into the history of reception is enhanced through the inclusion

---

[89] Professor Dr. August Kirsch (1925-1993) was director of the German FRG's Institute for Sports Science from 1973 until 1990. He was also president of the German Athletics Association from 1970 until 1985, IAAF Council member from 1975 until 1993 and vice-president of the FRG's National Olympic Committee from 1977. Between 1983 and 1990 August Kirsch was president of the International Council of Sport Science and Physical Education (ICSSPE). Ansgar MOLZBERGER, Caroline MEIER, Stephan WASSONG, Heike SCHIFFER and Ute GÖßNITZER, *Abgestaubt und Neu Erforschbar* (Cologne: Sportverlag Strauß, 2014), 246. This publication gives an overview of the archival collections of the DSHS and is part of a project at the Institute of Sport History of the DSHS that aims to professionalise the archival strategies of the DSHS.

[90] CARL UND LISELOTT DIEM ARCHIV, ed., *Nachlaß August Kirsch* (Aachen: Verlag Mainz, 1998).

[91] Professor Dr. Don H. Catlin (born 1938) became a member of the IOC Medical Commission in 1989. He is a medical doctor and was head of the IOC accredited anti-doping laboratory at the UCLA. For his contribution to the IOC's fight against doping until 1992 and his professional background, see Chapters 6 and 7. INTERNATIONAL OLYMPIC COMMITTEE, *Commission Médicale du C.I.O.* (Lausanne: International Olympic Committee, 1994), 18.

[92] Professor Dr. Jordi Segura (born 1949) became a member of the IOC Medical Commission in 1991. He is a chemical engineer and was head of the IOC accredited anti-doping laboratory in Barcelona. For his contribution to the IOC's fight against doping until 1992, see Chapter 6 and 7. INTERNATIONAL OLYMPIC COMMITTEE, *Commission Médicale*, 18.

[93] Eckhard MEINBERG, "Hermeneutische Methodik," in: *Zwischen Verstehen und Beschreiben. Forschungsmethodologische Ansätze in der Sportwissenschaft*, eds. Karl-Heinrich BETTE, Gerd HOFFMANN, Carsten KRUSE, Eckhard MEINBERG and Jörg THIELE (Köln: Bundesinstitut für Sportwissenschaft, 1993), 63.

of the experiences of contemporary witnesses. By employing a relatively open, yet pre-structured, interview guideline, such recommendations were followed to try to get as close as possible to the world of experience of the interviewed person. However, as in the study undertaken by KRÜGER et al., the first interviews resulted in the finding that only a few new insights could be discovered.[94] On the contrary, the analysed written sources presented the researcher much more detail that the contemporary witnesses could not provide. Moreover, it was the aim of this book to provide an academic and objective account of the involvement of anti-doping laboratory experts, but the interviews with the contemporary witnesses showed that one could not categorise their statements as "objective." Therefore, the hermeneutics of texts was the only analytical tool used within this book. Few statements of Don Catlin and Jordi Segura have been included to highlight key points that have resulted from the historical document analysis, but they were never the only source of information.

---

[94] KRÜGER et al., *Doping und Anti-Doping*, 17ff.

CHAPTER 2

Establishing Preconditions (until 1967)

EARLY EFFORTS OF SPORT MEDICINE AND ANTI-DOPING IN THE
OLYMPIC MOVEMENT

The involvement of medical doctors within the Olympic Movement goes back to
the beginning of the twentieth century.[1] The German Dr. Arthur MALLWITZ's[2]
dissertation entitled "Körperliche Höchstleistungen mit besonderer
Berücksichtigung des Olympischen Sportes [Physical high performance with
special attention to the Olympic sport]" (1908) surely must have been one of the
first medical studies conducted on Olympic athletes.[3] MALLWITZ had undertaken
his experiments at the 1906 Intercalated Olympic Games in Athens.[4] John A.
LUCAS gives an excellent detailed account of the first gathering of sport scientists

---

[1] It is not attempted to give a complete detailed overview on the history of the involvement
of sport medicine in the Olympic Movement. For a comprehensive summary, see: HEGGIE,
"Volunteers." Furthermore, also see the works of Roberta J. PARK. Some of her most
notable writings have been published in: James A. MANGAN and Patricia VERTINSKY, eds.,
Gender, Sport, Science. Selected Writings of Roberta J. Park (Abingdon: Routledge,
2009).

[2] Dr. Arthur Mallwitz (1880-1968) was appointed the first official sport medicine specialist
by the Committee of the German Reich for Scientific Research on Sport and Physical
Activity, which is considered to be the first sport medical organisation in the world, in
1913. For a concise historical review of organised sport medicine, see the chapter "Zur
Entwicklung der organisierten Sportmedizin," in: Wildor HOLLMANN and Heiko K.
STRÜDER, *Sportmedizin. Grundlagen für körperliche Aktivität, Training und
Präventivmedizin* (Stuttgart: Schattauer, 2009), 659ff.

[3] Arthur MALLWITZ, *Körperliche Höchstleistungen mit besonderer Berücksichtigung des
Olympischen Sports*, Dissertation (Halle an der Saale, 1908).

[4] Until today, the 1906 Athens Olympic Games are not officially recognised by the IOC.
They have their origin in the dispute between Pierre De Coubertin and the Greek, who
developed the plan to host the Modern Olympic Games permanently in Athens after the
successful Games in 1896. Karl LENNARTZ, "The 2nd International Olympic Games in
Athens 1906," *Journal of Olympic History* 10 (2001/2002), 10-27.

and medical doctors at the 1904 St. Louis Olympic Games.[5] These Olympic Games were incorporated into the Louisiana Purchase Celebration and Universal Exposition, involving a world fair, an athletic competition for the youth, the Olympic Games and scientific-educational-cultural symposia. LUCAS argues that the latter part, the "Olympic Lecture Course," was the beginning of physical education science.[6] Bill MALLON lists the different lectures given and shows that the participants discussed medical topics.[7] In 1913, Pierre De Coubertin organised an Olympic Congress entitled "Psychology and Physiology of Sports."[8] However, because Pierre de Coubertin felt threatened by the criticism of medical experts that excessive training would lead to health problems, he drew the attention to more psychological questions. Interestingly, Arthur Mallwitz attended the Congress as German representative.[9] Alison WRYNN reports that the potential of science, medicine and the Olympic Games was first realised at the 1928 Winter Olympic Games in St. Moritz, where a Medical-Scientific Congress was organised in the St. Moritz City Hall.[10] At the Congress, the FIMS was founded.[11] The general secretary of the Swiss Olympic Committee, Dr. Francis-Marius

---

[5] John A. LUCAS, "The Great Gathering of Sport Scientists: The 1904 St. Louis Olympic Games Exposition Fair Physical Education Lecturers," *Journal of Olympic History* 12, no. 1 (2002), 6-12.

[6] Ibid., 12.

[7] Bill MALLON, *The 1904 Olympic Games. Results for All Competitors in All Events, with Commentary* (Jefferson, Carolina: McFarland, 1999), 32.

[8] MÜLLER, *Olympism*, 449. It is also emphasised that the term "sports psychology" is not used by Pierre de Coubertin as we understand it today. For him "sports psychology" rather deals with his concept of the Pédagogie Sportive. Already at the Olympic Congress in Le Havre in 1897, Pierre de Coubertin had put a focus on this issue. Norbert MÜLLER, *One Hundred Years of Olympic Congresses 1894-1994* (Lausanne: International Olympic Committee, 1994), 49.

[9] Arthur MALLWITZ, "25 Jahre sportärztlicher Forschung," in: *Sportmedizin und Olympische Spiele 1936. Festschrift der Sportärzteschaft*, ed. Arthur MALLWITZ (Leipzig: Verlag Georg Thieme, 1936), 15.

[10] WRYNN, "The Human Factor," 213.

[11] The FIMS was founded under the name "Association Internationale Médico-Sportive" and changed its name to FIMS in 1934. Its first president was Professor Dr. Wilhelm Knoll. Kurt TITTEL and Howard G. KNUTTGEN, "The development, objectives and activities of the International Federation of Sports Medicine (FIMS)," in: *The Olympic Book of Sports Medicine*, eds. Albert DIRIX, Howard G. KNUTTGEN and Kurt TITTEL (Oxford: Blackwell, 1988), 7.

Messerli[12], who was a close friend of Pierre De Coubertin, had proposed the foundation.[13] Francis-Marius Messerli was a medical doctor himself and at the time occupied the position of the City of Lausanne's head doctor of health, whilst at the same time teaching at the Medical Faculty of the University of Lausanne. As he writes in a letter to the IOC about the organisation of the congress during the 1928 Winter Olympic Games in St. Moritz, the students of the Olympic Institute[14] were already subject to medical controls in 1917 and medical controls were discussed at the eighth Olympic Congress in Prague in 1925.[15] The Swiss NOC had already made an approach to conduct medical controls at the 1924 Paris Olympic Games. Ahead of the 1936 Winter Olympic Games in Garmisch-Partenkirchen, it was again Arthur Mallwitz who edited an informative publication on the involvement of sport medicine and the Olympic Games.[16] At the 1936 Berlin Olympic Games international sport medicine specialists

---

[12] Dr. Francis-Marius Messerli (1888-1975) was appointed by Pierre de Coubertin as the executor of his estate. They met for the first time, when Pierre de Coubertin visited a gymnasium in Lausanne in 1908. He was also the chair of the Greco-Swiss Friendship Association of Lausanne where Pierre de Coubertin participated actively. Francis-Marius Messerli was the director of the International Bureau of Sports Pedagogy after the death of Pierre de Coubertin and organised two congresses on sports pedagogy in Lausanne in 1944 and 1948. In 1946, he became the historian of the IOC and wrote several books on the history of medicine and the Olympic Games. Norbert MÜLLER, ed., *Olympism. Selected Writings* (Lausanne: International Olympic Committee, 2000), 248f. Also see: "The 80 years of Dr. Messerli. Ardent Disciple of Coubertin," *Olympic Review* 9 (1968), 225.

[13] Letter, "Francis-Marius Messerli to the IOC, Invitation à une conférence internationale convoquée à St. Moritz, le 20 février 1928, en vue de discuter de l'organisation du côntrole médical des sports," archive collection "Summer and Winter Olympic Games: Medical Files,", File 200484 "Medical tests during the 1928 Winter Olympic Games in St. Moritz: Correspondence," IOC Archive, Lausanne.

[14] The Olympic Institute was founded by Pierre de Coubertin in Lausanne in 1917. It offered practical education in sport and other subjects to Belgian and French prisoners of war. Pierre de COUBERTIN, "Olympisme," in: *Pierre de Coubertin: textes choisis. Vol. II*, ed. Norbert MÜLLER (Zürich: Weidmann, 1986), 592-593.

[15] Letter, "Francis-Marius Messerli to the IOC, February 13, 1928," archive collection "Summer and Winter Olympic Games: Medical Files," folder "Medical tests during the 1928 Winter Olympic Games in St. Moritz: Correspondance," IOC Archive, Lausanne.

[16] Arthur MALLWITZ, ed., *Sportmedizin und Olympische Spiele 1936. Festschrift der Sportärzteschaft*, (Leipzig: Verlag Georg Thieme, 1936).

discussed various scientific topics on a congress organised by Arthur Mallwitz.[17] Following the Second World War, the IOC Session during the 1948 Winter Olympic Games in St. Moritz raised doping and sport medical issues in an Olympic context. At this meeting, the IOC member and surgeon Sir Arthur Porritt[18] from New Zealand, reported about the usage of doping for the very first time, arguing that

> any direct action in this connection would but lead the Committee into spheres where it is neither justified nor equipped to enter... as a corporate body we have neither the right nor the machinery to play any direct or practical part.[19]

The statement serves as an example for the neglect to deal with doping issues at the time.

The official cooperation between the IOC and the FIMS began during the 1952 Winter Olympic Games in Oslo.[20] A direct consequence from the collaboration between FIMS and the IOC was the installation of a Medical Commission at the 1956 Winter Olympic Games in Cortina d'Ampezzo.

---

[17] Roberta J. PARK lists as the most important topics: metabolism, circulation and respiration, nutrition and training, injuries, medicine and sport, medicine and aviation, psychology and sport. This militates for a wide range of participants from various medical and scientific backgrounds. However, almost half of the presenters came from Germany. Roberta J. PARK, "Physicians, Scientists, Exercise and Athletics in Britain and America from the 1867 Boat Race to the Four-Minute Mile," *Sport in History* 31, no. 1 (2011), 18.

[18] Lord Arthur Espie Porritt (1900-1994) won a bronze medal at the 1924 Paris Olympic Games in the 100-metre race. After his athlete career, he studied medicine and became a surgeon to the Royal Household. Porritt was also the manager of the New Zealand team at the 1936 Berlin Olympic Games and chair of the British Empire (Commonwealth) Games Federation from 1948 to 1967. In 1967, he was appointed the governor of New Zealand and subsequently resigned from all his position in the sport and medical fields. He was knighted in 1957 and raised to Peerage in 1973 for his services to medicine. "The Biographies of all IOC members, No. 168 Lord Arthur Espie Porritt," *Journal of Olympic History* 19, no. 3 (2011), 55.

[19] WRYNN, "The Human Factor," 213.

[20] Ibid., 228n17.

President of the Medical Commission was Giuseppe La Cava[21], who later became
president of the FIMS. The 1956 Medical Commission worked as a sector of the
Organising Committee, but was coordinated jointly by the Italian Sport Medicine
Federation (Federazione Medico-Sportiva Italiana, FMSI) and the Alpine
Department of the Rizzoli Orthopaedic Institute at Bologna.[22] However, the 1956
Medical Commission did not concern itself with performance-enhancing
substances but focused entirely on health and first aid services in three categories:
aid during training and competition, aid in ambulatory and at home as well as
hospital aid.[23] Evidently, medicine and the Olympic Movement therefore have a
long-lasting relationship, although some projects, such as the attempt to create an
Olympic Medical Archive, were short-lived.[24]

Whilst HOBERMAN argues that doping was not condemned in the 1950s,[25]
there is evidence that based on their involvement in sport and the Olympic
Movement, medical experts began to promote anti-doping initiatives shortly after
the end of the Second World War. The most outspoken medical experts adopted a
critical perspective on the usage of performance-enhancing substances even
though many ambiguous comments were made on several occasions.[26] In
February 1952, a conference in Oslo under the auspices of the Organising
Committee of the 1952 Winter Olympic Games in Oslo and the Norwegian

---

[21] Prof. Dr. Giuseppe La Cava (1908-1988), a surgeon, was head of Surgery and health
director at the Civil Hospital in Ceccano from 1952 until 1972. Having a great interest in
sport medicine, he founded the FMSI and served as its first president from 1947 until
1959. He was also first general secretary and then president of the FIMS from 1968 until
1976. A. OLIARO, "Giuseppe La Cava (1908-1988)," *The Journal of Sports Medicine and
Physical Fitness* 28, no. 3 (1988), 313.

[22] ORGANISING COMMITTEE OF THE VIITH OLYMPIC WINTER GAMES, *Official Report of the
VIIth Olympic Winter Games in Cortina d'Ampezzo 1956,* (Cortina d'Ampezzo:
Organising Committee of the Games of the VIIth Olympic Winter Games, 1956), 334ff.

[23] Brochure, *VIIth Olympic Winter Games. Organising Committee. Health Committee.
Program of Medical Assistance,* archive collection "Summer and Winter Olympic Games:
Medical Files," File 201380 "Programme of medical assistance of the Health Commission
of the 1956 Winter Olympic Games in Cortina d'Ampezzo," IOC Archive, Lausanne.

[24] HEGGIE, "Volunteers," 101ff.

[25] John M. HOBERMAN, *Testosterone Dreams: Rejuvenation, Aphrodisia, Doping*
(Berkeley, CA: University of California Press, 2005), 186ff.

[26] DIMEO, *A History,* 87ff. He refers in particular to the case of the former British Olympic
team doctor Adolphe Abrahams, who argued in 1958 that if all athletes had access to
stimulants, then there would be no argument to forbid them. Yet, DIMEO disagrees with
other researchers, who argue that Adolphe Abrahams' statements are proof for a general
acceptance for the usage of performance-enhancing substances.

Olympic Committee addressed general questions of health and sport and participants spoke about doping. The official conference publication reveals many details about the content of the debates. The Norwegian medical doctor Karl Evang[27] reported of injections of anaesthetics during the just finished 1952 Winter Olympic Games and requested severe punishments: "All forms of dope must be banned. It should never be tolerated in any form. The strictest rules must here be introduced."[28] In addition to the previously known illnesses of speed skaters, suffering from amphetamine usage,[29] there seems therefore to be more indications for drug use at the event. Importantly, Karl Evang did not give any evidence how he wanted to control athletes, possibly because such measures went beyond his area of expertise. However, his contribution highlights that medical doctors were aware and concerned about the dangerous health effects of certain performance-enhancing substances. In fact, Karl Evang argued that one athlete was "treated in a way which every responsible doctor normally would regard as damage to the individual and against the ethical rules of the profession."[30] He thereby already touched on the ethical responsibility of medical doctors and demonstrates awareness that athletes could only gain from performance-enhancing substances with the help of a medical expert, something he personally opposed. The brief statement in the conference resolution, that "dope in any form should be strictly prohibited" addresses the matter,[31] although the participants did not make any pragmatic recommendations to control drug use in sports. Other conference speakers did not mention doping in their speeches. Rather, they highlighted the close relationship between sport medicine and athletic performance, because these fields were linked to their areas of interest and expertise.

---

[27] Karl Evang (1902-1981) was director of the Norwegian Directorate for Health from 1938 to 1972 and co-founder of the World Health Organisation (WHO) in 1948. He was the Norwegian delegate at the First World Health Assembly in June 1948 and presided over the Second World Health Assembly from June to July 1949. Knut RINGEN, "Karl Evang: A Giant in Public Health," *Journal of Public Health Policy* 11, no. 3 (1990), 360-367.

[28] Karl EVANG, "Health Authorities and Sport," in: *Sport and Health. International Conference on Sport and Health Oslo 1952*, ed. Otto JOHANSEN (Oslo: The Royal Norwegian Ministry of Education State Office for Sport and Youth Work, 1952), 36. EVANG argued that he heard over the broadcasting system a statement about an athlete who was to get an injection of anesthetic in order to help him deal with the pain of an infection.

[29] HOULIHAN, *Dying*, 34.

[30] EVANG, "Health Authorities," 35. It is important to note that Evang decribes the athlete as being ill and therefore requiring medical treatment.

[31] JOHANSEN, *Sport and Health*, 17.

It evolves from the events at the conference that neither was there a serious debate about suggested solutions, nor were there any other scientific experts from outside sports medicine consulted. Sports medicine specialists also undertook first attempts to control athletes for the usage of performance-enhancing substances independently from other sciences. As DIMEO explains, the first anti-doping initiatives based on doping tests of any kind were conducted by Professor Dr. Antonio Venerando[32], a medical doctor of the FMSI.[33] In 1963, he reported to the Council of Europe Committee for Out-of-School Education about his analysis of urine samples during cycling races that led to first suspensions of cyclists in 1956 and 1958.[34] For this purpose, the FMSI did also establish an anti-doping laboratory at the Sporting Medicine Centre in Florence to analyse the samples.[35] This was the first anti-doping testing institution. Significantly, the analytical procedures were conducted by medical experts under the leadership of Dr. Giuliano Marena, who was director of the institution from 1962 until 1997.[36] Besides establishing a basic understanding for the widespread use of doping in sport, they wanted to prove that doping was a danger for the health of the athletes because of their interest in medical questions. Likewise, the medical debates were mainly focusing on how to make a distinction between the legal usage of nutrition supplements and the usage of substances only used to enhance athletic performances.[37] Similar initiatives, which took place in Austria under the leadership of Ludwig Prokop, also point towards this development. Ludwig Prokop reported about spot-checking the dressing rooms at the 1952 Winter Olympic Games in Oslo and the increasing consumption of performance-

[32] Professor Dr. Antonio Venerando (1923-1990) was a member of the medical and scientific committee of the 1960 Rome Olympic Games. In 1963, he became commissary officer of the Italian Institute of Sports Medicine and became its head in 1966. From 1961 to 1970, he was president of the FMSI. In the 1980s, he was vice-president of FIMS.
[33] DIMEO, *A History*, 90ff.
[34] Antonio VENERANDO, "Italian Experiments on the Pathology of Doping and Ways to Control It," *Appendix to Council of Europe for Out-of-School Education, Doping of Athletes: Reports of the Special Working Parties* (Strasbourg: Council of Europe, 1964), 49.
[35] DIMEO, *A History*, 90ff.
[36] Sergio CALIFANO, *Istituto di Medicina dello Sport di Firenze. Il "Centro delle Cascine": 1950-2005 Oltre Mezzo Secolo al Servizio dello Sport* (Florence: Commune di Firenze, 2005), 73ff.
[37] REINOLD, "Arguing," 10. In there, REINOLD draws on several articles published in the *Olympic Review* in the 1950s in which different substances and their effect on athletic performance are debated.

enhancing substances in cycling.[38] DIMEO suggests that Ludwig Prokop's involvement in doping matters was mainly motivated by his concerns about the health of the athletes but also because he thought doping was against the "ideal of pure sporting competition."[39] The same attitude can be found in Great Britain, where investigations into the usage of stimulants at the 1958 Empire and Commonwealth Games took place, although there was no proof for these suspicions.[40] HOBERMAN attests that medical experts prompted also anti-doping initiatives in the United States of America (USA).[41] In 1957, the American Medical Association (AMA) reacted to the increasing usage of stimulants in sport by adopting an anti-doping resolution. Erik EGGERS identifies sport medicine specialists in the FRG that dealt with the effect of performance-enhancing substances in the 1950s.[42] A number of doctoral studies and diploma thesis were conducted in which doping practices and several substances are discussed and analysed.[43] Furthermore, there were medical doctors such as Werner Ruhemann and E. Fischbach who pushed for a list of banned substances and a national doping commission of medical experts to cooperate with international medical organisations.[44] The Association of German Sport Physicians[45] had already defined doping as "the intake of any pharmaceutical - regardless of its activity - with the intention to enhance performance during a competition."[46] EGGERS also

---

[38] PROKOP, "Zur Geschichte," 128.

[39] DIMEO, *A History*, 94.

[40] R.G. FISHER and H.E. ROBSON, "'Doping' in the 1958 Empire and Commonwealth Games," *British Journal of Sports Medicine* 4, no. 2 (1969), 163-181.

[41] John M. HOBERMAN, "Sports Physicians and the Doping Crisis in Elite Sport," *Clinical Journal of Sports Medicine* 12, no. 4 (2002), 203-208.

[42] Erik EGGERS, "Geschichtliche Aspekte des Dopings in der präanabolen Phase," in *Doping in Deutschland: Geschichte, Recht, Ethik. 1950-1972*, ed. Giselher SPITZER (Cologne: Sportverlag Strauß, 2013), 65.

[43] Ibid., 47ff. EGGERS refers specifically to the medical doctoral thesis by Oskar Wegener entitled "The effect of doping substances on blood circulation and on physical performance". Furthermore, EGGERS argues that a diploma thesis by Jürgen Bliesener from 1958/1959 reveals the widespread usage of performance-enhancing substances in cycling. According to the thesis, the German Cycling Federation (Bund Deutscher Radfahrer, BDR) was aware of the doping practices.

[44] EGGERS, "Geschichtliche Aspekte," 63f.

[45] Today: German Society for Sports Medicine and Prevention.

[46] The definition had been made following a controversy surrounding the German medical doctor Dr. Martin Brustmann, who had handed medical substances to rowers ahead of a qualification race for the 1952 Helsinki Olympic Games. However, the pills did not have a positive effect and Martin Brustmann was accussed of "negative doping". KRÜGER et al., *Doping und Anti-Doping*, 53ff.

mentions the account of German pharmacologist Klaus Soehring. He had demonstrated at the Sport Medicine Congress in Hamburg in 1957 that the detection of doping substances could be done with paper chromatography.[47] This is notable because one cannot find any other such early mention of the detection of doping substances in bodily fluids within a sporting context. There is, however, no evidence that Klaus Soehring´s proposal had an impact on anti-doping. Thus, in contrast to the efforts made in Italy, with the establishment of an anti-doping laboratory, the initiatives in the FRG were of much more superficial nature in the 1950s, even though several actors were dealing with the question of how to combat doping.

The short overview of early anti-doping initiatives in the 1950s confirms the claim that medical experts due to their links to sport and the Olympic Movement laid the foundation for the legitimacy of anti-doping, since they thought (some) performance-enhancing substances to be a health risk and a contradiction to the sense of fair play. The intensified consumption of substances can partly be attributed to the increasing politicisation of sport in the 1950s.[48] The 1950s were the pioneer phase in doping controls with the first involvements of medical doctors. However, there is no evidence for medical experts asking chemists or pharmacologists to assist them in implementing analytical procedures at the time. They appear to be convinced that their professional competencies were sufficient in order to install and maintain a doping control system. The German pharmacologist Klaus Soehring was an exception in this regard. His involvement points towards the fact that there was much scientific advancement made within pharmacology and chemistry to detect and analyse substances in human bodily fluids by the 1950s. As presented in Chapter 1, Alfred Bukowski had developed the first method to detect alkaloids in saliva due to the increasing application of performance-enhancing substances in horseracing in 1910.[49] THEVIS gives a detailed description about how this method has advanced and argues that the earliest assay to determine benzedrine in human urine was cultivated in 1938 by

---

[47] EGGERS, "Geschichtliche Aspekte," 63.

[48] REINOLD et al., "Die 1960er," 154. The authors outline that due to the increased interest of politics in sport and the accompanying pressure to be successful had an effect on the usage of performance-enhancing substances in several countries. This can also be attributed to the beginning of the East-West conflict. In the FRG, Martin Brustmann argued that chemical substances are necessary in order to remain a competitive nation in international sport. Furthermore, the foundation for the doping system in the GDR was also laid in the 1950s according to the authors.

[49] POKRYWKA et al., "In memory," 540.

Derek Richter.[50] With his method, it was possible to detect several amines such as ephedrine and amphetamine, which were also widespread amongst athletes in the 1950s. It took until 1943 before separation of substances through chromatography became as advanced so that it could be used in practice.[51] This method was then developed further with around 10,000 references on paper chromatography published until 1956.[52] Hence, the detection of substances in the body of athletes could have been developed much earlier than it was actually done. The historical account given by THEVIS is also evidence for this.[53] According to him, several researchers dealt with the separation of alkaloids and stimulants along with diuretic agents. These aimed to assist the detection of drug usage in general.[54] Two articles published by the two pharmacologists Hans KAISER and Heinz JORI from Stuttgart (Germany) 1954 about the toxicological detection of several compounds with the support of paper chromatography are of particular importance and Klaus Soehring must have been aware of them.[55] In fact, together

---

[50] THEVIS, *Mass Spectrometry*, 4ff.

[51] Joseph C. TOUCHSTONE, "History of Chromatography," *Journal of Liquid Chromatography* 16, no. 8 (1993), 1648. The author refers to the research work by CONSDEN, GORDON, Archer J.P. MARTIN and Richard L.M. SYNGE, who worked for the *Wool Industries Research Association* in Leeds. They published two articles, in which they outline their methods based on usage of filter paper as inert support, making the acetylation irrelevant. Therefore they developed the foundation for all paper partition chromatography. The original research articles are: A.H. GORDON, Archer J.P. MARTIN and Richard L.M. SYNGE, "Partition Chromatography in the Study of Protein Constituents," *Biochemical Journal* 37, no. 1 (1943), 79-86. A.H. GORDON, Archer J.P. MARTIN and Richard L.M. SYNGE, "The Amino-Acid Composition of Gramicidin," *Biochemical Journal* 37, no. 1 (1943), 86-92. R. CONSDEN, A.H. GORDON and A.J.P. MARTIN, "Qualitative analysis of proteins: a partition chromatographic method using paper," *Biochemical Journal* 38, no. 3 (1944), 224-232.

[52] TOUCHSTONE, "History of Chromatography," 1649.

[53] THEVIS, *Mass Spectrometry*, 10.

[54] Ibid., 11.

[55] Hans KAISER and Heinz JORI, "Beiträge zum toxikologischen Nachweis von Dromoran 'Roche', Morphin, Dilaudid, Cardiazol Coramin und Atropin mit Hilfe der Papierchromatographie," *Archiv der Pharmazie und Berichte der Deutschen Pharamzeutischen Gesellschaft* 287, no. 4 (1954), 224-242; contd. Hans KAISER and Heinz JORI, "Beiträge zum toxikologischen Nachweis von Dromoran 'Roche', Morphin, Dilaudid, Cardiazol Coramin und Atropin mit Hilfe der Papierchromatographie," *Archiv der Pharmazie und Berichte der Deutschen Pharamzeutischen Gesellschaft* 287, no. 4 (1954), 253-258.

with Werner DIETZ, Klaus SOEHRING had already published his only research article on detection with paper chromatography in the same journal in 1957.[56]

Consequently, even though there were researchers with competencies in the detection of substances in bodily fluids in the 1950s, there was no apparent interest in drug detection in sport. Medical doctors did not consult such experts for the purposes of doping analysis as they appeared to be convinced that they could deal with the issue of doping controls independently at the time. This belief stems partly from the fact that medical doctors were involved in sport and the Olympic Movement through various organising committees, research projects conducted at the Olympic Games, team doctors of Olympic team and through their participation in Olympic related, scientific conference. The Olympic Games enabled them to apply their professional competencies in a sport setting, which experts in drug analysis did evidently not do in the 1950s.

CREATING SYNERGIES IN THE 1960S

The field of anti-doping was essentially established in the 1960s, when more interest groups became increasingly involved with the issue.[57] It is generally reported that the death of the Danish cyclist Knud Jensen on the opening day of the 1960 Rome Olympic Games triggered the beginning of the IOC's anti-doping initiatives,[58] this being the first death at an Olympic competition since the 1912

---

[56] Werner DIETZ and Klaus SOEHRING, "Experimentelle Beiträge zum Nachweis von Thiobarbitursäuren aus dem Harn mit Hilfe der Papierchromatographie," *Archiv der Pharmazie und Berichte der Deutschen Pharamzeutischen Gesellschaft* 290, no. 2 (1957), 80-97.

[57] REINOLD et al., "Die 1960er," 154.

[58] Verner MØLLER, "Knud Enemark Jensen's Death During the 1960 Rome Olympics: A Search for Truth?" *Sport in History* 25, no. 3 (2005), 452ff. The diagnosis of the attending doctor as well as the official report of the Danish Olympic Committee state that Knud Jensen's cause of death was a brain injury, caused by a fall from his bike. The fall was triggered by a heatstroke. Dissident from this report, the IOC ascribes Knud Jensen's death the ingestion of amphetamines. Point of reference for this is the examination of Ludwig Prokop. He claims that traces of amphetamines were found during Jensen's autopsy. However, his findings are disputable. Although the Danish team doctor admitted that he gave his athletes ronicol to expand their blood vessels, no amphetamine abuse could be proved. It is, however, suspicious that Ludwig Prokop's documentation is not accessible anymore.

Stockholm Olympic Games.[59] However, HUNT attests that IOC president Avery Brundage had already been confronted with the issue by Professor Dr. Henry K. Beecher[60], a medical professor from Harvard University, in 1959, and again in early 1960.[61] As a result, Avery Brundage addressed the issue at the IOC Session in San Francisco in February 1960. Yet, HUNT asserts that Avery Brundage still took a passive approach to the doping matter, and according to the minutes of the IOC Session that he only urged the IOC members to speak about the forbidden usage of pharmaceutical substances in their countries but did not pledge for doping tests or preventive measures.[62] However, there is further evidence that the IOC planned to address the issue of doping even before the fatality of Knud Jensen. In an article published on August 15, 1960 in Lausanne, the French medical doctor Dr. Stanislas BURSTIN remarked that the IOC would address the doping matter in connection with the professionalization of sport during its next "Congress."[63] Although it remains unclear whether BURSTIN refers to the next IOC Session or indeed an Olympic Congress, [64] he must have had inside information. Moreover, he had already presented another paper in early 1960.[65]

---

[59] At the 1912 Stockholm Olympic Games, the flag bearer of the Portuguese team Francisco Lazaro died during the marathon race. The 21-year old suffered from a heat stroke eight kilometres before the finish line and collapsed. Ansgar MOLZBERGER, *Die Olympischen Spiele in Stockholm. Zwischen Patriotismus und Internationalität* (Sankt Augustin: Academia Verlag, 2012), 189n58.

[60] Henry K. Beecher (1904-1976) was a medical expert in anesthesiology, becoming the first to hold a chair in the subject in the USA. His main research focused on the placebo effect of drugs. In 1966, he published a groundbreaking study on unethical clinical research, which resulted in the introduction of requirements concerning informed consent and review processes through human subject review boards. Mark BEST and Duncan NEUHAUSER, "Henry K. Beecher: pain, belief and truth at the bedside. The powerful placebo, ethical research and anaesthesia safety," *Quality Safety in Health Care* 19 (2010), 466-468.

[61] HUNT, *Drug Games*, 10.

[62] Minutes, "56th Session of the IOC in San Francisco, February 15-16, 1960," archive collection "IOC Sessions 1894-2009," IOC Archive, Lausanne, 9.

[63] Stanislas BURSTIN, "Le dopage, ce 'mal' du Sport," *Vivre. Revue mensuelle d'information médicale, scientifique et de loisirs* 4 (1960), 10-14. A German translation of the text can be found in the CuLDA: "Manuscript translated by Alfred Schoenen - Das Doping, dieses Übel des Sports," archive collection "Nachlass Carl Diem," 1.3. "Korrespondenz," CuLDA, Cologne.

[64] No Olympic Congress was in the planning at this period and the subsequent X[th] Olympic Congress was to take place in Varna in 1973. MÜLLER, *One Hundred Years*, 149ff.

[65] Stanislas BURSTIN, "Le 'Dopage' Sportif," Paper presented at the Congress of the *Union Sportive Travailliste Du Nord et Du Pas-de-Calais*, Lens, March 20, 1960.

Therein he referred to the study of Henry K. Beecher, demonstrating that he was
informed about other academics researching the topic of doping in sport. In
contrast to the other medical experts, however, Stanislas Burstin claimed that
athletes needed to be educated about the negative effects of performance-
enhancing substances, thereby pledging for a more educational anti-doping
approach.[66]

Several sport historians have detailed the processes to inaugurate an IOC
anti-doping policy and it is not the focus of this book to echo these researchers.
Nevertheless, concerning the involvement of sport medicine specialists and anti-
doping laboratory experts, certain developments must be emphasised. First, when
at the IOC Executive Board Meeting in June 1961 the French IOC member
Comte Jean de Beaumont[67] affirmed the need for a "system of control over
doping,"[68] there appears to be no indication that more medical information on the
usage and effect of performance-enhancing substances was necessary. Instead, the
approach was of a political nature because forms of control should be installed in
order to combat doping. At the following 58th IOC Session, Avery Brundage
explained, "on the first instance, the I.O.C. should be informed as to what
constitutes a doping, and that we need medical advice."[69] HUNT claims that he
sought guidance in particular concerning a definition of doping being aware that
the medical sciences had already dealt with the issue due to the information he

[66] Manuscript translated by Alfred Schoenen, "Das Doping, dieses Übel des Sports," 3.
[67] Comte Jean Robert Bonnin de la Bonninière de Beaumont (1904-2002) was a World
Champion in shooting and participated in the 1924 Paris Olympic Games. He became an
IOC member in 1950 and served on its Executive Board from 1967 to 1971 and from 1976
to 1980, occupying the role of IOC vice president from 1970 to 1974. His most notable
contribution to the Olympic Movement was his proposal to found an Olympic Aid
Commission in order to support countries in Africa and Asia. Interestingly, this proposal
was made at the same Executive Board Meeting in which he proposed a doping control
system. In 1968, the Committee became a Commission and was later renamed into
Olympic Solidarity Commission. "The Biographies of all IOC members, No. 223 Jean
Bonnin de la Bonninière Count de Beaumont," *Journal of Olympic History* 20, no. 2
(2012), 70. More information on the establishment of Olympic Solidarity and the political
thinking behind the decision to support African and Asian countries can be found in: Ian
HENRY and Mansour AL TAUQI, "The Development of Olympic Solidarity: West and Non-
West (Core and Periphery) Relations in the Olympic World," *The International Journal
for the History of Sport* 25, no. 3 (2008), 355-369.
[68] Minutes, "Executive Board, June 15, 1961", archive collection "IOC Executive Board
Meetings 1921-1982," IOC Archive, Lausanne, 2.
[69] Minutes, "59th Session of the IOC in Athens, August 22-24, 1961", archive collection
"IOC Sessions 1894-2009," IOC Archive, Lausanne, 3.

had received prior to the 1960 Rome Olympic Games.[70] Consequently, he decided to install an IOC doping subcommittee, which consisted of IOC members with a medical background. This is not surprising because it allowed dealing with the problem internally and relates to the close relationship between medicine and sport. Arthur Porritt became its head.[71] Several researchers agree that his contribution as head of the IOC doping subcommittee was limited.[72] The other members of this inaugural committee were Dr. Ryotaro Azuma[73] from Japan, Professor Dr. Josef Gruss[74] from Czechoslovakia and Dr. Agustin Sosa[75] from Panama.[76] Despite the composition of the IOC doping subcommittee outlined in the minutes of the IOC Executive Board meeting of March 1962, it remains

---

[70] HUNT, *Drug Games*, 12.

[71] Minutes, "Executive Board, March 2/3, 1962", archive collection "IOC Executive Board Meetings 1921-1982," IOC Archive, Lausanne, 4.

[72] WRYNN, "The Human Factor," 219 and HUNT, *Drug Games*, 12ff.

[73] Dr. Ryotaro Azuma (1893-1983) was IOC member from 1950 onwards and honorary member until his death in 1983. In 1960, he became the first Asian on the IOC Executive Board. Ryotaro Azuma was president of the Japanese National Olympic Committee as well as president of the Japanese Amateur Athletics Association from 1947 to 1958, vice-president of the Organising Committee of the 1964 Tokyo Olympic Games and member of the Organising Committee of the 1972 Winter Olympic Games in Sapporo. Besides his sport political activities, Ryotaro Azuma was Tokyo's governor during the time of the 1960 Tokyo Olympic Games and became head of the Japanese Red Cross in 1968. "The Biographies of all IOC members, No. 221 Ryotaro Azuma," *Journal of Olympic History* 20, no. 2 (2012), 69.

[74] Dr. Josef Gruss (1884-1968) from Czechoslovakia was IOC member from 1946 to 1965. He replaced Jiři Guth-Jarkovsky, who was an IOC member right from the establishment of the IOC at the Sorbonne Congress in 1896. He participated in the tennis event at the 1908 London Olympic Games and was a member of the Czecheslovak fencing team in 1920 although he did not compete in Antwerp. Josef Gruss was president of the Bohemian/Czechoslovakian National Olympic Committee from 1929 until 1951. During his medical career, he specialised in gynaecology and surgery, occupying his medical profession at the Prague Hospital. "The Biographies of all IOC members, No. 194 Josef Gruss," *Journal of Olympic History* 20, no. 1 (2012), 57.

[75] Dr. Agustin Arturo Sosa (1905-1990) was opted onto the IOC at the 47th IOC Session in Helsinki in 1952 and resigned from the IOC in 1967. He was a medical doctor and became member of the Panama Olympic Committee in 1952. His specific aim on the IOC was to strengthen its position in Latin American, which is the reason why at the same Session Julio Gerlein-Comelin from Colombia and Julio B. Bustamente from Venezuela were voted onto the IOC. "The Biographies of all IOC members, No. 236 Agustin Arturo Sosa," *Journal of Olympic History* 20, no.3 (2012), 66.

[76] Minutes, "Executive Board, March 2/3, 1962," archive collection "IOC Executive Board Meetings 1921-1982," IOC Archive, Lausanne, 4.

unclear whether there was originally a fifth member, namely Dr. José Joaquim Ferreira Santos[77] from Brazil. Avery Brundage listed him in a letter to IOC chancellor Otto Mayer in January 1962, when informing the chancellor that he wanted to establish a doping subcommission.[78] Moreover, José Joaquim Ferreira Santos replaced Arthur Porritt during the 1962 IOC Session in Moscow and reported about a study he conducted with his Brazilian colleague Dr. Mario de Carvalho Pini.[79] Therefore, it is likely that his exclusion in the IOC minutes was a mistake,[80] especially as José Joaquim Ferreira Santos was briefly appointed head of the IOC doping subcommittee in November 1962.[81] However, he died a month later, only being able to contribute a short report on the doping issue in the February 1963 edition of the *Olympic Review*.[82] After his death, the chair of the IOC doping subcommittee returned to Arthur Porritt. Furthermore, one must emphasise that none of the members contributed to the work of the IOC doping

---

[77] Dr. José Joaquim Ferreira Santos (1892-1962), a medical doctor, became an IOC member in April 1923. He was secretary general of the first ever Brazilian Olympic team, who participated at the 1920 Antwerp Olympic Games and Head of the Brazilian delegation of the 1936 Berlin Olympic Games. After the Second World War, he became president of the Brazilian National Olympic Committee and Head of the 1963 Pan American Games in São Paulo. However, Ferreira Santos died one year before the Games were supposed to take place. "The Biographies of all IOC members, No. 119 José Joaquim Ferreira Santos," *Journal of Olympic History* 18, no. 3 (2010), 54.

[78] WRYNN, "The Human Factor," 218.

[79] Minutes, "59th Session of the IOC in Moscow, June 5-8, 1962," archive collection "IOC Sessions 1894-2009," IOC Archive, Lausanne, 4. The original study was published in 1964 by Dr. Mario de Carvalho Pini after the death of Ferreira Santos and can be found in the archive of the IOC: "Étude Critique du Dopage," archive collection "IOC Medical Commission," folder "Medical commission: studies and reflexion," IOC Archive Lausanne.

[80] There is also different information in academic literature regarding this issue. For example, in their otherwise very well researched chronological overview on the most important events in the IOC's dealings with doping, Jan TODD and Terry TODD only list Arthur Porritt, Ryotaro Azuma, Josef Gruss and Joaquim Ferreira Santos as members of the IOC doping subcommittee. However, it is unclear where exactly they got their information from. Jan TODD and Terry TODD, "Significant Events in the History of Drug Testing and the Olympic Movement: 1960-1999," in: *Doping in Elite Sport: The Politics of Drugs in the Olympic Movement*, eds. Wayne WILSON and Edward DERSE (Champaign, Illinois: Human Kinetics, 2001), 67.

[81] Letter, Otto Mayer to José Joaquim Ferreira Santos, November 8, 1962, archive collection "IOC Medical Commission," folder "Medical Commission: Alphabetical correspondence 1960-1967," IOC Archive, Lausanne.

[82] José Joaquim Ferreira SANTOS, "Doping," *Olympic Review* 81 (1963), 56-57.

subcommittee and their efforts on the IOC are also negligible.[83] Only Ryotaro Azuma attended the majority of the IOC meetings although he was occupied with his decisive role in the Organising Committee of the 1964 Tokyo Olympic Games. In addition, the very specific medical expertise of the IOC doping subcommittee members such as the gynaecologist Josef Gruss and the surgeon Arthur Porritt do not point towards great interest into the doping issue either. Hence, the installation needs to be regarded as a compromise in terms of turning towards sport medicine in doping matters but at the same time the installation did not allow external experts – chemical or medical with competencies in anti-doping – to enter the IOC.

Furthermore, through the installation of the IOC doping subcommittee, Avery Brundage wanted the members to cooperate with organisations rather than individuals and he integrated the FIMS into the discussions about a doping definition.[84] One result of this was a publication by FIMS President Giuseppe La Cava in the *Olympic Review* in May 1963.[85] Even so, the decision of IOC president Avery Brundage to install an IOC doping policy was unsuccessful, because there appeared to be no urgency. Moreover, the installation cannot be considered as the start of the collaboration between sport medicine, anti-doping laboratory experts, of which there was none within the IOC, and the organisation itself. Rather, it was only an attempt by the IOC to define doping and position the organisation against the usage of performance-enhancing substances during the Olympic Games.

These developments do not mean that medical experts stopped their research on doping and the detection of bodily fluids. Quite the contrary, they also began to create a transnational network at the beginning of the 1960s,[86] and made an important contribution to the most notable international meeting dealing with doping in the early 1960s, organised by the Council of Europe Committee for Out-of-School Education. This meeting, held in Strasbourg in January 1963, resulted in the first international report on the topic and was the first international

---

[83] Agustin Sosa was present at 4 out of 18 IOC Sessions during his membership and José Joaquim Ferreira Santos was also not a very active IOC member, having attended only 11 out of 38 IOC Sessions.

[84] Minutes, "Executive Board, March 2/3, 1962," archive collection "IOC Executive Board Meetings 1921-1982," IOC Archive, Lausanne, 4.

[85] Giuseppe LA CAVA, "The Use of Drugs in Competitive Sport," *Olympic Review* 78 (1962), 52–53.

[86] REINOLD et al., "Die 1960er," 156.

collaboration against doping in sport.[87] A key person in the committee was FMSI president Antonio Venerando, who reported to the Committee about the anti-doping laboratory in Florence. By 1965, a medical committee under his leadership consisting only of medical experts agreed on analytical techniques to detect banned substances.[88] The techniques listed were different chromatographic methods, and the specialists emphasised that an international working group was needed in order to exchange information on the technical advancements of methods of detection and analysis.[89] Remarkably, these methods should be dealt with by medical experts. Hence, they remained convinced that they could deal with doping analysis without consultation of experts from other scientific fields. The results of the meeting were eventually concluded in a resolution against doping by the CoE in 1967,[90] and the FIMS along with the IOC adopted the definition of doping in 1964.[91]

One reason for the inclusion of more precise analytical testing methods is that by 1963, the testing methods – although still not specifically developed for sports drug testing – had also made progress. There were 8,292 references dealing with paper chromatography in 1960 alone.[92] This indicates towards the increased interest and a fast development of the testing technique. In addition to the progress in paper chromatography, the capability of GC to separate compounds relevant for doping controls was acknowledged in the late 1950s also.[93] Importantly, the techniques could be adapted more specifically to detect substances in bodily fluids, which made testing procedures also more attractive for the world of sport.[94] Hence, more useful methods for sports drug testing were developed in the 1960s.

---

[87] Kathryn HENNE, "WADA, the Promises of Law and the Landscapes of Antidoping Regulation," *Political and Legal Anthropology Review* 33, no. 2 (2010), 311.

[88] Report, "Report of the Medical Committee to the Conference Doping des Athletes by the *Council of Europe Committee for Out-of-School Education,* September 23-25, 1965," archive collection "Avery Brundage Collection, 1908-1975," film 54, folder 0007 "Medical Amphetamines used in Athletics 1937-1969," IOC Archive, Lausanne, 143.

[89] Ibid.

[90] COMMITTEE OF MINISTERS OF THE COUNCIL OF EUROPE, *Resolution on the Doping of Athletes (67/12), adopted by the Ministers' Deputies on 29th June 1967* (Strasbourg: Council of Europe, 1967).

[91] HOULIHAN, *Dying to Win,* 130.

[92] TOUCHSTONE, "History," 1649.

[93] THEVIS, *Mass Spectrometry,* 11.

[94] For references on the most important research conducted on gas chromatography and an overview of the historical development, including the technical details, see THEVIS, *Mass Spectrometry,* 11ff. and TOUCHSTONE, "History," 1649ff.

Ultimately, the involvement of scientific experts into the anti-doping initiatives in sport was achieved because of developments made in Great Britain along with an accidental meeting. One of the institutions researching on scientific methods to find amounts of substances and drugs in human fluids was the Department of Pharmacy at the Chelsea College of the University of London.[95] Later publications of researchers working at Chelsea College reveal that they had already started dealing with the issue in 1958.[96] Supported by his colleagues, the research on drug detection was led by Professor Dr. Arnold Beckett. An early curriculum vitae found at the KCL (of which the Chelsea College is a part today) discloses that Arnold Beckett received his Ph.D. from the University of London in 1950 for his work on synthetic analgesics.[97] Hence he was already confronted with substances that could potentially be misused during sporting competitions in the formative years of his academic career. In the mid-1950s, he continued to work on the same issue, later arguing that the work in the field of sympathomimetic amines and narcotic drugs "necessitated the development of analytical techniques for determining very small amounts of drugs and metabolites in biological fluids."[98] Arnold Beckett and his co-workers published their earliest and most important scientific articles on the detection of substances with paper chromatography in 1960[99] and 1962.[100] The eventual involvement into sport, however, happened almost by accident. BECKETT and COWAN describe the events as follows:

> We presented some of our earlier work, in which we chose amphetamines and related compounds as our examples, to an International Research Symposium on "Medicinal Chemistry" at Chelsea College in the Easter of 1965. During the Conference, a friend of A.H.B.

---

[95] DIMEO, *A History*, 106ff.

[96] Arnold BECKETT and David A. COWAN, "Misuse of Drugs in Sport," *British Journal of Sports Medicine* 12 (1979), 185.

[97] Curriculum Vitae, "Arnold Heyworth Beckett", archive collection "CDPM/FPA2 Beckett," King's College London Archives, London, 1. Also see: Claire TAYLOR and Gwyn WILLIAMS, eds., *King's College London. Contributions to biomedicine a continuing story* (King's College London: London, 2006), 64f.

[98] BECKETT and COWAN, "Misuse," 185.

[99] Arnold BECKETT, M.A. BEAVAN and Anne E. ROBINSON, "Some Factors Involved in Multiple Spot Formation in the Paper Chromatography," *Journal of Pharmacy and Pharmacology* 12 (1960), 203-216.

[100] Arnold BECKETT and D.F. CASY, "The Testing and Development of Analgesic Drugs," in: *Progress in Medicinal Chemistry*, eds. G.P. Ellis and G.B. West (London: Butterworths, 1962), 43-87.

[Arnold Beckett] from Belgium expressed interest in the work and said that obviously we now had sensitive methods of analysis for drugs such as amphetamines. He further asked for how long we could detect amphetamines in man after an oral dose had been given. When told about 48 hours he said that A.H.B. [Arnold Beckett] should notify sports authorities of our important sensitive methods because in many countries a very serious problem of drug misuse in sport was developing.[101]

The meeting between Arnold Beckett and his "friend," who DIMEO has identified as the Belgian scientist Dr. Paul Janssen[102], caused Arnold Beckett to become involved in sports drug testing. Consequently, this meeting was of major significance for the history of anti-doping laboratory experts, as their involvement in sport appears to begin with this encounter. Furthermore, it is equally important to emphasise that it was not the IOC, who Arnold Beckett worked for first. In fact, he undertook doping controls and doping analysis at the Tour of Britain[103] in 1965,[104] and applied most recent advancements made in MS.[105] Eventually, four

---

[101] BECKETT and COWAN, "Misuse," 185.

[102] Dr. Paul Janssen (1926-2003) was a medical doctor and pharmaceutical expert, who founded the Belgian company Janssen Pharmaceutica in 1953. Together with his team, he developed over 80 pharmaceutical compounds for usage in human, botanical and veterinary medicine. Theodore H. STANLEY, Talmage D. EGAN and Hugo VAN AKEN, "A Tribute to Dr. Paul A.J. Janssen: Entrepreneur Extraordinaire, Innovative Scientist, and Significant Contributor to Anaesthesiology," *Anesthesia & Analgesia* 106, no. 2 (2008), 451-462.

[103] From 1958 onwards, the Tour of Britain was known as the Milk Cup because it was sponsored by the Milk Marketing Board, a British government agency that controlled the milk production and distribution. The Milk Marketing Board celebrated its 25th year of existence through the sponsorship and at the same time saved the cycling competition as in 1956 and 1957 it did not take place because no sponsor could be found. Peter A. CLIFFORD and John BUTFIELD, *The History of the Tour of Britain* (London: The International Cyclists Saddle Club, 1967), 41.

[104] BECKETT and COWAN, "Misuse," 185.

riders were disqualified as their tests proved to be positive.[106] Certainly, this highlights that Arnold Beckett´s involvement had an immediate - if little - impact and signified a new age for sports drug testing because his professional competencies in the field of doping analysis were essential for the slowly evolving doping control system. Consequently, he could later argue, "the new methods were beginning to have an effect."[107] The successful tests at the cycling events caused the English Football Association to contact Arnold Beckett to conduct tests at the 1966 World Cup,[108] held in Britain, yet it remains unclear

---

[105] Remarkably, the first attempts to combine mass spectrometry and gas chromatography (GC-MS) were made at the end of the 1950s, thus coinciding with the first attempts by sport organisations to combat doping. Arguably, the first application of MS to characterise complex matrices - still independently from sports drug testing - was made by Carl-Ove ANDERSSON in Sweden in 1958. In the article, Carl-Ove ANDERSSON argues the application has been used in order to analyse amino-acids and peptides. He states that the high resolution of the mass spectrometer used offers interesting possibilities for further research on the analysis of amino-acids and peptides. Carl-Ove ANDERSSON, "Mass Spectrometric Studies on Amino Acid and Peptide Derivatives," *Acta Chemica Scandinavia* 12 (1958), 1353. Shortly after, in 1959, Roland S. GOHLKE reported in a journal article in *Analytical Chemistry* that he successfully combined GC with MS although he had already presented a paper on the issue together with his colleague Fred MCLAFFERTY at the 129th North American Chemical Society in 1956. It is most interesting within the Olympic context that the two chemists worked at time for the Dow Chemical Company in Chicago, Michigan. The Dow Chemical Company is today one of The Official Worldwide Partners (TOP) of the IOC and the official chemistry company of the Olympic Movement. O. David SPARKMAN, Zelda E. PETON and Fulton G. KITSON, *Gas Chromatography and Mass Spectrometry. A Practical Guide* (Burlington, MA: Elsevier, 2011), 5. The original research paper is: Roland S. GOHLKE, "Time-of-flight mass spectrometry and gas-liquid partition chromatography," *Analytical Chemistry* 31 (1959), 535-541. The Virginia-based researchers Joseph C. Holmes and Francis A. Morell also accomplished GC-MS in the late 1950s and presented their efforts in a paper in 1957. SPARKMAN, PETON and KITSON, *Gas Chromatography*, 5.

[106] Three of the four disqualified racers were Spanish riders, the other one the British cyclist Ken Hill. Amongst the Spanish racers was also the, on the morning of the last stage, leader of the Tour, Luis Pedros Santamarina. However, he was disqualified together with the other three cyclists and consequently the British cyclist Lesley West eventually won the Tour of Britain in 1965 as he won the race on the final stage. In the subsequent investigations, the Spaniards were cleared by their Federation. The British Cycling Federation, however, imposed an 18-month ban on Ken Hill, which was reduced to 12 months after an appeal. CLIFFORD and BUTFIELD, *The History*, 80ff.

[107] BECKETT and COWAN, "Misuse," 185.

[108] Martin NOLTE, "Dopingbekämpfung anlässlich der FIFA Fußball-Weltmeisterschaft England 1966," in *Doping. Kulturwissenschaftlich betrachtet*, eds. Eckhard MEINBERG and Swen KÖRNER (St. Augustin: Academia Verlag, 2013), 117f.

how the federation approached him. In the final report, the scientists in charge reasoned that the detection and analytical methods were implemented based on the experience made at the two editions of the Tour of Britain.[109]

The developments within pharmaceutical and biochemical research remained unnoticed by the IOC at first and there is no proof that the IOC doping subcommittee was aware of Arnold Beckett's work and tests. Even though, at the 62nd IOC Session in Tokyo in 1964, Arthur Porritt finally introduced four interconnected policies. These foresaw an official declaration against the usage of performance-enhancing substances, the creation of regulations for sanctions, the implementation of testing and an anti-doping declaration form for the athletes.[110] At the 1964 Tokyo Olympic Games, unofficial doping controls took place during the team race of the cycling event.[111] These were no real "controls" because they fulfilled research purposes. The tests consisted of the search for drugs before the start, search for proof for injections and urine samples. No incidents were reported.[112] The Belgian Dr. Albert Dirix[113], the official doctor of the Tour de France Dr. Pierre Dumas[114] and Ludwig Prokop conducted the tests on riders from Holland, Italy, Sweden, Argentina, France and the USSR.[115] Albert DIRIX

---

[109] Report, "Report on the Testing for Artificial Substances in Urine Samples from Football Players in the World Championship by A.H. Beckett, G.T. Tucker and R.D. James," 1966, archive collection "CDPM/FPUB4 Prof. Beckett 1965-1966," King's College London Archives, London, 114.

[110] Minutes, "62nd IOC Session in Tokyo, October 6-8, 1962," archive collection "IOC Sessions 1894-2009," IOC Archive, Lausanne, 11.

[111] WRYNN reports that Avery Brundage was not in favour of cycling being an Olympic sport because of such "professional" elements as prize money and sponsorship. Furthermore, the UCI was unhappy about its sport being the only one tested, however, due to the experiences with Knud Jensen's death at the 1960 Rome Olympic Games and further suspicions of drug use in cycling, it made perfect sense to conduct tests in the sport. WRYNN, "The Human Factor," 219.

[112] Albert DIRIX, "The Doping Problem at the Tokyo and Mexico City Olympic Games," *Journal of Sports Medicine and Physical Fitness* 6 (1966), 184ff.

[113] Dr. Albert Dirix (1914-1999) was a Belgian sports medicine specialist and vice-president of the Belgian National Olympic Committee from 1966 until 1981. He became secretary of the IOC Medical Commission in 1967 and remained in this position until 1992. "Obituaries," *Olympic Review* XXVI, no. 27 (1999), 85.

[114] Dr. Pierre Dumas (1921-2000) was the third official medical doctor of the Tour de France and succeeded Dr. Pierre Mathieu (1949-1951) and René Berthy (1952-1954) in 1955. He occupied this position until 1968, when he became the responsible person to conduct the doping tests at the Tour de France. Jean-Pierre DE MONDENARD, *Tour de France. Histoires extraordinaires des géants de la route* (Paris: Hugo Sport, 2012), 133ff.

[115] DIRIX, "The Doping Problem," 184ff.

reports that Japanese medical doctors analysed the urine samples.[116] However, it remains unclear which analytical methods they applied and which individuals were in charge of the analysis. Furthermore, due to unexplained circumstances, several tests could not be carried out "and this led the Japanese doctors to abandon the project."[117] None of the members of the IOC doping subcommittee was involved in the testing. This, once again, points towards the inactivity of the IOC doping subcommittee members. Furthermore, during the 1964 Congress of the FIMS, the organisation had established an Interfederal Medical Commission, listing amongst its main tasks the dealings with doping.[118] Via the Official Bulletin of the FIMS, the IFs were asked to send their medical supervisor onto the Committee.[119] Eighteen of 27 federations replied, and the list of the individuals involved included some of the later influential doping experts, such as Ludwig Prokop (sleigh), Dr. Pieter van Dijk[120] (cycling), Dr. Max Danz[121] (athletics) and Albert Dirix (cycling).[122] Consequently, medical experts that were involved in IFs had yet another forum to exchange strategies against doping.

By the mid-1960s, Arthur Porritt along with Avery Brundage increasingly adopted the stance that the International Federations (IFs) were responsible for the execution of the doping tests. As a result, IFs were more active concerning anti-doping measures. FIFA and the UCI introduced tests at their World Championships. The increased efforts of the UCI also enabled the first doping tests at the Tour de France in 1966, where doping inspectors woke up cyclists at

---

[116] Ibid.

[117] Ibid.

[118] "Minutes of the Meeting of the Interfederal Medical Commission," *Official Bulletin of the Fédération Internationale de Médicine Sportive* 7, no. 2 (1967), 10.

[119] "Circular letter No. 5," *Official Bulletin of the Fédération Internationale de Médicine Sportive* 5, no. 4 (1965), 10.

[120] Dr. Pieter van Dijk was the president of the Royal Dutch Cycling Union (Koninklijke Nederlandsche Wielren Unie, KNWU) from 1954 until 1971. Despite various attempts, it was not possible to find out his biographical data throughout this research project.

[121] Max Danz (1908-2000) was the founder and first president of the German Athletics Association (Deutscher Leichathletik Verband, DLV) from 1949 until 1970. He was a member of the IAAF from 1952 and its honorary vice-president from 1981.

[122] "Minutes of the Meeting of the Interfederal Medical Commission," 11.

night to give urine samples.[123] Pierre Dumas supervised these doping controls. The UCI also became the first sport organisation to establish a Medical Committee in 1964, dealing with anti-doping issues such as the evaluation of the doping analysis reports.[124] The Committee consisted of the sport medicine specialists Dr. Robert Boncour (France), Dr. Roland Marlier (Belgium) and Professor Dr. Michele Montanaro (Italy),[125] which highlights that also in the UCI medical experts attempted to deal with doping analysis. Finally, governments saw a need for involvement. For example, in 1965 France and Belgium introduced anti-doping laws, marking the beginning of the criminalisation of doping.[126]

By 1965, the IOC doping subcommittee presented results of undertaken research. However, it was none of its original members but the new IOC member and IOC doping subcommittee member Prince Alexandre de Mérode from Belgium, who provided the results.[127] In contrast to the other members, Alexandre de Mérode was not a medical doctor, but a graduate in classics, philosophy, arts and law and a practising lawyer. As the other members of the IOC doping subcommittee either had passed away or had resigned from the IOC, Alexandre de Mérode was the only other member on the IOC doping subcommittee, along with Arthur Porritt. Due to the absence of Arthur Porritt at the IOC Session in 1965, Alexandre de Mérode reported to the IOC, while relying

---

[123] As a reaction to the doping control measures, the riders decided to go on a strike at the beginning of the following stage. The tour organisation then negotiated that doping tests would continue, but that the urine samples were taken ahead of the start instead of in the night. The following athletes were tested positive during the Tour de France of 1966: Gilbert Bellone (France), Julien Delocht (Belgium), Jean Dupont (France), Roger Millot (France), Guido Neri (Italy), Hermann van Springel (Belgium). In the same year, the Dutch amateur Huub Heiligers died of pervitin consumption at a cycling race in the Netherlands and the Italian amateur Giovanni Gatti collapsed and died during a tour in Italy. KRÜGER, "Doping in Cycling," 335.

[124] Ibid., 339.

[125] Report, Medical Commission of the International Cycling Union by Dr. Roland Marlier, January 13, 1968, archive collection "IOC Medical Commission," folder "Medical Commission: Reports with the Sessions and the EC and report on the program of the tests anti-doping to the Pan American plays of 1968," IOC Archive, Lausanne, 1.

[126] John M. HOBERMAN, "'Athletes in handcuffs?' The criminalization of doping" in: *Doping and Anti-Doping Policy in Sport: Ethical, Legal and Social Perspectives, eds.* Mike MCNAMEE and Verner MØLLER (New York, NY: Routledge, 2011), 100.

[127] Alexandre de Merode was elected onto the IOC at the 62nd IOC Session in Tokyo in October 1964 and replaced Prince Albert of Liège. Minutes, "62nd IOC Session in Tokyo, October 6-8, 1962", archive collection "IOC Sessions 1894-2009," IOC Archive, Lausanne, 4.

on medical reports compiled by Albert Dirix.[128] Significantly, following the meeting, Avery Brundage contacted Alexandre de Mérode, asking him to explore the composition of a possible Control Committee for doping, together with Albert Dirix.[129] Such intent to install a new committee dealing with doping controls in a more pragmatic way is the first indication of foreseeable changes within the organisation of the IOC's doping fight. Furthermore, it reveals the increased emphasis on doping tests to be the only anticipated solution combating doping in sport. This was the outcome of Alexandre de Mérode's report and therefore his entry into the IOC's anti-doping efforts marks the beginning of an anti-doping policy based on doping testing.

Another report by Arthur Porritt at the 1966 IOC Session followed Alexandre de Mérode's appearance.[130] Interestingly, this report built on Alexandre de Mérode's communication and included for the first time not only recommendations concerning testing possibilities but also stated that educational measures should be introduced by the NOCs in order to implement a "long-term educational policy."[131] However, at the same time, the report presented a more aggressive approach in terms of testing procedures: NOCs should include a statement by the athletes to refrain from doping in their entry forms, IFs should establish their own anti-doping rules, the IOC should issue a statement against doping, and establish sanctions against athletes and their NOCs in the case of positive tests. Importantly, it also stressed that preparations for doping test during the upcoming Olympic Games in Grenoble and Mexico City should be initiated.[132] For this reason, Arthur Porritt remarked that a list of prohibited drugs and artificial stimulants had been established and that these substances would be

---

[128] Avery Brundage thanked Albert Dirix in a letter for his efforts to compile the report together with the Council of Europe. Letter, "Avery Brundage to Dr. Albert Dirix, January 4, 1966," archive collection "IOC Medical Commission," folder "Medical Commission: Alphabetical correspondence 1960-1967," IOC Archive, Lausanne.

[129] Letter, "Avery Brundage to Alexandre De Mérode, January 5, 1966," archive collection "IOC Medical Commission," folder "Medical Commission: Alphabetical correspondence 1960-1967," IOC Archive, Lausanne.

[130] Minutes, "64th IOC Session in Rome, April 24-30, 1966," archive collection "IOC Sessions 1894-2009," IOC Archive, Lausanne, 49.

[131] Ibid.

[132] Ibid.

particularly dangerous in Mexico City due to the high altitude.[133] At the following IOC Executive Board Meeting in October 1966, it was eventually decided that doping and gender tests[134] had to be introduced for the 1968 Mexico City Olympic Games, and the matter was again put on the agenda for the following IOC Session in Tehran in 1967, mainly to determine the list of banned substances.[135] There, the IOC members decided that alcohols, amphetamine and ephedrine, cocaine, vaso dilators, opiates (opium, morphine, heroin, pethedrine, methadin) and cannabis (hashish) constituted "dope."[136] In addition to these substances, the IOC emphasised that anabolic steroids were doping. However, because no testing method for steroids existed at the time, they were not officially listed.[137] This highlights the need for an integration of more experts with professional competencies in doping analysis. However, the IOC did not included them yet, and instead international specialists from FIMS together with local specialists foreseen to conduct the doping controls at the 1968 Olympic Games.

Nevertheless, the decision to establish tests officially points towards the now prevalent knowledge by Arthur Porritt and Alexandre de Mérode about reliable testing procedures for the listed substances. Otherwise, the distinction concerning anabolic steroids would not have been made. This was a result of the early influence of Alexandre de Mérode, who always argued that only substances that could be completely reliably tested for, should be added to the list of banned substances.[138] This is even more important because at the time of the IOC Session

---

[133] Minutes, "64th IOC Session in Rome, April 24-30, 1966," 21. The altitude question ahead of the 1968 Mexico City Olympic Games, with which the medical experts in the IOC dealt extensively, has been addressed in detailed by WRYNN. In fact, it had already been attempted by the rival bids of Lyon, Detroit and Buenos Aires to point out this issue prior to the vote. The IOC in particular debated whether athletes should be granted more time to prepare for the extreme setting in Mexico City. However, although several studies by NOCs outlined that this would be a necessary change, the IOC ignored the recommendations because it was against the amateur rules. Ultimately, the IOC allowed the athletes two more weeks to prepare for the Games. However, only two weeks were allowed to be training weeks at high altitudes. WRYNN, "The Human Factor," 215ff.
[134] For a conclusive summary on gender testing at the Olympic Games, see: Lindsay P. PIEPER, "Sex Testing and the Maintenance of Western Femininity in International Sport," *International Journal of the History of Sport* 31, no 13 (2014), 1563.
[135] Minutes, "Executive Board, October 22, 1966," archive collection "IOC Executive Board Meetings 1921-1982," IOC Archive, Lausanne, 11.
[136] Minutes, "65th IOC Session in Tehran, May 3-9, 1967," archive collection "IOC Sessions 1894-2009," IOC Archive, Lausanne, Annex 11a.
[137] Ibid.
[138] DIMEO et al., "Saint or Sinner?," 932ff.

in Tehran, Arthur Porritt was not officially head of the IOC doping subcommittee anymore. Already in summer 1966, Arthur Porritt had announced his resignation from the IOC to become governor of New Zealand. In April 1967, IOC general secretary Johann Wilhelm Westerhoff invited Alexandre de Mérode to head the Committee,[139] with him accepting his new position only a couple of days later.[140] In his acceptance letter, he referred to a possible expansion of the committee, which he wanted to discuss in Tehran. DIMEO et al. write that this decision was most likely due to Alexandre de Mérode's political skills and his previous engagement in doping matters at IOC Sessions.[141] Expert or not, it was eventually Alexandre de Mérode, who was about to constitute a new IOC Medical Commission, who included anti-doping laboratory experts into the Committee and therefore instigated their actual involvement in the IOC's fight against doping.

INTERIM RESULTS FOR THE PERIOD UNTIL 1967: SPORT MEDICINE SPECIALISTS LAY FOUNDATION FOR OLYMPIC DOPING CONTROL SYSTEM

The brief investigation into early efforts of medical experts to define and find ways to combat doping reveals that they were at the forefront of these processes since the early 1950s. In sport medical conferences, medical experts debated about the effects of performance-enhancing substances on the health of athletes and undertook experiments to investigate into the exact impact of the substances. Others, such as Pierre Dumas, even led campaigns to raise awareness about the health risks of doping that eventually led to the introduction of anti-doping laws.[142] Some medical experts were beginning to apply testing and verification procedures for the usage of doping and established the first anti-doping laboratory in Florence in 1956. Together with governments and sport organisations, the experts were also involved in the first installations of anti-doping laws in European countries and the first doping definition by the CoE. Due to the long-

---

[139] Letter, "Johann Wilhelm Westerhoff to Alexandre De Mérode, April 6, 1967," archive collection "IOC Medical Commission," folder "Medical Commission: Alphabetical correspondence 1960-1967," IOC Archive, Lausanne.

[140] Letter, "Alexandre De Mérode to Johann Wilhelm Westerhoff, April 13, 1967," archive collection "IOC Medical Commission," folder "Medical Commission: Alphabetical correspondence 1960-1967," IOC Archive, Lausanne.

[141] DIMEO et al., "Saint or Sinner?," 929.

[142] Neil CARTER, *Medicine, Sport and the Body. A Historical Perspective* (London: Bloomsbury, 2012), 117.

lasting relationship between the IOC and medicine, medical experts constituted the first IOC doping subcommittee in 1961. However, the integrated IOC members with a medical background did not contribute extensively to the committee.

Parallel to the processes in sport medicine and sport organisations, pharmaceutical and biochemical experts were making fast progress in the development of testing techniques to detect the usage of drugs in bodily fluids by the 1960s. It is important to understand these technical advancements as they coincide with the increased efforts of medical experts and sport organisations to establish doping definitions and anti-doping regulations. This is despite the fact that the pharmaceutical and biochemical experts did not have a focus on sports drug testing. No such organised scientific expertise as "sports drug testing" existed due to the lack of a doping control system. Consequently, sport administrators did not need their professional competencies, yet. However, Vanessa HEGGIE highlights that the increased interest in and funding for sport medicine by the mid-1960s, "began to attract the attention of researchers who might not otherwise have become involved with athletes."[143] One of them was Arnold Beckett. By applying his expertise to the area of sports drug testing, initially mainly in Great Britain, Arnold Beckett became the first anti-doping laboratory expert and the first chemical expert to establish a knowledge base concerning the topic. His expertise did have an immediate impact as the positive doping controls at the Tour of Britain revealed and soon individuals began to recognise the value of his scientific competencies for the world of sport.

Finally, one has to ascertain that no network of anti-doping laboratory experts with a biochemical or pharmaceutical background existed until 1967. As demonstrated, one can relate this to the lack of intention to implement testing procedures and the strong involvement of medical experts who had also conducted doping tests. Arnold Beckett appears to have been an isolated pioneer in the development of doping analysis procedures at the time. However, the work related to sport was not his specific focus as numerous publications related to other chemical issues, published in the 1960s, reveal. In contrast, a core group of medical anti-doping experts dealt with the issue more intensively and therefore laid the foundation for the anti-doping laboratory network to build on in subsequent years.

---

[143] Vanessa HEGGIE, *A history of British sports medicine* (Manchester: Manchester University Press, 2011), 113.

CHAPTER 3

Individual Consultancy (1967-1972)

INCLUSION OF ARNOLD BECKETT ON THE IOC MEDICAL
COMMISSION

The installation of the IOC Medical Commission resulted in a major reconstruction on the individual level of the IOC's fight against doping. As in the case of the IOC doping subcommission, it is important to consider the different professional backgrounds of the future members because they had decisive effect on its work.[1]

Alexandre de Mérode had already worked on the set-up of the Commission prior to his official appointment. Written exchanges to invite the new potential members reveal that Alexandre de Mérode and Johann Wilhelm Westerhoff had been informed about the work of Arnold Beckett. Curiously, however, they still lacked sufficient knowledge about him. One can recognise this by the letter Johann Wilhelm Westerhoff sent to the secretary of the BOA, Sandy Duncan, in which he was trying to find out the correct name of Arnold Beckett:

> As you know, the IOC has decided that a new medical commission is to be set up under the chairmanship of Prince Alexandre de Mérode. We have been asked to write to all those who have been chosen to be members in order to find out if they are willing to serve on this commission. Amongst these nominations is an English doctor who is a specialist in questions of doping and whose name is Professor Plaskett or Basckett. We would be most grateful if you could give us the correct

---

[1] For example, HENNE touches briefly on the professions of the inaugural members of the IOC Medical Commission and argues that the members were mainly outspoken advocates on the issue of doping. She also identifies Arnold Beckett and Alexandre de Mérode as the two central figures of the IOC's fight against doping. However, she does not go into detail about the background of the other members. HENNE, "The Origins," 11.

name, initials and address of this gentleman so that we can write to him as requested.[2]

An immediate response to the letter came from David Burghley who clarified Arnold Beckett's name, whilst stating that he was a "great football expert on doping" because he had undertaken the doping controls at the 1966 World Cup.[3] Furthermore, it is noteworthy that Johann Wilhelm Westerhoff does not refer to Arnold Beckett as a pharmacologist or a chemist, but a "doctor". This is an important detail as it suggests that he did not distinguish between different scientific fields to deal with the doping issue. In his response, Sandy Duncan therefore also emphasised Arnold Beckett's profession:

> He is not a medical doctor but a scientist (chemist) who has had great experience in dope testing in this Country [sic]. He would seem to be a most suitable member of your commission.[4]

This episode reveals how IOC administrators were ignorant about the composition of the IOC Medical Committee. In fact, Arnold Beckett was invited to be a member of the IOC Medical Commission, despite the IOC's general secretary appearing to have had no knowledge about his exact profession, his contribution to the anti-doping initiatives, or indeed shockingly his name. Notwithstanding, when Arnold Beckett accepted the membership on the IOC Medical Commission, the first anti-doping laboratory expert from outside the medical sciences began to occupy a role within a decision-making IOC body. One has to consider this the start of a new phase in the IOC's efforts to combat doping in sport.

In contrast to the problems the IOC administration faced in tracing Arnold Beckett, establishing contact with the other potential members of the IOC Medical Commission turned out to be significantly easier. This was mainly because these persons already had close contact to the IOC through prior

---

[2] Letter, "Johann Wilhelm Westerhoff to Sandy Duncan, July 11, 1967," archive collection "IOC Medical Commission," folder "Medical Commission: Alphabetical correspondence 1960-1967," IOC Archive, Lausanne.

[3] Letter, "Lord David Burghley to Johann Wilhelm Westerhoff, July 11, 1967," archive collection "IOC Medical Commission," folder "Medical Commission: Alphabetical correspondence 1960-1967," IOC Archive, Lausanne.

[4] Letter, "Sandy Duncan to Johann Wilhelm Westerhoff, July 14, 1967," archive collection "IOC Medical Commission," folder "Medical Commission: Alphabetical correspondence 1960-1967," IOC Archive, Lausanne.

involvements. As no other IOC members from the former IOC doping subcommittee were available, Hungarian IOC member Árpád Csánadi[5] became vice-chairman. This was in line with the IOC strategy to keep IOC members at the forefront of its commissions since Árpád Csánadi´s medical knowledge, according to his own admission, did not "surpass the level of average sports-expert´s knowledge."[6] Furthermore, Alexandre de Mérode also included medical experts who had coined the first phase of anti-doping efforts from a medical perspective and were involved in the FIMS. He invited Ludwig Prokop to work on the Commission. Ludwig Prokop´s determination to deal with the doping issue in a more rigorous manner comes to the fore in his response, when he argued, "there are many urgent and difficult problems to clear up."[7] Interestingly, he also stated that he knew all the proposed members personally, which emphasises the previously introduced network of sport medicine specialists. Ludwig Prokop certainly had permanent knowledge exchange with the second prominent medical doctor to become a member, Albert Dirix. Due to his leading role in the superficial doping controls at the 1964 Tokyo Olympic Games and his involvement in anti-doping initiatives of the UCI and FIMS, Albert Dirix seemed to be an obvious choice. In order to strengthen the links to the FIMS, Alexandre de Mérode asked the FIMS president, Giuseppe La Cava, to become a permanent member of the IOC Medical Commission. Finally, Alexandre de Mérode nominated Pieter van Dijk in order to integrate international and national sport federations. Apart from being president of the KNWU, Pieter van Dijk had a proven record in sports medicine and was involved in the Medical Commission of the UCI.[8]

---

[5] Árpád Csánadi (1923-1983) was a graduate of the Budapest University Law School and the Hungarian College of Physical Education and had a Ph.D. in history. In 1968, he became chairperson of the Sports Commission and served as the IOC´s honorary sports director until his death in 1983. He was elected onto the IOC Executive Board twice from May 1979 to May 1979 and from May 1982 to March 1983. He was a very engaging IOC member and did not miss any IOC Session during his membership. "The Biographies of all IOC members, No. 262 Árpád Csánadi," *Journal of Olympic History* 2, no. 1 (2013), 63.

[6] Letter, "Árpád Csánadi to Johann Wilhelm Westerhoff, August 15, 1967," archive collection "IOC Medical Commission," folder "Medical Commission: Alphabetical correspondence 1960-1967," IOC Archive, Lausanne.

[7] Letter, "Ludwig Prokop to Johann Wilhelm Westerhoff, August 9, 1967," archive collection "IOC Medical Commission," folder "Medical Commission: Alphabetical correspondence 1960-1967," IOC Archive, Lausanne.

[8] Press Release, "IOC Medical Commission, September 27, 1967," archive collection "IOC Medical Commission," folder "Medical Commission: Alphabetical correspondence 1960-1967," IOC Archive, Lausanne.

In addition to permanent members, Johann Wilhelm Westerhoff also wrote to the Organising Committees of the 1968 Olympic Games to name representatives that would work on the IOC Medical Commission until the end of their respective Games. The representative of the 1968 Mexico City Olympic Games became Professor Dr. Eduardo Hay,[9] who served as coordinator for International Congresses and chief of protocol on the Organising Committee. The Organising Committee of the 1968 Winter Olympic Games in Grenoble also appointed a medical doctor. Originally, this was Dr. Roger Genin,[10] who is listed in the letter sent out to all anticipated members in July 1967[11] as well as in the official announcement about the establishment of the Medical Commission in August 1967.[12] However, from December 1967 onwards, Dr. Jacques Thiebault[13] replaced Roger Genin because CNOSF, for whom Jacques Thiebault worked, attempted to have a permanent member on the body.[14]

The first composition of the IOC Medical Commission therefore reveals several strategies that were beginning to take shape after the takeover of the IOC´s fight against doping through Alexandre de Mérode. The approach towards external medical experts shows that he wanted to have much more experienced and specialised experts on the Commission. One can attribute this to the fact that Alexandre de Mérode was not a medical doctor himself and therefore had no *professional* interest in the topic. He was an outstanding networker and had connections to the key players from the medical field through his previous

---

[9] Professor Dr. Eduardo Hay (1915-2005) was also Professor of gynaecology and obstetrics at the National University of Mexico City as well as director of the American British Cowdray Hospital and the Ampero Maternity Hospital in Mexico City. "The Biographies of all IOC members, No. 306 Dr. Eduardo Hay," *Journal of Olympic History* 22, no. 1 (2014), 60.

[10] ORGANISING COMMITTEE OF THE XXTH WINTER OLYMPIC GAMES, *Official Report of the 10th Winter Olympic Games in Grenoble* (Genoble: Organising Committee of the XXth Winter Olympic Games, 1969), 18.

[11] Letter, "Johann Wilhelm Westerhoff, July 6, 1967," archive collection "IOC Medical Commission," folder "Medical Commission: Alphabetical correspondence 1960-1967," IOC Archive, Lausanne.

[12] Information Letter, "Johann Wilhelm Westerhoff to the Members of the IOC Medical Commission, n.d." archive collection "IOC Medical Commission," folder "Medical Commission: Alphabetical correspondence 1960-1967," IOC Archive, Lausanne.

[13] It was not possible to obtain additional biographical data on Dr. Jacques Thiebault, neither from the archival sources nor through additional resources.

[14] Letter, "French National Olympic Committee to Johan Wilhelm Westerhoff, December 15, 1967," archive collection "IOC Medical Commission," folder "Medical Commission: Alphabetical correspondence 1960-1967," IOC Archive, Lausanne.

involvement in anti-doping. This strategy was a dramatic change in comparison to the previous policy under Sir Arthur Porritt, who was a medical doctor himself. Pragmatic issues resulted from this. For example, financial issues now had to be resolved prior to the eventual composition of the Commission. Alexandre de Mérode was aware that the external advisors would expect their travel expenses to be paid by the IOC and he addressed this matter when he first spoke to Johann Wilhelm Westerhoff about a possible expansion of the then still IOC doping subcommittee.[15]

HUNT claims that after the resignation of Arthur Porritt from the IOC, a shift from "doping" to "medicine" took place within the Olympic Movement.[16] However, after the reconsideration undertaken in this chapter, it seems necessary to regard this as an even more particularised shift. It is certainly correct that the main debate until 1967 was to define doping. However, these debates were only being held by *internal* medical experts, who relied heavily on external advisors. Yet, the IOC did not integrate these advisors until 1967. Their role was reduced to the publication of articles and as agents of the IOC. The change that occurred after 1967 was caused by the attitude that the IOC only added testable substances to the banned list. In combination with the takeover of Alexandre de Mérode, this allowed *external* medical experts to get more actively involved and started the collaboration with anti-doping laboratory experts. The change is therefore more a shift from internal to external medical expertise in the 1960s, when considering the different actors dealing with doping in the IOC.

Finally, the set-up of the original IOC Medical Commission reveals that Alexandre de Mérode was in favour of a strict testing policy, for which he needed the inclusion of an expert in the analytical procedures of doping controls. Consequently, bringing together medical experts and a scientist with anti-doping laboratory experience and competencies in doping analysis appeared to be the logical solution.

ARNOLD BECKETT STARTS CONSULTING THE IOC's FIGHT AGAINST DOPING

The IOC informed the public about the formation of the IOC Medical Commission in a press release in September 1967. Therein it outlined its composition (at the time still including Roger Genin) and stated that both doping

---

[15] WRYNN, "The Human Factor," 220.

[16] HUNT, *Drug Games*, 23.

and gender controls were its main concerns.[17] The press release also reveals that the focus of the first meeting of the IOC Medical Commission had been on the establishment of official doping testing procedures:

> After having drawn up a list of drugs, the Commission analysed and prepared point by point all the various stages which must be followed from the moment a sample is taken to the moment that a laboratory has carried out its analysis. The Commission took great care to lay down a procedure for these tests which will be as efficient as possible. Details of the procedure will later be made known by the International Olympic Committee. The procedures will be put into use in during International Competitions in Mexico.[18]

HUNT argues that the introduction of this very specific protocol points towards Alexandre de Mérode´s care for athlete´s rights but also a reduction of possible legal proceedings from participant´s perspective.[19] Moreover, the weight given to the single steps of doping controls, from the sample taking to the result of the laboratory test, was also a result of the individuals now working together on the body. The medical experts had firsthand experience about the conduction of doping controls and dealt with the single steps at various sporting events. One has to assume that Arnold Beckett had an influence on the first mentioning of a standardised "laboratory" for the analytical procedures of the samples in an official IOC publication. Furthermore, ahead of the first preliminary meeting of the Medical Commission in August 1967, Arnold Beckett proposed to add the issue "Organisation of Sampling Procedures and the General Protocol of Anti-Doping Control" onto the meeting agenda.[20] This point is a first indication for the establishment of a systematic guideline for doping controls and shows his pragmatic concern for the matter beyond doping analysis. Just two days after the meeting, he provided Johann Wilhelm Westerhoff with the report on the doping controls at the 1966 World Cup, along with a specific research report on the

---

[17] Press Release, "IOC Medical Commission, September 27, 1967."

[18] Ibid.

[19] HUNT, *Drug Games*, 25.

[20] Letter, "Arnold H. Beckett to Johann Wilhelm Westerhoff, August 24, 1967," archive collection "IOC Medical Commission," folder "Medical Commission: Alphabetical correspondence 1960-1967," IOC Archive, Lausanne.

testing methods.[21] He sent the documents to all members of the IOC Medical Commission and Arnold Beckett supplied them with a first draft to adopt the analytical methods for usage at the Olympic Games.[22]

The other members and IOC general secretary Johann Wilhelm Westerhoff regarded Arnold Beckett as the person to establish guidelines for doping analysis. When Johann Wilhelm Westerhoff informed Arnold Beckett about a further IOC Medical Commission meeting, he asked Arnold Beckett to compile "a report concerning laboratory methods for doping tests." [23] Such details confirm the assertion that Arnold Beckett instantly occupied a leading role within the IOC Medical Commission.[24] In retrospect, this principal function must be contributed to Arnold Beckett's specific professional competencies. He had firsthand experience in the development of the analytical procedures and was best equipped to advise the medical experts and the IOC on these matters. Arnold Beckett himself also left no doubt that he was responsible for this aspect of the doping analysis.[25] Hence, he aimed to standardise anti-doping laboratory techniques from the very beginning of his activities on the IOC Medical Commission. Clearly, he was encouraged in his intentions by the frequent occurrence of ambiguous results such as at the International Sports Week in Mexico, where three analysed samples contained unidentified substances.[26] Similar problems occurred during the 1967 Pan American Games in Winnipeg, where the Department of Medicine of the Manitoba Clinic and the School of Pharmacy of the University of Manitoba

[21] Letter, "Arnold H. Beckett to Johann Wilhelm Westerhoff, September 29, 1967," archive collection "IOC Medical Commission," folder "Medical Commission: Alphabetical correspondence 1960-1967," IOC Archive, Lausanne.

[22] Letter, "Arnold H. Beckett to Members of the Medical Committee of the International Olympic Committee, November 10, 1967," archive collection "IOC Medical Commission," folder "Medical Commission: Alphabetical correspondence 1960-1967," IOC Archive, Lausanne.

[23] Letter, "Johann Wilhelm Westerhoff to Arnold H. Beckett, November 1, 1967," archive collection "IOC Medical Commission," folder "Medical Commission: Alphabetical correspondence 1960-1967," IOC Archive, Lausanne.

[24] DIMEO et al., "Saint or Sinner?," 930.

[25] Letter, "Arnold H. Beckett to Johann Wilhelm Westerhoff, November 6, 1967," archive collection "IOC Medical Commission," folder "Medical Commission: Alphabetical correspondence 1960-1967," IOC Archive, Lausanne.

[26] Report, "Chemical control and laboratory report, Eduardo Hay, October 1967," archive collection "IOC Medical Commission," folder "Medical Commission: Alphabetical correspondence 1960-1967," IOC Archive, Lausanne.

conducted the doping tests.[27] The reports of these events stressed the need for the development of more rapid and precise laboratory methods.

The medical expert the most engaged in the discussions and first steps of the IOC Medical Commission was Ludwig Prokop. As mentioned above, in his response to the invitation to be part of the new body, Ludwig Prokop demonstrated great urgency towards finding a solution to the doping problem. A second letter confirms this attitude. Therein, he provided Johann Wilhelm Westerhoff with a "basis for discussion," where he argued that the list of banned substances should consist of substances that could be tested for, but also those for which detection was not yet available.[28] This contradicted Alexandre de Mérode´s point of view and the basis for anti-doping laboratory work, namely to rely only on scientific evidence. Ludwig Prokop was also of the opinion that the substances should not be made public, so the athletes and officials could not substitute their drugs for other substances. Furthermore, Ludwig Prokop suggested different steps of the sampling procedure, and voiced his opinion on the role of the IOC Medical Commission members, which included the randomly chosen controlling of the urine sampling and the analytical procedures. [29] However, he already distinguished clearly between medical responsibilities and those of Arnold Beckett. Whereas Ludwig Prokop discussed in detail the possible substances to be banned, and gave suggestions on the sampling of doping controls, he only referred to the analytical procedures very briefly whilst maintaining that Arnold Beckett should coordinate them.[30]

Since the 1968 Winter Olympic Games in Grenoble began on February 6, 1968, it seems reasonable that the IOC Medical Commission met for a second time in December 1967 in order to determine the exact procedures and rules for

---

[27] Report, "Report on the Drug Testing Programme (Cycling Event) Fifth Pan American Games, M.F. McInnes and J.W. Steele, 1967," archive collection "IOC Medical Commission," folder "Medical Commission: Alphabetical correspondence 1960-1967," IOC Archive, Lausanne.

[28] Letter, "Ludwig Prokop to Johann Wilhelm Westerhoff, December 6, 1967," archive collection "IOC Medical Commission," folder "Medical Commission: Meeting in Lausanne on September 26-27 and on December 20, 1967 and Mexico City on 1968," IOC Archive, Lausanne.

[29] Ibid.

[30] Ibid.

the doping tests.[31] The results of the meeting essentially demonstrate the main contents of the written exchanges in autumn 1967. This may also be because Ludwig Prokop's "basis for discussion" paper had been translated into English. At the end of the meeting, the IOC Medical Commission made decisions on the sanctioning of athletes, the methods of doping analysis, the list of banned substances, the collection of the urine sample and the selection of the athletes. It is particular interesting that TLC and GC, but also "any other methods which could prove to be necessary, according to the circumstances" could be used for the analysis of the urine samples.[32] The clause reveals that the IOC Medical Commission attached value to the fast-developing testing techniques and left open the possibility for even more sophisticated analytical methods. The strategy was quite clearly one of testing as much as possible and as specific. But such a policy also left a high degree of flexibility to the staff of the anti-doping laboratory at the Olympic Games, which was not provided with clear guidelines.

In addition to Alexandre de Mérode's attempts to centralise the IOC's anti-doping efforts to the IOC Medical Commission, the significance of Arnold Beckett's role becomes once again evident at the meeting. He proposed that in the case of a positive finding, an international commission under his supervision should carry out a second analytical test.[33] Therefore, he created a key role for himself and assured that the IOC Medical Commission had control over possible positive cases. Moreover, Arnold Beckett took over the responsibility of finding out whether the anti-doping laboratories at the upcoming Olympic Games in Grenoble and Mexico City were in a position to carry out the testing procedures. This was a very important aspect of the entire doping control procedure. In order to ensure the operational readiness of the laboratory, Arnold Beckett could further make use of technical equipment given free of charge by an American firm, which had already supplied laboratory equipment at the International Sports Week.[34] In agreement with the medical authorities of the Organising Committee, he could also employ further staff members for technical assistance.[35]

---

[31] This meeting was the first appearance of Dr. Jacques Thiebault as representative of the Organising Committee of the 1968 Winter Olympic Games in Grenoble. Minutes, "IOC Medical Commission, December 20, 1967," archive collection "IOC Medical Commission," folder "Medical Commission: Meeting in Lausanne on September 26-27 and on December 20, 1967 and Mexico City on 1968," IOC Archive, Lausanne.

[32] Ibid.

[33] Ibid.

[34] Ibid.

[35] Ibid.

Consequently, Arnold Beckett had a large amount of responsibility from the very beginning of the IOC Medical Commission. The essential partial aspect of the analytical procedures, now necessary due to Alexandre de Mérode´s testing policy, was covered by the involvement of anti-doping laboratory expert Arnold Beckett, who had the professional competencies in the field of doping analysis. The authority given to Arnold Beckett in the initial meetings highlights that Alexandre de Mérode did not consider the medical experts able to ensure completely reliable analytical methods like Arnold Beckett could. His appointment reflects Alexandre de Mérode´s hope to provide more reliability in the doping controls and the possibility to test for more substances.

DOPING CONTROLS AT THE 1968 WINTER OLYMPIC GAMES IN GRENOBLE

Preparations for the Anti-doping Laboratory

Researchers have paid little attention to the doping controls at the 1968 Winter Olympic Games in Grenoble. For example, HEMMERSBACH claims that they were a "pilot project"[36] and Craig KAMMERER does not list doping controls at Winter Olympic Games at all.[37] It is surprising that despite the lack of an official doping protocol, researchers did not illustrate the different steps and the analytical methods, especially considering their significance as the first official doping controls at any Olympic Games. This mirrors the general lack of research focus on Winter Olympic Games.[38]

---

[36] Importantly though, HEMMERSBACH focuses his article only on the history of MS at the Olympic Games, which was not used in Grenoble. HEMMERSBACH, "History," 839.

[37] R. Craig KAMMERER, "What Is Doping and How Is It Detected?," in: *Doping in Elite Sport. The Politics of Drugs in the Olympic Movement*, eds. Wayne WILSON and Edward DERSE (Champaign, Ill: Human Kinetics, 2001), 5.

[38] Most authors argue that their reluctance to deal with the Olympic Winter Games is rooted in the limited length of their articles, in other historical reviews on event specific subjects, they are not mentioned at all. For a general chronological review on the Winter Olympic Games, see Volker KLUGE´s publication: Volker KLUGE, *Olympische Winterspiele – Die Chronik* (Berlin, Sportverlag, 1994). Otto SCHANTZ analyses the general attitude towards the Winter Olympic Games and argues that they are influenced by the Olympic Movement´s interpretation of Olympism. Otto SCHANTZ, "The Olympic Ideal and the Winter Games: Attitudes Towards the Olympic Winter Games in Olympic Discourses – from Coubertin to Samaranch," in: *From Chamonix to Turin. The Winter Games in the Scope of Olympic Research*, eds. Norbert MÜLLER, Manfred MESSING and Holger PREUß (Kassel: Agon Sportverlag, 2006), 39-57.

Past approaches and assumptions should not hide the fact that the doping controls conducted in Grenoble were being implemented based on the decisions made by the IOC Medical Commission in December 1967. As previously mentioned, the main drug testing policy was to only test for substances that could reliably be detected and therefore anabolic steroids were not found on the list of banned substances that Alexandre de Mérode presented to the IOC Executive Board in January 1968.[39] The IOC Medical Commission's clarified this also at an Executive Board meeting on February 6, 1968, where Jacques Thiebault gave an overview of the planned doping control mechanism.[40] Responding to a query from Avery Brundage about whether the proposed tests are reliable, Jacques Thiebault answered that with the GC and the infrared spectrophotometer one could practically give a guarantee of 100%.[41] Later on, he reaffirmed this position, when once again questioned by Avery Brundage. The IOC president appeared to be very concerned about the reliability of the test, an attitude, which he would maintain for the entire time of his presidency.[42] It was also discussed extensively whether medals could be awarded before the results of the doping analysis became available. As the IOC Medical Commission members estimated that this procedure took between half an hour and three hours, there was great concern that the medal ceremony would be postponed. Nothing was decided, but it appears that the Executive Board agreed with the suggestion by Soviet IOC

---

[39] The substances on the definitive list were: 1) sympathomimetic amines (for example amphetamines), ephedrine and similar substances; 2) stimulants of the central nervous system (strychnine) and analeptics; 3) narcotics and analgesics (for example morphine), similar substances; 4) anti-depressants, imipramine and similar substances; 5) major tranquillisers (for example phenothiazine). Minutes, Executive Board, January 26 and 27, 1968, archive collection "IOC Executive Board Meetings 1921-1982," IOC Archive, Lausanne, Annex 3.

[40] It appears that not all members of the IOC Medical Commission were present at the meeting because besides Jacques Thiebault and Alexandre de Mérode only Giuseppe La Cava, Eduardo Hay and Ludwig Prokop make an appearance in the official minutes of the meeting. Arnold Beckett is not mentioned and questions concerning the analytical procedures are answered by Jacques Thiebault.

[41] Minutes, "Executive Board, February 6, 1968," archive collection "IOC Executive Board Meetings 1921-1982," IOC Archive, Lausanne, 11.

[42] Without referring to the above-discussed minutes of the IOC Executive Board meeting in February 1968, HUNT outlines that the IOC's reluctance to test for more substances had indeed been activated by the attitude to protect the IOC and the IOC Medical Commission legally. This can be linked to Avery Brundage's position that the IFs should be responsible for the actual conduction of the tests with the IOC Medical Commission members only occupying a supervisor role. HUNT, *Drug Games*, 25.

member Nikolay Andrianov to only withhold the medals in such "doping endangered sports" as biathlon, speed skating and skiing.[43] Clearly, the IOC administration did not favour such a regulation, whilst the discussion also illustrates the need for faster analytical procedures. Moreover, Jacques Thiebault gave information on the profile of the laboratory, where the analytical parts of the control were conducted and thus a first indication of the profile of the inaugural, still very basic, anti-doping laboratory at any Olympic Games. He argued that France had experience in conducting doping tests:

> Nous avon mise sur pied, à la Faculté de Médecine de Paris, un laboratoire specialisé qui est dote du matériel le plus moderne et qui se tient au courant des techniques et des produits employés, ainsi que des recherches. Ce laboratoire a été transporté en entier à Grenoble pour travailler au profit des Jeux Olympiques. Lorsqu'on parle de toxicologie les instruments sont une chose, mais les techniciens sont aussi importants.

> [We have established a specialised laboratory at the Faculty of Medicine in Paris, which is equipped according to the most modern standards and always up-to-date concerning the applied techniques and products as well as research. This laboratory has been completely transported to Grenoble in order to work for the profit of the Olympic Games. If we speak about toxicology, the instruments are one thing but the technicians are also important.][44]

In contrast to the tests in 1964, an entire laboratory team, relocated to Grenoble from the University of Paris, worked on the doping controls. Three analytical gas chromatographs, one preparative gas chromatograph and an infrared spectrophotometer were used for the analytical procedures and transported from Paris to Grenoble.[45] The analytical methods applied were the ones described by

---

[43] Minutes, "Executive Board, February 6, 1968," 14.

[44] Ibid., 9f.

[45] Report, "Jacques Thiebault on the work of the Medical Commission at the 1968 Grenoble Olympic Winter Games, 1968," archive collection "Avery Brundage Collection, 1908-1975," film 54, folder 0005 "Medical Commission IOC 1966-1969," IOC Archive, Lausanne, 19.

Arnold BECKETT et al. in their article from 1967,[46] again displaying the significance of the groundwork that Arnold Beckett had made. The main equipment, plus further appliances, was installed at the Grenoble Armies' Hospital one week ahead of the Olympic Games.[47] It was anticipated to analyse ten samples per day and that the "analytical methods employed must be indisputable and leave no hold for criticism."[48] Furthermore, Arnold Beckett was supposed to supervise the analysis but the technicians from the laboratory in Paris were in charge of undertaking the analytical parts of the tests.[49] Ludwig Prokop criticised this detail after the Olympic Games:

> For fundamental reasons, a laboratory working on sex and dope controls cannot be entirely occupied by experts from the host country, but must work with International experts or be supervised by two international experts.[50]

Consequently, the controls at the 1968 Winter Olympic Games in Grenoble were an opposed process to the developments surrounding the IOC Medical Commission. Whereas its members attempted to develop international standards for doping analysis, the implementation of the analytical procedures in Grenoble were of national character. Hence, while the circumstances point towards more inclusion of anti-doping laboratory expertise, this was not yet realised. At the same time, the used equipment and applied methods reflect the advancements made in doping analysis.

First Athletes Tested at Olympic Games

As intended, the laboratory staff analysed 86 urine specimens in Grenoble. These 86 samples were the first ever officially IOC-sanctioned doping controls at any Olympic Games. The first controls took place on February 7, 1968, following the men's 30km cross-country skiing race. This was the first medal competition of

---

[46] Arnold H. BECKETT, G.T. TUCKER and A.C. MOFFAT, "Routine Detection and Determination of Ephedrine and its Congeners in Urine by Gas Chromatography," *Journal of Pharmacy and Pharmacology* 19 (1967), 273-294.

[47] ORGANISING COMMITTEE OF THE X[TH] WINTER OLYMPIC GAMES, *Official Report*, 276ff.

[48] Ibid.

[49] Report, "Jacques Thiebault on the work of the Medical Commission at the 1968 Grenoble Olympic Winter Games, 1968," 21.

[50] Letter, "Ludwig Prokop to Alexandre de Mérode, March 14, 1968," archive collection "IOC Medical Commission," folder "Medical Commission: Alphabetical correspondence L-Z 1968," IOC Archive, Lausanne.

the entire Games, staged in Autrans.[51] The athletes occupying the first six places, along with four randomly selected competitors underwent the first doping control. According to the historical files in the IOC archive, the Finish athlete Eero Mäntyranta[52], who came third in the race, was the first ever athlete to be controlled for a banned substance at any Olympic Games.[53] In the presence of a Finish official, Eduardo Hay and Alexandre de Mérode, Eero Mäntyranta gave his urine sample on February 7, 1968, at 11.30am. The IOC Medical Commission members labelled the urine bottle with the number "one," which does not point towards a sophisticated system to protect the anonymity of the athlete.[54] In retrospect, the fact that he was the first athlete to be tested has to be considered ironic: in 1972, Eero Mäntyranta became the first ever Finish athlete to be tested positive for doping, and throughout his career he was suspect to blood doping because of his genetically high amount of red blood cells.[55] Besides Eero Mäntyranta, his teammate Kalevi Laurila, who finished in sixth place, and the race winner Franco Nones (Italy), gave their samples in the first round. However, due to the serial number "one" given to Eero Mäntyranta's sample, there is sufficient evidence to argue that his test was the first. The other athletes, who underwent the doping controls following the 30km race were Odd Martinsen (Norway, 2nd place), Vladimir Voronkov (USSR, 4th place) and Giulio de Florian (Italy, 5th place) as well as the anonymously drafted Arto Tiainen (Finland, 16th

---

[51] Autrans was the site of the cross-country skiing, biathlon, nordic combined and the ski jumping events. ORGANISING COMMITTEE OF THE XTH WINTER OLYMPIC GAMES, *Official Report*, 218.

[52] Eero Mäntyranta (1937-2013) had won a total of three Olympic gold medals at the 1960 and the 1964 Winter Olympic Games. After the 1968 Olympic Games, he had ended his career but started a successful comeback in 1971. After the 1972 Sapporo Winter Olympic Games, it was announced that he has used stimulants during the qualification event for the Games on January 16, 1972. However, no punishment was given. KLUGE, *Olympische Winterspiele*, 247n1.

[53] "Epreuve des Trente KMS (Fond), February 7, 1968," archive collection "IOC Medical Commission," folder "Grenoble 1968 Medical Files," IOC Archive, Lausanne.

[54] Ibid.

[55] Eero Mäntyranta was born with a genetic mutation, called myostatin mutation, which increases the production of oxygen-rich red blood cells. In order to prove this, 200 of Eero Mäntyranta's family members were tested in the 1990s, 50 of them turned out to be born with the mutation. Due to the performance-enhancing effect, Eero Mäntyranta is assumed to have had a great advantage over his competitors during his sporting career. However, the positive doping test in 1972 cannot be contributed to the mutation because at the time no testing procedures for blood doping had been developed yet. Torbjörn TÄNNSJÖ, "Commentary," *Journal of Medical Ethics* 3, no. 2 (2005), 113.

place), Jan Fajstavr (Czechoslovakia, 22nd place), Ernst Pühringer (Austria, 38th place) and Roger Pires (France, 43rd place).[56]

The minutes of the IOC Medical Commission do not reveal other events chosen for doping controls. Rather it is stated that "the events will be selected by the drawing of lots on the morning of the competition is given."[57] However, the control sheets proved to be very revealing in this regard. Other than the cross-country skiers on the first day of the Olympic events, control sheets are available for: men's ice hockey match between the USA and the USSR (February 9, 1968), men's downhill skiing race (February 9, 1968), women's 1,500m speed skating race (February 10, 1968), men's nordic combined skiing race (February 11, 1968), men's giant slalom race (February 12, 1968), men's 500m speed skating race (February 14, 1968), men's ice hockey match between Canada and Sweden (February 15, 1968) and women's 3x5km cross country skiing race (February 16, 1968).[58] The first female athlete who underwent a doping control at Olympic Games was Christina "Stien" Kaiser from the Netherlands, who finished third in the 1500m speed skating race. The other selected female athletes were Kaija Mustonen (Finland, 1st place), Carolina "Carry" Geijssen (Netherlands, 2nd place), Sigrid Sundby (Norway, 4th place), Lasma Kouniste (USSR, 5th place), Kaijsa Keskivitikka (Finland, 6th place), Christina Lindblom (Sweden, 9th place), Jeanne Ashworth (USA, 16th place), Sachiko Saito (Japan, 18th place), and Arja Kantola (Finland, 22nd place).[59]

Whereas these facts are revealing for the overall history of the doping at the Olympic Games, it is important to emphasise that there was no positive testing result. In light of the increased efforts of the IOC Medical Commission, and the more advanced analytical procedures, this shows that the effect of the efforts was still extremely limited at the time.

[56] "Epreuve des Trente KMS (Fond)." The official results of the race can be found in: ORGANISING COMMITTEE OF THE X[TH] WINTER OLYMPIC GAMES, *Official Report*, 378.

[57] Minutes, "IOC Medical Commission, December 20, 1967."

[58] Consequently, not all Olympic sports were subject to doping test in Grenoble yet. No controls took place in the biathlon, bobsleigh, luge/tobogganing and figure skating events. "Doping Control Sheets, February 7, 1968," archive collection "IOC Medical Commission," folder "Grenoble 1968 Medical Files," IOC Archive, Lausanne.

[59] "Doping Control Sheets, February 7, 1968." The official results of the race can be found in: ORGANISING COMMITTEE OF THE X[TH] WINTER OLYMPIC GAMES, *Official Report*, 387.

Role of the Members of the IOC Medical Commission

Apart from the revelation of the first Olympic athletes subject to doping controls, it is necessary to emphasise that a medical doctor from the IOC Medical Commission signed all doping control sheets. In addition to this, Alexandre de Mérode was present at most of the doping controls. When he was not available, Eduardo Hay and Giuseppe La Cava signed the control sheet on behalf of the IOC. Since Arnold Beckett was not a medical doctor, it seems obvious that he was not involved in the sampling procedures. However, there is also no evidence that he was involved with the analytical procedures either. As explained earlier in this chapter, the members of the IOC Medical Commission were absent from the anti-doping laboratory, absence which Ludwig Prokop criticised.[60] Therefore, despite the major influence of Arnold Beckett in the preparations of the doping tests in general and the analytical procedures more specifically, he was not actively involved. Since there were officially no positive results, the procedure proposed by Arnold Beckett to carry out a second analytical test under his auspices did not require any implementation.

Giuseppe La Cava raised doubts about the analytical procedures. In his own report on the doping and gender controls, he proposed to implement "occasional counter-tests" to assure the functionality and reliability of the gas chromatographic instruments used.[61] In order to assure this, a person not engaged in the Olympic Games should take a substance from the banned list and then be tested by the Olympic Games apparatus. Giuseppe La Cava reported that he was thereby in agreement with Arnold Beckett, who had originally raised this idea.[62] This shows that Arnold Beckett insisted on the standardisation of the doping controls, especially the technical equipment. As a result, the IOC applied this measure from the 1968 Mexico City Olympic Games onwards.

Moreover, the report, with Jacques Thiebault's written notations, gives some very significant indications of the future tasks of the IOC Medical Commission.[63] Most importantly, he criticised that no official doping protocol, including an outline of all the different steps had been established. Hence, Jacques Thiebault

---

[60] Letter, "Ludwig Prokop to Alexandre de Mérode, March 14, 1968."

[61] Report, "Report on the Activity of the Medical Commission of the C.I.O. at the Winter Games of Grenoble, Giuseppe La Cava, April 4, 1968," archive collection archive collection "IOC Medical Commission," folder "Medical Commission: Alphabetical correspondence L-Z 1968," IOC Archive, Lausanne, 3.

[62] Ibid.

[63] Report, "Jacques Thiebault on the work of the Medical Commission at the 1968 Grenoble Olympic Winter Games, 1968," 16.

recommended, "our Commission could perhaps carry out the dispatch of a sort of memorandum, which could be widely circulated by the IOC to all those concerned with these questions."[64] Furthermore, he suggested that the IOC should take the samples not immediately after the event, due to the tiredness and emotiveness of the athletes. This had led to problems, and instead he proposed to leave one to two hours between the end of the competition and the sampling procedure, which would also mean that the medical staff would need to have more time on site to conduct the test.

Consequently, medical specialists on the IOC Medical Commission played central roles during the doping controls at the 1968 Winter Olympic Games in Grenoble. In reality, they dealt with all aspects of the controls. Arnold Beckett only had limited influence because he did not ultimately supervise the anti-doping laboratory. As a result, the doping analysis was still of an exploratory nature, and there was no active involvement of any anti-doping laboratory expert in the doping controls.

Doping Controls at the 1968 Mexico City Olympic Games

HUNT gives a detailed overview of the time period between the 1968 Winter Olympic Games in Grenoble and the 1968 Mexico City Olympic Games, arguing that the main dealings of Alexandre de Mérode were to discuss with Avery Brundage the responsibilities of doping controls.[65] Therefore, this is not the focus of this chapter. Avery Brundage was a stern believer that the doping controls were a technical matter and should thus be the responsibility of the IFs. However, after complaints by Alexandre de Mérode, who protected the relevance of "his" IOC Medical Commission, he backpedalled and eventually, the members of the IOC Medical Commission were allowed to direct the doping and gender tests at the 1968 Mexico City Olympic Games.[66] The only meeting of the IOC Medical Commission took place in July, after the IOC Finance Commission had caused the cancellation of an earlier meeting. Alexandre de Mérode had already addressed the reimbursement of the travel expenses prior to the establishment of the IOC Medical Commission, making it a requirement to gather the best international specialists. However, the IOC Finance Commission objected to the reimbursement because IOC members had to pay their own travel expenses. This issue could only be solved by Alexandre de Mérode's efforts to emphasise that

---

[64] Ibid., 18.

[65] HUNT, *Drug Games*, 33f.

[66] Ibid.

the members of the IOC Medical Commission were working voluntarily, and that only members from Europe were selected in order to be able to meet more frequently and more cost-efficiently.[67] Both incidents illustrate that despite their reputation in their respective scientific fields, the IOC Medical Commission members had no standing within the IOC, yet, although Alexandre de Mérode followed the policy to integrate them.

However, the financial difficulties were not the sole issue up for discussion within the IOC Medical Commission as it continued to approach scientific problems. Its members decided that athletes from all sports had to be tested, with the specific events to be randomly drawn at the beginning of each day. The recommendation of Jacques Thiebault in his report to give the athletes more time following the events was also put in place. Moreover, Eduardo Hay had proposed that the alcohol test should be taken with breathalyzers as used by police for testing alcohol consumption.[68] However, the other members opposed this because they did not consider this method a scientific test. Consequently, they decided that only a blood test would be appropriate for testing alcohol, and that the International Modern Pentathlon Union (UIPM), the only federation that demanded alcohol tests, would have to be informed about this decision.[69]

The anti-doping laboratory facilities in Mexico City were considerably bigger than those in Grenoble, which is understandable considering the significantly higher number of tests conducted. In addition to the sixteen competition site staff members, who collected the samples and coordinated the laboratory and site personnel, ten professional chemists and two laboratory technicians undertook the analytical tests during the duration of the Games.[70] The analytical apparatus used in Mexico City was very similar to the one used in Grenoble. The laboratory staff also applied the same methods. Along with the analysis via GC, the laboratory team also systematically conducted tests with

---

[67] Minutes, "IOC Medical Commission, July 13 and 14, 1968," archive collection "IOC Medical Commission," folder "Medical Commission: Meeting in Lausanne July 13-14, 1968 and January 25-26, 1969," IOC Archive, Lausanne.

[68] Minutes, "IOC Medical Commission, October 12, 1968," archive collection "IOC Medical Commission," folder "Doing at the 1968 Summer Games in Mexico City: Results of medical tests, report," IOC Archive, Lausanne, 3.

[69] Ibid.

[70] The official letters by the chemical laboratory to the IOC Medical Commission are written on the letterhead of the Control Quimico Company where the two chemists Guillermo Cortina Ancolia (chemical engineer) and Manuel Madrazo Garamendi were employed. However, the historical documents do not reveal whether the other laboratory staff were also from this company, or hired from elsewhere.

paper chromatography, thereby applying of a clause in the IOC regulations that other methods could be used if necessary. But, it is important to note that the results of the paper chromatography, even if it displayed a different result, only served as an experimental method to the IOC Medical Commission. It was argued that the analytical procedures had to be conducted employing Arnold Beckett´s method.[71] This is a significant result because it shows that alternatives would have been available. Eventually, the entire apparatus consisted of four gas chromatographs, one spectrometer with graphometer, a computer, a Polaroid camera with a trinocular microscope, four cameras for chromatography on paper, one chromatograph paper dryer, three refrigerators and two ultraviolet lamps.[72]

In contrast to the files found in relation to the 1968 Winter Olympic Games in Grenoble, the medical files of the Mexico Games do not reveal which Olympic athletes were the first ones tested for doping at Olympic Summer Games. However, it can be traced back that the first doping controls took place at the volleyball event, held on October 13, 1968, because the information sheets are available.[73] The doping controllers took 670 urine samples in total, and analysed them during the 1968 Mexico City Olympic Games. Most of them came from the swimming events, where 136 athletes were tested.[74] Importantly, the total number also includes control samples mixed by members of the IOC Medical Commission in order to test the laboratory team and its machines according to the suggestion made by Arnold Beckett and Giuseppe La Cava. In addition to this, the IOC Medical Commission took 48 analyses for alcohol in blood samples, amongst them the only declared positive test by the Swedish pentathlete Hans-Gunnar Liljenwall in the team competition, resulting in the disqualification of the Swedish team.[75] However, as DIMEO stresses, the inclusion of alcohol tests was vague and arguably legally not valid.[76]

---

[71] Report, "General Report on the Work of the Medical Commission of the International Olympic Committee During the Games of the XIXth Olympiad, Eduardo Hay, 1968," archive collection "IOC Medical Commission," folder "Doping tests at the 1968 Summer Olympic Games in Mexico City: Results of medical tests, report," IOC Archive, Lausanne, 12.

[72] Ibid.

[73] Note, "Informe Sobre Investigacion de Drogas, October 13, 1968," archive collection "IOC Medical Commission," folder "Doping tests at the 1968 Summer Olympic Games in Mexico City: Results of medical tests, report," IOC Archive, Lausanne.

[74] Report, "General Report, Eduardo Hay," 5ff.

[75] Minutes, "Executive Board, March 22 and 23, 1968," archive collection "IOC Executive Board Meetings 1921-1982," IOC Archive, Lausanne, 6.

[76] Dimeo, *A History,* 114.

Controversial Role of Arnold Beckett in Mexico City

When focusing on the role of anti-doping laboratory experts, it is important to investigate more in-depth into the role of Arnold Beckett during the 1968 Mexico City Olympic Games. The report by Eduardo Hay along with a letter by the two heads of the anti-doping laboratory shed light into this issue.[77] It has already been outlined that the analytical procedures were based on Arnold Beckett's experience with GC. However, the analysis did not run smoothly as the laboratory staff summarised the doping tests and the undertaken analytical work as follows:

a) For gaseous phase chromatography eighteen samples presented abnormal peaks, without being able to identify the drug.

b) For chromatography on paper, eighty-four samples presented abnormal stains.

c) Of the eighty-four samples that produced abnormal results in chromatography on paper, only three were abnormal in gaseous phase chromatography.

d) Of the eighty-four abnormal samples, twenty-two presented an absorption curve in ultraviolet light with abnormal peaks, without being able to identify the nature of the chromophoric grouping.

e) Of the eighty-four samples of chromatography on paper, twenty produced stains and reactions characteristic of nitrogenised substances (tertiary bases) of high molecular weight.

f) Of the eighty-four samples, eight presented reactions to that indicated the presence of tranquilizing drugs.78

This summary illustrates that there had been 18 suspicious samples discovered through the official analytical method using GC and even 48 suspicious samples according to the paper chromatography method, not regarded as official. One can also find these comments at the bottom of the sheets outlining the analytical

---

[77] Letter, "Guillermo Cortina Anciola and Manuel Madrazo Garamendi to Eduardo Hay, October 18, 1968," archive collection "IOC Medical Commission," folder "Doping at the 1968 Summer Games in Mexico City: Results of medical tests, report," IOC Archive, Lausanne.

[78] Report, "General Report, Eduardo Hay," 13.

results.[79] Clearly, the Olympic Games in Mexico City were not as clean as they were presented. Eduardo Hay did not refrain from criticising the choice of analytical method for the inaccuracies. He claimed that due to the publication of Arnold Beckett´s method in an international magazine, it had been easy for athletes to turn to alternative substances, undetectable by GC.[80] However, even during the Olympic Games, Arnold Beckett instructed the laboratory staff that the results from the paper chromatography should remain unofficial.[81] Ultimately, this was the first controversy on analytical methods at Olympic doping controls, indicating that Arnold Beckett had the last word on the analytical methods despite possibly more techniques being available. Importantly, Arnold Beckett had Alexandre de Mérode´s backing, who wished to have scientifically waterproof methods employed. He wanted to avoid the conviction of innocent athletes. In his final report, Eduardo Hay contested this policy, arguing:

> It is indispensable to use several techniques and to adopt criteria for those cases where a drug is indisputable present can be identified through analysis. A positive result may be obtained even though the chemical product is not specified, but rather the group to which the product belongs.[82]

Hence, whereas Arnold Beckett followed Alexandre de Mérode´s strict policy in preferring reliability to the possibility to mistakenly convict an innocent athlete, other members of the IOC Medical Commission were of different opinion. Another attitude could have led to many more disqualifications.

Other than being in control of the official analytical method, the IOC Medical Commission appointed Arnold Beckett to instruct the laboratory. However, he displayed a lack of communication with the laboratory staff. On

---

[79] For example, the analytical results obtained from the volleyball event on October 13, 1968, read: "En las muestras 13-Vo-2, 13-Vo-5 y 13-Vo-8 se encontré per cromatografiá en papel, un componente que no es normal en la erina y que no es una de las drogas estandar usadas en le relación de la Federación de Ciclisme [In the samples 13-Vo-2, 13-Vo 5 and 13-Vo-8 we found with the paper chromatography method, a component, which normally cannot be found in urine and which is not one of the standard substances used by the International Cyclist Union]." "Informe Sobre Investigacion de Drogas, October 13, 1968," archive collection "IOC Medical Commission," folder "Doing at the 1968 Summer Games in Mexico City: Results of medical tests, report," IOC Archive, Lausanne.

[80] Report, "General Report, Eduardo Hay," 12.

[81] Letter, "Guillermo Cortina Anciola and Manuel Madrazo Garamendi to Eduardo Hay, October 18, 1968."

[82] Report, "General Report, Eduardo Hay," 12.

October 18, 1968, five days after the start of the Olympic Games, staff members informed Eduardo Hay that Arnold Beckett had visited the laboratory on only two occasions: October 11 and October 15.[83] This appears to be the first time that Arnold Beckett had established contact with the laboratory at all, since the laboratory technicians reported about several failed attempts to contact him from 1966 onwards. Only during his two visits to the laboratory, he informed about the analytical methods, some of which the staff needed to implement for them to become effective for the analysis. Furthermore, the staff argued that Arnold Beckett provided them with a list of more than 80 doping substances, compiled by the UCI, that they should investigate for during the analytical process.[84] However, among these drugs, there were plenty of substances that did not appear in the scientific article by BECKETT et al. Therefore, it was almost impossible to identify these products.

Finally, during Arnold Beckett 's visit to the laboratory, he informed for the first time about possible additional analytical procedures for the "control samples," of the artificial substances mixed by members of the IOC Medical Commission.[85] The laboratory staff confirmed the lack of communication about the additional tests prior to Arnold Beckett's appearance and that extra controls went beyond their capacities. In contrast to this, Arnold Beckett reported to the Medical Commission on October 12 that the laboratory agreed to adopt the additional checks of the control samples.[86] Clearly, communication was vague in this matter. Eventually, the laboratory report named the samples, but declared that the samples were taken "under irregular conditions" because "no laboratory personnel was present at the taking of the samples nor to verify the respective reports."[87]

Clearly, Arnold Beckett was the leading advisor behind the analytical procedures and scientific aspects of the doping controls. Although his personal communication with the laboratory staff does not appear to have been sufficient, he attempted to give them appropriate guidance for the conduction and implementation of the GC, which he had developed together with his colleagues from the KCL. However, some of the letters sent to him by the laboratory staff date back to 1966, when he was not yet working for the IOC Medical

---

[83] Letter, "Guillermo Cortina Anciola and Manuel Madrazo Garamendi to Eduardo Hay, October 18, 1968."

[84] Ibid.

[85] Ibid.

[86] Ibid.

[87] Report, "General Report, Eduardo Hay," 10.

Commission. This might explain why he did not reply to the letters. But it is important to emphasise that Arnold Beckett was in charge of the only counter-examination at the Games, when the Swedish NOC and the UIPM challenged the positive test of Hans-Gunnar Liljenwall in the presence of a Swedish team doctor and a medical expert of the IF.[88] This was in line with official IOC regulations, which foresaw his involvement in the analysis of the second sample, in case of a positive first result. However, his engagement was not enough to convince the other IOC Medical Commission members to give more attention to the quality of the laboratory. Considerable flaws were the results.

INCREASED EMPHASIS ON DOPING ANALYSIS

First Personal Changes in the IOC Medical Commission

In contrast to the aftermath of the 1968 Winter Olympic Games in Grenoble, few written exchanges on the IOC Medical Commission's members' feedback over the doping controls in Mexico City exist. In addition to this, despite the controversy depicted in Eduardo Hay's final report, the discussions within the IOC Medical Commission in its first meeting after Mexico City Games in January 1969 focused again on the relationship with the IFs.

Importantly, there were personal changes within the IOC Medical Commission that are significant when investigating the development of the different scientific expertise. Earlier in October 1968, Alexandre de Mérode had announced that he had accepted a medical doctor from the USA and a medical doctor from the USSR as members.[89] At the time, Jacques Thiebault had criticised this decision since he considered the decision merely a reflection of the increasing political nature of the Olympic Movement.[90] However, he had also raised these doubts because he was not a permanent member of the IOC Medical Commission but only a representative of an Organising Committee with long-term membership ambitions. In fact, he even maintained that whilst his country France did not have a permanent representative on the IOC Medical Commission,

---

[88] Minutes, "IOC Medical Commission, January 25 and 26, 1969," archive collection "IOC Medical Commission," folder "Medical Commission: Meeting in Lausanne July 13-14, 1968 and January 25-26, 1969," IOC Archive, Lausanne.

[89] Minutes, "IOC Medical Commission, October 12, 1968," 1ff.

[90] Ibid.

Alexandre de Mérode should not accept other members on grounds of their nationality.[91]

When considering the expertise of the two newly adopted members, his criticism seems reasonable. The Soviet medical doctor asked to join the Commission was Dr. Nina Grashinskaya[92], who did not have any experience in the conduction of doping controls. Instead, her research focused on the medical effect of sport onto the cardiovascular system. But she did have a standing within the sport medical profession, having presented a lecture at the World Congress for Sports Medicine in 1966.[93] In addition to Nina Grashinskaya, the American Dr. Daniel Hanley[94] joined. He had been the official team doctor of the USA Olympic Committee (USOC) at the 1964 and 1968 Olympic Games. He also appeared to have had an interest in the doping issue but from a medical perspective. In a letter following the 1968 Winter Olympic Games, he pointed Alexandre de Mérode's attention to the amphetamine detection method, based on

---

[91] Ibid.

[92] Dr. Nina Danilovna Grashinskaya or Graevskaja (1919-2008) (throughout the research, the correct spelling of her name remained unclear. Even in official IOC publications, she is sometimes referred to as Nina Grashinskaya and sometimes as Nina Graevskaja) was from 1947 until 1976 employed at the All-Union Scientific Research Institute of Physical Culture. She started there as a graduate student and reached the deputy director chair at the end of this period. In 1976, she became head of Department of Sports Medicine at the Moscow State Academy of Physical Culture. The majority of her work is devoted to the influence of physical culture and sports on human health and specifically on the cardiovascular system. For example, in 1975, she was the first Soviet researcher who collected, analysed, edited and published an extensive data (collected through long-term observations) on ex-elite athletes' health issues. She published more than 250 academic papers in the field of sports medicine in the USSR and in Russia. She was also the first person to implement the EchoKG method. P.K. LYSOV, T.I. DOLMATOVA and G.A. GONCHAROVA, "Graevskaya Nina Danilovna - physician, scientist, educator," *Journal of Russian Association for Sports Medicine and Rehabilitation of Sick and Disabled People* 30, no. 3 (2009), 12-14.

[93] Nina GRAEVSKAJA, "The significance of the active motor regime for the preservation of health of the former leading sportsmen," in: *Funktionsminderung und Funktionsertüchtigung im modernen Leben*, ed. Günter HANEKOPF (Hamburg: Deutscher Sportärztebund, 1966), 454-458.

[94] Daniel F. Hanley (1916-2001) earned a medical doctorate from Columbia University in 1943. In World War II, he was an Army physician in the China-Burma-India Theater. Following the end of the war, he became active in the Olympic Movement and was involved in the 1960 Rome Olympic Games for the first time, when he served as an assistant for the medical USOC staff. Frank LITSKY, "Dan Hanley, 85, U.S. Olympic Doctor, Dies," *New York Times*, May 10, 2001.

ultraviolet spectrophotometry developed by Dr. Jack Wallace, and claimed that the test results could be obtained within one hour.[95] Daniel Hanley concluded that the method allowed testing all athletes at the Olympic Games. However, he also had only a partial understanding of the doping detection techniques. In a letter sent to Daniel Hanley by Jack Wallace a couple of days after his written approach to Alexandre de Mérode, Jack Wallace corrected Daniel Hanley arguing that to conduct 250 amphetamine tests per day would be a "hearty task."[96] Additionally, Daniel Hanley did not have any proven record in anti-doping matters.[97] Therefore, neither of the two new members can be regarded as an anti-doping laboratory expert, because they did not have competencies in doping analysis. The same applies for the decision to make Jacques Thiebault a permanent member in 1969.[98] Due to the discussion surrounding the adoption of Daniel Hanley and Nina Grashinskaya, it was made very clear that Jacques Thiebault was chosen based on his competence in medical matters, experience and his young age.[99] The IOC Medical Commission also determined that not every medical representative appointed by an Organising Committee would eventually become a member.

In preparation of the upcoming Summer and Winter Olympic Games in 1972, the medical doctors Professor Dr. Herbert Reindell (Germany, Munich) and Professor Dr. Yoshio Kuroda[100] (Japan, Sapporo) represented their respective Organising Committee in the IOC Medical Commission. Due to their more general tasks in organising and coordinating the entire medical services at the Olympic Games, it seems understandable that they did not have a proven record

---

[95] Letter, "Daniel Hanley to Alexandre de Mérode, March 8, 1968," archive collection "IOC Medical Commission," folder "Medical Commission: Alphabetical correspondence A-K 1968," IOC Archive, Lausanne.

[96] Letter, "Jack Wallace to Daniel Hanley, March 13, 1968," archive collection "IOC Medical Commission," folder "Medical Commission: Alphabetical correspondence A-K 1968," IOC Archive, Lausanne.

[97] HOBERMAN argues that Daniel Hanley had a conservative viewpoint on doping. In contrast to the IOC Medical Commission's general opinion, he stated in an interview in 1969, "there is a time and place for certain drugs in sports but each situation has to be evaluated individually". HOBERMAN, "Sports Physicians," 205.

[98] Minutes, "IOC Medical Commission, January 25 and 26, 1969."

[99] Ibid.

[100] Professor Dr. Yoshio Kuroda (born 1925) was professor in sports medicine at the Department of Sports Science at the University of Tokyo from 1970, before he moved to the Juntendo University in Tokyo in 1988. From 2001 until 2004, he was president of the Japanese Anti-Doping Agency. INTERNATIONAL OLYMPIC COMMITTEE, *Commission Médicale*, 30.

in anti-doping campaigns. Herbert Reindell from the University of Freiburg was a proven expert in cardiology and had served as the team doctor of the German Olympic team from 1952 to 1972. He was the first physiologist to demonstrate the heart volume of humans and proved that particular forms of training had a specific effect on the volume of the human heart. [101] At the time of his appointment to the IOC Medical Commission, he was also president of the Association of German Sport Physicians and a member of the FIMS. [102]

In consideration of the personnel changes that occurred within the IOC Medical Commission in 1968, only a year after its establishment, one must conclude that the original set-up of proven experts in medical and analytical doping aspects had been markedly widened. This development was in contrast to Alexandre de Mérode´s intention to keep the body as small and specific as possible. Arnold Beckett raised this point in the discussion on the new additions and "pointed out that the Commission is constituted on a basis of individual merit and not on national representation."[103] However, through the calculated decision to include a member from the USA and the USSR, this attitude has to be regarded naïve. It remains unclear whether Alexandre de Mérode had faced political pressure to adopt a member from the Eastern bloc when putting forward the idea to make Daniel Hanley a member. However, when considering the increasing (sport) political tensions at the end of the 1960s,[104] this appears to be a logical conclusion. Hence, the personnel changes in the IOC Medical Commission reflect the inevitable link between the intensification of nationalism and the usage of performance-enhancing substances. But on this basis, no support for the anti-doping laboratory work was to be expected from the new members, since they had no professional competencies in the field of doping analysis.

---

[101] Arnd KRÜGER, "Viele Wege führen nach Olympia. Die Veränderungen in den Trainingssystemen für Mittel- und Langstreckenläufer (1850-1997)," in *Sportliche Leistung im Wandel* (Jahrestagung der DVS-Sektion Sportgeschichte), ed. Norbert GISSEL (Hamburg: Czwalina Verlag, 1998), 50.

[102] Wilfried KINDERMANN, "Der Vater des Sportherzens – Herbert Reindell 100 Jahre," *Deutsche Zeitschrift für Sportmedizin* 59, no. 3 (2008), 73-75.

[103] Minutes, "IOC Medical Commission, October 12, 1968."

[104] An excellent study on the struggle of the Olympic Movement in light of political tensions at the end of the 1960s is: Cesar R. TORRES and Mark DYRESON, "The Cold War Games," in: *Global Olympics. Historical and Sociological Studies of the Modern Games*, eds. Kevin YOUNG and Kevin B. WAMSLEY (Bingley: JAI Press, 2007), 59-82.

Recognising the Steroid Problem

HUNT shows that the period in between the 1968 and the 1972 Olympic Games was also defined by IOC president Avery Brundage´s continuous attempt to restrict the possibilities of the IOC Medical Commission.[105] According to Avery Brundage and the Executive Board, the IOC Medical Commission should only hold a supervisory role and not be responsibility for the testing. However, Avery Brundage did not discourage Alexandre de Mérode, who continued to centralise the anti-doping efforts by strengthening the position of the IOC Medical Commission. Eventually, as discussed at the meeting of the Medical Commission in July 1971, the IFs had the technical responsibility for the tests, such as the number of taken samples, the selection of athletes and the time of the samples taken.[106] In contrast, the IOC Medical Commission would have the overall responsibility for the doping tests and make proposals for the elimination of an athlete from the Olympic Games to the IFs. Importantly, this also included the supervision of the doping analysis.

In addition to the personnel changes, Alexandre de Mérode envisaged a broader approach of the IOC Medical Commission following the 1968 Mexico City Olympic Games. In January 1969, he proposed that the body´s work should go beyond the doping fight and gender testing, and asked the members to contribute ideas. Jacques Thiebault suggested focusing on the danger of young elite sport and Giuseppe La Cava made the proposal to investigate into the problem of eliminatory series.[107] Both suggestions were of a medical nature. However, in contrast to Alexandre de Mérode´s original plan to widen the working field, he eventually decided to give priority to a third proposal by Arnold Beckett, namely to study in detail the dangers, effects and detection methods of anabolic steroids. As mentioned above, the IOC Medical Commission did consider anabolic steroids doping substances, but because no testing method existed, it had not added them to the list of banned substances. Competitors such as Tom Waddell, who had participated in the decathlon event at the 1968 Mexico City Olympic Games, claimed that athletes had made use of anabolic steroids in training camps ahead of the Olympic Games.[108] Hence the decision to concentrate

---

[105] HUNT, *Drug Games*, 39f.

[106] Minutes, "IOC Medical Commission, July 29, 1971," archive collection "IOC Medical Commission," folder "Medical matters at the 1972 Summer Olympic Games in Munich: Doping and gender tests," IOC Archive, Lausanne.

[107] Minutes, "IOC Medical Commission, January 25 and 26, 1969," 7.

[108] Terry TODD, "Anabolic steroids: the Gremlins of Sport," *Journal of Sport History* 14 (1987), 95.

even more on this issue reflects a rising awareness about the undetected usage of steroids. In addition, one must verify that Arnold Beckett's attempt to make the IOC Medical Commission focus even closer on doping issues was therefore successful.

Another incident in Mexico City supported the decision to focus on anabolic steroid testing. The KNWU, of which IOC Medical Commission member Pieter van Dijk was president, sent a Dutch physiotherapist home because he had treated a cyclist with an anabolic steroid injection.[109] In contrast to the federation's reaction, however, the IOC did not penalise the competitor, since its list of banned substances did not contain anabolic steroids. The UCI criticised this attitude, although an exchange of information took place during the Games. According to the minutes of the IOC Medical Commission meeting, "the immediate or long-range secondary effects" of anabolic steroids were unknown and "difficult or even impossible to determine."[110] Furthermore, the incident started a debate about the methods and detection possibilities of hormone usage. During the discussion, where Arnold Beckett featured prominently, the members appeared still anxious to test for steroids, because of the physiological variations in human bodies and because there was no effective measurement tool in place.[111] Moreover, Arnold Beckett, who continuously appeared to be at the forefront of all testing methods, had no expertise in anabolic steroid testing and was more specialised in the detection of amphetamines. Therefore, an initial distinction of very specific expertise within the group of anti-doping laboratory experts becomes obvious for the first time. As reported by Manfred DONIKE a couple of years later, publications on testing methods for anabolic steroids had already existed since 1963.[112]

Notwithstanding, Alexandre de Mérode reported to the IOC Session even two years later:

> Professor Beckett of Great Britain, had studied this subject [anabolic steroids] and was the most eminent world specialist. However, he had

---

[109] Minutes, "IOC Medical Commission, January 25 and 26, 1969," 4.

[110] Ibid., 5.

[111] The same attitude had already been provided by Arthur Porritt, when he presented the results of steroid use by the medical doctor and former shot putter Martyn Lucking in 1963. DIMEO, *A History*, 113f.

[112] Manfred DONIKE, "Zum Problem des Nachweises der anabolen Steroide: Gas-chromatographische und massenspezifische Möglichkeiten," *Sportarzt und Sportmedizin* 1 (1975), 1-6.

not gone far enough in his research for the Medical Commission to use any control in this field.[113]

Alexandre de Mérode's statement reveals how highly he valued Arnold Beckett's opinion and knowledge. Yet, he did seem to be unaware of Arnold Beckett's lack of expertise in anabolic steroid testing compared to testing amphetamines. Although Arnold Beckett knew about the extent of the steroid problem, and showed serious concern for the issue, the problem actually demonstrated the need for more anti-doping laboratory experts to support him in analytical questions. While there were indeed particular advancements in the development of MS and TLC combinations at the end of the 1960s,114 there were no applications of steroid testing techniques within the field of sport, yet. In view of the usage of such substances at the time, the fact that no scientist other than Arnold Beckett was included to conduct research on the matter appears to have been a major mistake. Instead, Alexandre de Mérode deemed the inclusion of an American and a Soviet representative more important than steroid testing. This is despite the reality that in addition to a lack of sophisticated testing methods, the IOC Medical Commission had to face the problem that most athletes used anabolic substances only in the weeks prior to the competition, so that detection during the Olympic Games became less likely. The restriction of the IOC Executive Board to allow testing only during the Games time as well as the time immediately before and after it, made successful testing for anabolic steroids impossible.[115]

First Exchanges of Knowledge amongst Anti-doping Laboratory Experts

As highlighted in Chapter 2, no exchange of information between chemical experts in doping tests had taken place until the late 1960s because no such specific scientific field existed. A first attempt to bring together experts in doping analysis was the "Doping Technicians" symposium in Rome from October 31 to November 1, 1969. The meeting was organised by the FIMS in collaboration with the IOC Medical Commission. Amongst the people addressed were Herbert

---

[113] Minutes, "71st Session of the IOC in Luxembourg, September 11-18, 1971," archive collection "IOC Sessions 1894-2009," IOC Archive, Lausanne, 23.

[114] Holger ALFES and Dirk CLASING, "Identifizierung geringer Mengen Methamphetamins nach Körperpassage durch Kopplung von Dünnschichtchomatographie und Massenspektrometrie," *Deutsche Zeitschrift für die gesamte gerichtliche Medizin* 64 (1969), 235-240.

[115] HUNT, *Drug Games*, 41.

Reindell, Yoshio Kuroda, Nina Grashinskaya, Daniel Hanley, Pieter Van Dijk, Arnold Beckett, Eduardo Hay and Robert Boncour. [116] Significantly, FIMS president Antonio Venerando requested in the invitation for the attendance of chemical experts who actually dealt with the development of testing techniques and had professional competencies in the field of doping analysis. This was an entirely new approach at the time. Most addressees complied with the request. For example, Yoshio Kuroda sent two highly ranked directors of Japanese pharmaceutical institutes: Takeshi Matsumoto and Tsuyoshi Kittaka. [117] Arnold Beckett obviously attended the symposium and brought along two other experts in pharmaceutical chemistry from Great Britain: Dr. Fish from the Department of Pharmaceutical Chemistry of the University of Strathclyde and J.H. McAndrew from his own department at the KCL. [118] Herbert Reindell sent three experts on his behalf: Dr. Hermann Weidemann, medical doctor and expert for the effects of high altitude training, Dr. Gerhard Hauck, toxicologist (both from the University of Freiburg), [119] and most importantly the chemist Dr. Manfred Donike from the University of Cologne. [120] He had been a successful professional cyclist and had participated at the Tour de France in 1960 and 1961. Besides his cycling career, Manfred Donike had also obtained a university degree from the Institute for Anorganic Chemistry at the University of Cologne in 1963. Only two years later, he finished his dissertation on the topic "Contribution to the Analysis of Acylitated Anthocyanes." which he wrote under the supervision of Professor Dr. Leonhard Birkofer. In his dissertation, research on the detection of doping substances already played an important role because he had worked part-time for

---

[116] "Liste des Destinataires de la Lettre 'Symposium Antidopage'," archive collection "IOC Medical Commission," folder "Medical Commission: Alphabetical Correspondence A-G 1968-1969," IOC Archive, Lausanne.

[117] Letter, "Yoshio Kuroda to Antonio Venerando, October 7, 1969," archive collection "IOC Medical Commission," folder "Medical Commission: Alphabetical Correspondence A-G 1968-1969," IOC Archive, Lausanne.

[118] Letter, "Arnold Beckett to Alexandre de Mérode, October 10, 1969," archive collection "IOC Medical Commission," folder "Medical Commission: Alphabetical Correspondence A-G 1968-1969," IOC Archive, Lausanne.

[119] At the time of the symposium, Gerhard Hauck was director of the toxological-chemical department at the University of Freiburg. In 1970, he moved to the Ludwig Maximilian-University of Munich and established a toxicological-chemical department there. Letter, "Herbert Reindell to Alexandre de Mérode, October 20, 1969," archive collection "IOC Medical Commission," folder "Medical Commission: Correspondence alphabétique L-Z 1968," IOC Archive, Lausanne.

[120] Letter, Herbert Reindell to Alexandre de Mérode, October 20, 1969.

Professor Dr. Wildor Hollmann[121] at the Institute of Cardiology and Sports Medicine at the DSHS.[122] In the following years, by then employed at the Biochemical Institute of the University of Cologne with ambitions to habilitate, he dedicated his research entirely to doping analysis in sport.[123] Consequently, one has to categorise Manfred Donike into the group of anti-doping laboratory experts. In contrast to Arnold Beckett, who dealt with pharmacological research more generally, Manfred Donike worked only within the field of sports drug testing.

The body of source material from the various visited archives does not shed any light on the final list of participants at the symposium nor is there an official agenda or protocol available.[124] However, a report by the German attendees exists, revealing that the participants did not only exchange knowledge on doping analysis but made important agreements.[125] The congress started with opening presentations by Arnold Beckett on the diverse problems of doping. Following what has been described as a "lengthy discussion,"[126] the participants agreed on several guidelines of doping analysis. Primarily, they came to terms that the analytical procedure of the doping test should be conducted in three steps, namely screening, identification and confirmation. After the extraction of the urine samples, the preliminary screening process should be used in order to determine

---

[121] Professor Dr. Dr. h.c. mult. Wildor Hollmann (born 1925) is a German sport medicine specialist, who founded the Institute of Cardiology and Sports Medicine at the DSHS in 1958 after his promotion and habilitation in sports medicine at the University of Cologne. From 1969 until 1971 he was rector of the DSHS, from 1967 until 1969 respectively 1971 until 1982 its vice-rector. From 1984 until 1998, he was president of the Association of German Sport Physicians and from 1986 until 1994 president of the FIMS. Wildor HOLLMANN, *Ziel und Zufall - ein bewegtes Leben als Arzt, Universitätsprofessor, Forscher und Manager* (Cologne: Sportverlag Strauß, 2012).

[122] Wildor Hollmann reports that he was actually looking for a scientist, who was able to determine stress hormones during physical exercise. Wildor HOLLMANN, *Medizin – Sport – Neuland. 40 Jahre mit der Deutschen Sporthochschule Köln* (Sankt Augustin: Academia, 1993), 151.

[123] Wildor HOLLMANN and Kurt TITTEL, *Geschichte der deutschen Sportmedizin* (Gera: Druckhaus Gera, 2008), 65f.

[124] Minutes, "Meeting of the IOC Medical Commission with the Organising Committee of the 1972 Munich Olympic Games, June 12, 1970," archive collection "Olympische Spiele 1972," folder "21. Sanitätswesen," CuLDA, Cologne, 4.

[125] Report, "Dr. M. Donike, Dr. H. Weidemann and Dr. Hauck on the symposium on analytical aspects of doping in Rome on October 31 and November 1, 1969," archive collection "Olympische Spiele 1972," folder "21. Sanitätswesen," CuLDA, Cologne.

[126] Ibid.

whether the sample could possibly contain a doping substance.[127] Due to the experiences in Mexico City, the participants decided that GC was to be used to test a sample for volatile substances, and thin-layer or paper chromatography for non-volatile substances, allowing for the detection of more substances.[128] Therefore, the participants overruled Arnold Beckett, who had advanced a different opinion during the 1968 Mexico City Olympic Games. The majority of experts thought that paper chromatography for non-volatile substances was sufficient. In the case of the presence of a forbidden substance, the laboratory staff should start the identification process. The same methods would be used for the identification, however, different separation methods and derivative formation would be applied.[129] Finally, after the identification, the new guidelines foresaw a specific confirmation reaction with the mass spectrometer technique or by using micro infrared spectroscopy.[130]

These jointly agreed analytical methods were the first internationally standardised guidelines of their kind and therefore are of major significance for the history of anti-doping and doping analysis. In particular, the guiding principles aimed to avoid problems concerning the laboratory procedures, instantly leading to the general implementation of MS for sports drug testing on the international level. Moreover, the participants anticipated an increased exchange of knowledge. This was needed in order to coordinate more vigorously the information about used substances, the detection methods of such substances and their metabolism.[131] Arnold Beckett aimed to publish the presented papers and conclusions of the congress. As he reported, the methods and means of doping testing could be distributed to laboratories all over the world in this way.[132] This was a necessity in order to enable an increased communication between the involved individuals. Finally, there must have also been a discussion on the requirement of having certain standards for the anti-doping laboratory facilities to do official testing because the attendees decided to analyse the control

---

[127] Ibid.

[128] Ibid.

[129] Ibid.

[130] Letter, "Dr. G. Hauck to Professor Dr. med. H. Reindell, April 7, 1970," archive collection "Olympische Spiele 1972," folder "21. Sanitätswesen," CuLDA, Cologne.

[131] The first step of the newly planned international cooperation was to conduct a ring analysis about the stability of methyl amphetamine and ephedrine, when different storage conditions are used. Report, "Dr. M. Donike, Dr. H. Weidemann and Dr. Hauck on the symposium on analytical aspects of doping in Rome on October 31 and November 1, 1969."

[132] Minutes, "IOC Medical Commission, January 25 and 26, 1969," 7.

sample only in a "recognised" laboratory. However, it was not specified how they wanted to select laboratories.[133]

Due to the uniqueness of the event because of its specific orientation towards doping analysis, the "Doping Technicians" symposium in Rome in autumn 1969 has to be regarded as the first international exchange forum for anti-doping laboratory experts. Moreover, at the following IOC Session in Amsterdam in 1970, Alexandre de Mérode even reported about the symposium as "meeting of laboratory experts and well-known experts in the field of doping control."[134] In his report, he added:

> Last October in Rome we held a meeting with laboratory technicians, through the co-operation of the Italian Medical Federation. This meeting has made possible the standardization of working methods in the large European laboratories and to put this same question to the USSR and the USA.[135]

One can draw several conclusions from the "Doping Technicians" symposium. First, it stands for first decisions on international standards in doping analysis. Curiously, the FIMS played a passive but decisive role in this process because it invited to the symposium together with the IOC Medical Commission. Whereas prior to the meeting individuals were independently dealing with research and application on doping analysis, the assembly enabled an important exchange. This resulted in an agreement on the international standards and closer cooperation overall. Second, it is important to highlight that Arnold Beckett occupied the pioneering and leading role amongst the anti-doping laboratory experts. One can connect this to him giving the opening speech on the symposium and appearing to have led the discussions due to his involvement in the IOC Medical Commission. Third, Manfred Donike appeared internationally for the first time on the symposium. He played a central role within the anti-doping strategies of international sporting organisations from 1969 onwards. Finally, the discussions on doping analysis and its equipment were of different nature than the medical issues addressed by conferences in sports medicine.

---

[133] Ibid.

[134] Minutes, "69th Session of the IOC in Amsterdam, May 12-16, 1970," archive collection "IOC Sessions 1894-2009," IOC Archive, Lausanne, 145.

[135] Ibid., Annex 17.

Development of the *Doping* Brochure

HUNT describes the development of a doping control brochure, entitled *Doping*, by the IOC Medical Commission as another attempt by Alexandre de Mérode to gain control over the Olympic Movement's fight against doping. [136] The discussions and the contents of the publication reveal that the brochure was a first official systematic guide on the conduction of doping controls and doping analysis for major sporting events. Whereas the anti-doping laboratories at the Olympic Games in 1968 relied solely on Arnold Beckett's publication and did not have an official protocol, all future anti-doping laboratories could work according to the principles written in the *Doping* brochure. Moreover, organisations still apply many of the guidelines today. [137] Ultimately, the brochure contained articles on the doping problem in general, doping analysis and the technical organisation of the doping controls at the 1972 Olympic Games in Sapporo and Munich. [138] The chapter about the doping analysis in the *Doping* brochure is of particular importance because it recorded the principles on analytical aspects of doping controls as discussed and agreed upon at the "Doping Technicians" symposium in Rome in 1969. This again stresses the symposium's significance. The process to develop standardised analytical procedures, were the first combined efforts of anti-doping laboratory experts apart from the Rome meeting. Thus, it is important to chronicle the process and communications that eventually led to the publication of the brochure, with a particular focus on the chapter on doping analysis.

A reason to produce the brochure was the prognosis formed in 1968, which revealed the need for uniform procedures and an official doping protocol. Both Jacques Thiebault and Eduardo Hay had already suggested the development of general principles in their final reports of the 1968 Olympic Games. The latter recommended:

> Among its functions, the Medical Commission can officially establish the analysis techniques to be applied in all sports events controlled by the I.O.C. and provide the standards of the drugs to the laboratory

---

[136] HUNT, *Drug Games*, 40.

[137] HEMMERSBACH, "History," 841

[138] MEDICAL COMMISSION OF THE INTERNATIONAL OLYMPIC COMMITTEE, *Doping* (Lausanne: International Olympic Committee, 1972).

responsible for the analysis. It can also give counsel, as a form of collaboration, to those responsible for analysis in the future.[139]

Significantly, he made specific reference to doping analysis.

For the first time, the development of a brochure is mentioned in the official minutes of the meeting of the IOC Medical Commission with the Organising Committee of the 1972 Munich Olympic Games (OK) in June 1970.[140] This is not surprising since the purpose of the meeting was to determine the exact guidelines for the OK to install adequate doping controls, and it explains the presence of the two "visitors" Gerhard Hauck and Manfred Donike at the meeting. Therefore, other chemical experts besides Arnold Beckett were present for the first time at an IOC Medical Commission meeting, although without discretionary competencies. Alexandre de Mérode informed about the decision to publish the brochure at the IOC Session in Amsterdam in July 1970.[141] The IOC Medical Commission's report to the IOC Session clearly emphasised the need for standardised procedures again. Furthermore, the manual should not only be used during the Olympic Games, but also constitute the basic anti-doping regulations for "all important international sport competitions."[142] Thus, the intentions to develop international standards become apparent, which increasingly formed the self-conception of the IOC Medical Commission in the global fight against doping.

Arnold Beckett drafted the chapter on doping analysis in the brochure, whilst Ludwig Prokop wrote the introductory chapter on the general problem of doping and the historical context.[143] Arnold Beckett mainly relied on the decisions made at the "Doping Technicians" meeting in Rome in 1969, along with a personal proposal made after the 1968 Mexico City Olympic Games. In the proposal, he had already listed several organisational aspects of the doping controls, such as the responsibilities of the members of the IOC Medical Commission, the coding

---

[139] Report, "General Report, Eduardo Hay," 12.
[140] Minutes, "Meeting of the IOC Medical Commission with the Organising Committee of the 1972 Munich Olympic Games, June 12, 1970," archive collection "IOC Medical Commission," folder "Medical matters at the 1972 Summer Olympic Games in Munich: Doping and gender tests," IOC Archive, Lausanne.
[141] Minutes, "69th Session of the IOC in Amsterdam, May 12-16, 1970," 145.
[142] Ibid.
[143] Minutes, "Meeting of the IOC Medical Commission with the Organising Committee of the 1972 Munich Olympic Games, May 19, 1971," archive collection "Olympische Spiele 1972," folder "9.10. Doping," CuLDA, Cologne.

of the urine samples and the processes in case of a positive sample.[144] Most importantly, he highlighted that the second analysis should be undertaken only in an approved laboratory "with proved wide experience in dope testing in man."[145] This had also been one of the major outcomes of the Doping Technicians meeting. Arnold Beckett sent his first draft to Alexandre de Mérode in July 1971, and provided the technical director of the OK, Ernst Knoesel, with a copy because the OK was co-editor of the manual and responsible for the third chapter.[146] In line with his previous engagement on the IOC Medical Commission and his competencies in doping analysis, Arnold Beckett interpreted his task as only dealing with the analytical aspects of the doping controls, assuming that "(a) Classification of substances as dope, and (b) Method of sampling will have been dealt with already."[147] The IOC Medical Commission approved his first draft later in the same month whereas it revised Ludwig Prokop's part and slightly changed the information.[148]

Highly important for the developing network of anti-doping laboratory experts was the decision that the final version of the doping analysis chapter should be edited jointly by Manfred Donike and Arnold Beckett.[149] This is a clear indication of the appreciation of Manfred Donike's work, but also evidences the closer cooperation between the OK and Arnold Beckett in terms of the analytical procedures compared to the preparation of the laboratory in Mexico City four years earlier. They wanted to avoid another miscommunication between the laboratory staff and the IOC Medical Commission.

The IOC Medical Commission published 4,000 copies of the Doping brochure and distributed them to the IOC, the IFs and other stakeholders of the Olympic Movement.[150] Unquestionably, the brochure stands as an exemplar for

---

[144] Letter, "Arnold Beckett to the Medical Commission, n.d.," archive collection "IOC Medical Commission," folder "Medical Commission: Alphabetical correspondence 68-69," IOC Archive, Lausanne.

[145] Ibid.

[146] Letter, "Arnold Beckett to Alexandre de Mérode, July 9, 1971," archive collection "IOC Medical Commission," folder "Medical Commission: Correspondence: 1971-972," IOC Archive, Lausanne.

[147] Letter, "Arnold Beckett to Ernst Knoesel, July 9, 1971," archive collection "IOC Medical Commission," folder "Medical Commission: Correspondence: 1971-972," IOC Archive, Lausanne

[148] Minutes, "Meeting of the Working Group of the IOC Medical Commission with the Organising Committee of the 1972 Munich Olympic Games, July 29, 1971," archive collection "Olympische Spiele 1972," folder "9.10. Doping," CuLDA, Cologne.

[149] Ibid.

[150] HUNT, *Drug Games*, 40.

the continuing efforts to standardise all aspects of doping controls as well as the slowly growing influence of anti-doping laboratory experts. Arnold Beckett, their pioneer, continued to play a central role in this process. He developed – in the later stages together with Manfred Donike – the first official standards for doping analysis, which can be linked back to the "Doping Technicians" symposium and are an indirect outcome of it. One anticipated more reliable doping controls as a result of the increasing standardisation of the analytical procedures for which competencies in doping analysis were essential.

Manfred Donike's Preparations for the 1972 Munich Olympic Games

It is necessary to examine Manfred Donike's role in the preparations of the analytical procedures of the Munich doping controls, while analysing how he was approaching the task. In the final chapter of their article about the political impact of the 1972 Munich Olympic Games on the anti-doping policy in the FRG, Michael KRÜGER et al. have already briefly indicated the important milestones that led to Manfred Donike becoming the head of the doping analysis.[151] The researchers demonstrate that this had wide-reaching consequences because after the Olympic Games, the apparatus installed in Munich was used to establish a central doping analysis institution for the FRG in Cologne in 1974. However, where the focus of their work has entirely been on the effects on the *national* level, it is important to stress how Manfred Donike's work affected the history of the network of *international* anti-doping laboratory experts as well.

Herbert Reindell initially consulted Manfred Donike about the requirements and pre-conditions of the doping controls in May 1969. Significantly, this was before the meeting of "Doping Technicians" and before the OK officially chose Manfred Donike to lead the "Commission of Doping Analysis."[152] KRÜGER et al. demonstrate that apart from Manfred Donike, the Institute of Juridical Medicine and Insurance Medicine at the University of Munich was interested to conduct the doping analysis of the 1972 Olympic Games, and applied officially. The OK initially preferred this application because it offered to carry out the doping analysis within their facilities, but only if the head of the doping analysis would be a staff member the Institute. However, the sport medicine specialists Herbert

---

[151] Michael KRÜGER, Stefan NIELSEN and Christian BECKER, "The Munich Olympics 1972: Its Impact on the Relationship Between State, Sports, and Anti-Doping Policy in West Germany," *Sport in History* 32, no. 4 (2012), 540f.

[152] KRÜGER et al., *Doping und Anti-Doping*, 72ff.

Reindell, Professor Dr. Joseph Keul[153] and Wildor Hollmann who were involved, supported Manfred Donike's bid, because they wanted to keep the doping controls and doping analysis within the sport system. One reason for this must have been that its equipment could be used to establish a permanent central doping control centre for sport in the FRG, which Wildor Hollmann wanted to locate in Cologne.[154] In his first letter to Herbert Reindell, Manfred Donike emphasised that his proposal was based on his experience as head of a pharmaceutical laboratory with eleven staff members.[155] He claimed that this was an advantage over the rival application. He provided a brief overview on the sampling procedure and then focused mainly on doping analysis in his proposal. In the letter, Manfred Donike also referenced Arnold Beckett's study. However, he maintained that through an acceleration of the shaking process, the accomplishment of the derivate formation and the detection through specific detectors such as a nitrogen detector, the screening procedure could be considerably simplified. [156] The analysis of both, the screening and the identification procedure, in case of a positive test, could be done with a computer. Clearly, the significant advancement of previous doping analysis becomes obvious with this example. With this method, one could analyse up to 100 samples per day. He also pointed towards the necessity of testing the proposed analytical methods in the years ahead of the Olympic Games, because the large amount of tests to be conducted would not leave enough time to correct possible mistakes. Consequently, he proposed a time schedule, which had already started in 1969 by deciding which classes of substances should be tested. Following this decision, research on the exact constitution and metabolism of possibly used medications should be made. From 1970 onwards, the elaboration of the analytical methods should begin. In particular, Donike wanted to refine the following aspects: 1) assurance of the result 2) sensitivity and reproducibility 3)

---

[153] Professor Dr. Dr. h.c. Joseph Keul (1932-2000) was a German sport medicine specialists, who held a professorship for sports medicine at the University of Freiburg. He worked as medical support for the German Olympic team from the 1960 Olympic Games and became its chief doctor from 1980 onwards. From 1998 until 2000, he was commissioner for anti-doping of the German Olympic Olympic Committee, the German Sport Association and the BISp. Aloys BERG and Hans-Hermann DICKHUTH, "Nachruf auf Prof. Dr. Dr. h.c. Joseph Keul," *Deutsche Zeitschrift für Sportmedizin* 51, no. 7/8 (2000), 280.

[154] KRÜGER et al., *Doping und Anti-Doping*, 74.

[155] Letter, "Dr. M. Donike to Professor Dr. med. H. Reindell, May 14, 1969," archive collection "Olympische Spiele 1972," folder "21. Sanitätswesen," CuLDA, Cologne.

[156] Ibid., 4.

maximum capacity of the laboratory through simplification of the sample preparation procedure and automatic evaluation of the results.[157] The detailed proposal highlights his expertise in the field.

Without doubt, Manfred Donike´s intensive engagement and detailed preparations of the doping analysis were unique at the time. He had a clear conception on its implementation and did not require the same level of support and guidance from Arnold Beckett as the laboratory staff at the previous Olympic Games had needed. This degree of independence can be attributed to his focus on sports drug testing in his professional work. Significantly, most of his detailed preparation took place before he was officially selected to supervise the doping analysis at the 1972 Munich Olympic Games. But interestingly, this did not stop Manfred Donike from linking up with other anti-doping laboratory experts and he visited the doping centres in Rome, London, Paris and Ghent during the preparation phase. [158] This demonstrates the increased communication and collaboration amongst the leaders of the few existing anti-doping laboratories.

Manfred Donike´s preparations allowed him to raise the number of possible analysed doping tests during the period of the Olympic Games to a maximum of 200 analyses. He thought that no more than twenty laboratory staff members should work in the anti-doping laboratory at the same time to allow appropriate guidance.[159] He based his calculations on information received from each IFs about the number of doping tests planned for each sport.[160] In June 1970, there were also hints towards the IOC Medical Commission favouring Manfred Donike for the position of head of the anti-doping laboratory. The minutes disclose that although the IOC Medical Commission members wanted the analytical procedures to take place in a suitable laboratory in Munich, they stressed that the involvement of scientists with practical experience was necessary. Moreover, the IOC Medical Commission pressured the OK to make a decision about the laboratory in 1970.[161] Once Manfred Donike officially became "Commissioner

---

[157] Letter, "Dr. M. Donike to Professor Dr. med. H. Reindell, May 14, 1969," 10.

[158] Letter, "Professor Dr. med. H. Reindell and Dr. med. J. Keul to German Ministry of Interior, the principal Kroppenstedt, April 20, 1970," archive collection "Olympische Spiele 1972," folder "21. Sanitätswesen," CuLDA, Cologne.

[159] Remark, "Ernst Knoesel, May 4, 1970," archive collection "Olympische Spiele 1972," folder "21. Sanitätswesen," CuLDA, Cologne.

[160] Minutes, "Meeting of the IOC Medical Commission with the OK, June 12, 1970," archive collection "Olympische Spiele 1972," folder "21. Sanitätswesen," CuLDA, Cologne, 2.

[161] Ibid., 3.

for Doping Analysis" in December 1970,[162] he provided the OK with an even more detailed proposal on the preparation phase of the doping analysis.[163] He tested all the equipment and trained staff members in his laboratory at the Institute of Biochemistry of the University of Cologne for a total of two years.[164] According to Manfred Donike, this was essential because the testing of the equipment was an essential part of the controls.[165] He then aimed to transport all of the equipment from Cologne to Munich in July 1972, in order to have two more weeks of preparation on site. He also pointed out the importance of employing staff members for the preparation phase, since the OK had to finance them.[166] Compared to the IOC Medical Commission, who requested clarification on the number of analyses, Manfred Donike wanted to wait until the finalisation of the preparations.[167] Once again, his determination to guarantee scientific reliability for the doping analysis becomes evident. Nevertheless, he demonstrated that the targeted twelve laboratory assistants could work on a maximum of 144 urine samples at the same time (twelve each).[168] With this method, the 24-hour deadline for the results of the analysis could be reached independently from the final number of conducted tests. One year later, in February 1972, Donike eventually reported about successful preparations in Cologne, and provided the OK with the final time schedule for the doping analysis and the transportation of the equipment to Munich.[169] Notably, this was one year after the IOC had finalised the list of banned substances.

Despite Manfred Donike's detailed preparations, the IOC Medical Commission did not give full authority to the German laboratory staff team at the Munich Games. It regarded Arnold Beckett as the main supervisor of the laboratory. However, because Manfred Donike and Arnold Beckett had worked together closely and Manfred Donike had visited Arnold Beckett's laboratory in London prior to the doping controls in Munich, one has to consider the

---

[162] KRÜGER et al., "The Munich Olympics 1972," 542.

[163] Letter, "Dr. M. Donike to Organisationskomitee für die Olympischen Spiele der XX. Olympiade in München 1972, January 4, 1971," archive collection "Olympische Spiele 1972," folder "21. Sanitätswesen," CuLDA, Cologne.

[164] Ibid.

[165] Ibid.

[166] Ibid.

[167] Ibid.

[168] Ibid.

[169] Letter, "Dr. M. Donike to Organisationskomitee für die Olympischen Spiele der XX. Olympiade in München 1972, February 2, 1972," archive collection "Olympische Spiele 1972," folder "21. Sanitätswesen," CuLDA Cologne, 3.

relationship one of cooperation rather than supervision. Accordingly, Manfred Donike had to request Arnold Beckett to conduct a second doping analysis in the case of a positive doping test.[170] The procedure would take place in the same laboratory facilities and with the same equipment. This again points towards Manfred Donike´s awareness for objective analytical procedures, but also reflects the IOC Medical Commission´s policy to maintain control over potentially positive doping tests.

It is unsurprising that Manfred Donike was heavily involved in the development of the doping analysis chapter of the *Doping* brochure, together with Arnold Beckett, who already had international experience and an elevated position within the Medical Commission. Essentially, the documents that Manfred Donike had compiled to inform the OK about the preparation and conduction phases do reiterate the information in the brochure. These facts were combined with the decisions made on the "Doping Technicians" meeting in Rome in 1969, at which both Manfred Donike and Arnold Beckett participated. As stated in the final report, it had also been Manfred Donike´s aim to set "international standards" for doping analysis.[171] As a result, his national initiative for the 1972 Munich Olympic Games joined force with Arnold Beckett´s efforts to establish standards for doping analysis. In light of these developments and the increasing responsibility given to scientists outside the Medical Commission, it is not unexpected that the report to the 71st IOC Session in 1971 distinguishes between different scientific expertises. It states that:

> A number of medical experts, chemists and scientific institutions had invented methods and instruments in order to facilitate and accelerate the control against these extremely dangerous stimulants in sport.[172]

Alexandre de Mérode, who reported to the Session at the same meeting about an assembly of doping technicians in 1969, also made this change in rhetoric.[173] Such statements point towards the increasing acknowledgement for individuals with expertise in the domain field of doping analysis.

---

[170] Minutes, "Meeting of the IOC Medical Commission with the OK, June 12, 1970," 3.

[171] Dirk CLASING, Manfred DONIKE and Armin KLÜMPER, "Dopingkontrollen bei den Spielen der XX. Olympiade, München 1972 (III)," *Leistungssport* 4 (1975), 303-306.

[172] Minutes, "71st Session of the IOC in Luxembourg, September 11-18, 1971," Annex 17.

[173] Ibid., 23.

Significance of the Anti-doping Laboratory at the 1972 Munich Olympic Games

The Doping Controls at the 1972 Winter Olympic Games in Sapporo

Before detailing the significance of the doping controls at the 1972 Summer Games, it is necessary to outline the difficulties that arose during the Winter Olympic Games in Sapporo, held earlier in the same year. This allows a comparison between the two implementations of doping controls.

The regulations written down in the *Doping* brochure were already in place for Sapporo, and the Japanese Organising Committee made a financial contribution to its publication. However, despite the continuous presence of Yoshiro Kuroda during the preparatory meetings of the IOC Medical Commission, he did not have any decisive influence. Furthermore, whereas a permanent exchange of information between Manfred Donike and the IOC Medical Commission took place, there were no specific meetings between the doping control team in Sapporo and the IOC Medical Commission. Rather, all information was distributed in written form or via Yoshio Kuroda. One explanation for this could be the attitude of Alexandre de Mérode, who believed that doping was more widespread in the Summer Olympic Games. [174] Consequently, there is a considerable lack of sources related to the scientific aspects of the doping controls and analytical procedures of the 1972 Winter Olympic Games in Sapporo.

Despite these difficulties, two main sources, namely the minutes of the meetings of the IOC Medical Commission in Sapporo [175] and the *Official Report*,[176] give insights into work at the anti-doping laboratory and the role of the IOC Medical Commission members. Yoshio Kuroda supervised all doping and gender tests, although the *Official Report* mistakenly lists him as a "member of

---

[174] Another indication for this attitude can be seen by the fact that Alexandre de Mérode introduced tests for anabolic steroids only for the 1976 Montreal Olympic Games although it would have already been possible to test for steroids at the prior 1976 Winter Olmpic Games in Innsbruck (see Chapter 4).

[175] Minutes, "Meetings of the IOC Medical Commission, January 30 and February 3, 1972," archive collection "IOC Medical Commission," folder "Doping Controls at the Winter Games of Sapporo 1972, analysis reports, results and correspondence," IOC Archive, Lausanne.

[176] Organising Committee of the Games of the XITH Olympic Winter Games, *Official Report of the XIth Olympic Winter Games, Sapporo 1972, Part 1* (Sapporo: Organising Committee of the Games of the XIth Olympic Winter Games, 1972), 386.

the IOC Medical Commission." [177] The first official meeting took place on January 29, 1972, to exchange of information with representatives of the IFs. [178] In contrast to the preparation for the Munich Games, no agreement with the IFs concerning the number of doping tests had been in place until that point. Instead, the IFs had 24 hours to decide for their sport. Once the IOC Medical Commission met the next day to discuss the suggestions of the IFs, several problems arose. For example, it regarded a request of the UIPM (to take samples of *all* competitors of the biathlon events but then only conduct analytical tests with the samples of eight athletes) as impossible. [179] Because the International Ice Hockey Federation (IIHF) had left it open for the IOC Medical Commission to decide on the number of doping controls, this issue triggered a lengthy debate. Arnold Beckett wanted to test three competitors from each team, because he knew that the laboratory would have the capacity to do as many analyses. He even suggested that the analysis could be done on the day after the ice hockey games, if there was not enough time following the late evening ice hockey games. However, Alexandre de Mérode did not wish to postpone the doping analysis until the next day. He wanted to have a consistent approach of testing as many athletes as possible instead. In addition, Eduardo Hay stressed that testing for a different number of competitors following different matches would lead to suspicions. Consequently, the other members overruled Arnold Beckett and decided to test two randomly chosen athletes from each team. [180] Moreover, Yoshio Kuroda, as representative of the Organising Committee, had to assure that the laboratory would analyse all samples on the day of the sample taking. Hence, Arnold Beckett continued to vow for scientific reliability as the main priority whereas the majority of the IOC Medical Commission members preferred to have quick results. The result was less tests.

Furthermore, it appears from the meeting with the IFs, that despite the distribution of the *Doping* brochure, the federations were still unsure whether the second sample would also be analysed in the same laboratory under international supervision. Alexandre de Mérode and Arnold Beckett confirmed this and pointed out that a different laboratory team under Arnold Beckett´s guidance

---

[177] Ibid.

[178] The meeting was not considered an official meeting of the IOC Medical Commission.

[179] Minutes, "Meetings of the IOC Medical Commission, January 30 and February 3, 1972," 10.

[180] Ibid.

analysed the second sample.[181] Similar to the doping controls in Mexico City, when Arnold Beckett provided the laboratory with a list of possible doping substances a few days before the start of the competition, he suggested handing out a list of medicines containing forbidden substances.[182] Arnold Beckett thought that this would lead to a better relationship between the IOC Medical Commission and the Olympic team doctors, and that it would inform all doctors and athletes about which medical products they could use legally and which ones contained banned substances.[183] Albert Dirix also emphasised the need for such a list during the debate and pointed out that it could be useful to those competitors that did not have any medical support during the Olympic Games. Daniel Hanley remarked that in this way, athletes using medical reasons, such as epilepsy and asthma, could notify the IOC Medical Commission beforehand. The other members approved this medical argument, and Alexandre de Mérode sent out a circular letter to all Olympic team doctors, informing them to get in touch in case of the need for the usage of medicine due to illness.[184] However, the IOC Medical Commission never published a list of medical products. Instead, other members contested the attempted openness and supportive approach. For example, Jacques Thiebault stressed that athletes, who were tested positive, could use the list as an excuse and Alexandre de Mérode followed this line of argument. Thus, despite the introduction of analytical standards, members still had concerns about alternative ways to get around a positive doping test.

The Hokkaido Sanitation Institute hosted the anti-doping laboratory but the *Official Report* does not contain precise numbers of the laboratory staff and the used equipment.[185] Moreover, a note by the Sapporo Organising Committee discloses that no advancement in terms of the used methods had been made.[186]

[181] Minutes, "Meeting of the IOC Medical Commission with the representatives of the International Winter Sports Federations, January 29, 1972," archive collection "IOC Medical Commission," folder "Doping Controls at the Winter Games of Sapporo 1972, analysis reports, results and correspondence," IOC Archive, Lausanne.
[182] Minutes, "Meetings of the IOC Medical Commission, January 30 and February 3, 1972," 6.
[183] Minutes, "Meetings of the IOC Medical Commission, January 30 and February 3, 1972," 7.
[184] Minutes, "Meeting of the IOC Medical Commission with the representatives of the International Winter Sports Federations, January 29, 1972," Annex 2.
[185] ORGANISING COMMITTEE OF THE GAMES OF THE XITH OLYMPIC WINTER GAMES, *Official Report*, 386.
[186] Note, "Sapporo Organising Committee, n.d.," archive collection "IOC Medical Commission," folder "Doping Controls at the Winter Games of Sapporo 1972, analysis reports, results and correspondence," IOC Archive, Lausanne.

However, the laboratory staff carried out the analysis based on the general procedures listed in BECKETT et al. The argument brought forward by Eduardo Hay after the 1968 Mexico City Games about athletes being aware of the testing methods due to the publication of the methods, was subsequently not addressed. Furthermore, it is revealed that according to the standards decided upon during the doping technicians meeting in Rome, the samples were tested for volatile substances applying gas-liquid chromatography and for non-volatile substances with TLC. However, in contrast to the anticipated processes, the laboratory staff did not use mass-spectrometers. Instead, they attempted to identify possible doping substances with an infrared spectrophotometer. The reasons for this remain unclear but it shows that the doping controls were again not as good as they could have been.

During the 1972 Winter Olympic Games in Sapporo, the IOC Medical Commission made 211 doping tests. Amongst them was only one positive case, a significantly low number considering the public revelations by athletes to make extensive use of performance-enhancing drugs around the same time, if not in winter sports.[187] The positive doping test followed the FRG's 6:2 defeat over Yugoslavia in the preliminary ice hockey round, when the examination of the doping sample of FRG team captain Alois Schloder resulted in the detection of ephedrine.[188] The athlete denied the consumption of the substance, but the German Ice Hockey Federation eventually banned him for 18 months. Months later, however, it was explained that the German team doctor Dr. Franz Schlickenrieder had provided Alois Schloder with the substance "RR Plus," which contained ephedrine and therefore the federation lifted the ban.[189] Interestingly though, the IOC Medical Commission did not stick with its doping regulations in the case of Alois Schloder. Whereas the *Doping* brochure reads that if an athlete from within a team sports was tested positive, the entire team would be disqualified, this rule was not applied. Instead, Alexandre de Mérode argued during the IOC Session in summer 1972 that the IOC Medical Commission did

---

[187] HUNT describes in his book the case of the Amercian weightlifter Ken Patera, who openly admitted to use doping substances in order to keep up with super-heavyweight World Champion Vasily Alexeyev from the USSR. HUNT, *Drug Games*, 43.

[188] ORGANISING COMMITTEE OF THE GAMES OF THE XITH OLYMPIC WINTER GAMES, *Official Report*, 386.

[189] Curiously, Alois Schloder also returned to the Olympic stage and won the bronze medal with the German team at the 1976 Winter Olympic Games in Innsbruck.

not put the rule into effect due to "technical reasons".[190] However, it strongly recommended to the OK not to involve Franz Schlickenrieder in the doping controls of the 1972 Munich Olympic Games.[191]

It is difficult to filter out specific developments in the history of the anti-doping laboratory experts from the 1972 Winter Olympic Games in Sapporo. Certainly, the preparations for the anti-doping laboratory were not as detailed as for the Olympic Games in Munich in the same year. One reason for this was that no individual efforts, such as those by Manfred Donike, were undertaken. Hence it progressively emerges, that the quality of the anti-doping laboratory at Olympic Games depended on the initiative of responsible people in the host country during this period. The network of experts, still marginal at the time, and the IOC Medical Commission in form of Arnold Beckett could only create guidelines and a basic framework. Such steps were necessary, but without a proper implementation, there was little possibility to catch all doping offenders. Moreover, there was no communication between the anti-doping laboratory staff in Sapporo and Munich, which the IOC Medical Commission could have fostered. Consequently, the doping controls in Sapporo were very similar to the ones in Grenoble and Mexico City, although they took place in the transition period towards more harmonisation, during which anti-doping laboratory experts already consulted the IOC´s anti-doping activities.

Implementation of First Standardized Doping Controls

The IOC Medical Commission did not meet again before the Olympic Games in Munich in August 1972. In view of the frequent exchange, and the detailed preparations on the side of the laboratory by Manfred Donike this appears to be logical. However, this was a result of the dissatisfactory and palliative communication between the doping control commission of the Munich Games and the IOC Medical Commission. In order to arrive at this point, it is important to describe the efforts and actions of both sides.

During the IOC Medical Commission meeting in Sapporo, Dr. Wolfgang Hegels of the OK claimed that the anti-doping laboratory in Munich could in fact

---

[190] Minutes, "73rd Session of the IOC in Munich, August 21-24 and September 5, 1972," archive collection "IOC Sessions 1894-2009," IOC Archive, Lausanne, 32. This has also been outlined by HUNT, *Drug Games*, 43.

[191] In contrast to the IOC, German sport officials considered the incident to be only an individual slip-up by Alois Schlickenrieder and did not draw any further reaching conclusions. KRÜGER et al., "The Munich Olympics 1972," 539.

conduct as many as 1,000 doping controls per day (twelve hours) if necessary.[192] However, the IOC Medical Commission still decided to go with the planned 200 tests, because the eight Medical Commission members collecting the samples would not be able work any more hours. Wolfgang Hegels also disagreed with Manfred Donike, who regularly stressed that only a maximum of 200 analyses could guarantee scientific reliability, in this matter. This reflected the general standpoint of Arnold Beckett as demonstrated in various previous cases. In their final report, CLASING et al. write that the number of controls was – allegedly as KRÜGER et al. point out[193] – an "optimal compromise" between the number of tested competitors, the maximum laboratory capacity of 250 analyses per day and the total number of competitors.[194] In an attempt to justify the lack of tests for all medal winners, although Wolfgang Hegels suggested this could have been possible, CLASING et al. note that it would be an unjust assumption that doping would lead to medals and that doping would have a performance-enhancing influence in all cases.[195] Nevertheless, their usage of the word "compromise," points towards a possibility for more tests.

Manfred Donike used the months leading up to the Munich Olympic Games to test the technical equipment. In February 1972, he reported that the he had completed all plans for the organisation of the doping analysis.[196] As the OK had approved his methods, additional steps were only to be coordinated "in consultation with Prof. Beckett,"[197] which illustrates that Manfred Donike and Arnold Beckett were in charge of all doping analysis issues. The 1972 Munich doping control commission focused its efforts on the administrative, personnel and technical preparations. However, it would go beyond the scope of this book to detail these single steps, so only an overview of the main tasks and decisions with significance for the research question are given at this point.

---

[192] Minutes, "Meetings of the IOC Medical Commission, January 30 and February 3, 1972."

[193] KRÜGER et al., "The Munich Olympics 1972," 542.

[194] CLASING et al., "Dopingkontrolle", 131.

[195] Ibid.

[196] Minutes, "Sitzung der Dopingkontrollkommission des Organisationskomitees, February 16, 1972," archive collection "Olympische Spiele 1972," folder "9.10. Doping," CuLDA, Cologne, 3.

[197] Minutes, "Sitzung der Dopingkontrollkommission des Organisationskomitees, May 12, 1972," archive collection "Olympische Spiele 1972," folder "9.10. Doping," CuLDA, Cologne, 5.

First, Professor Dr. Gottfried Schönholzer[198] from Switzerland supervised the administrative part of the controls. The OK deemed it necessary to have an international expert as supervisor for all medical matters, rather than a team entirely consisting of staff from the FRG. Moreover, Gottfried Schönholzer had already published a paper on the issue in 1937.[199] This was one of the first important academic publications on the doping problem. Together with his deputy Dr. Bernhard Segesser[200], the team doctor of the Swiss Olympic team, he supervised the two sections "sampling" and "laboratory." Dr. Armin Klümper[201] and Dr. Dirk Clasing were responsible for the former sector, whereas Manfred Donike was in charge of the anti-doping laboratory. In his final report, Gottfried Schönholzer criticised the decision to appoint Armin Klümper as head of the sampling procedure, due to his involvement as medical expert of the German Olympic team.[202] He stressed that Armin Klümper occupied a "dangerous double function,"[203] and described that this led to an enormous work overload and emotional reactions. Gottfried Schönholzer even accused Armin Klümper of

---

[198] Professor Dr. Gottfried Schönholzer (1906-1979) was a medical doctor, who had specialised in sport medicine. Until 1972, was head of the medical institute at the Swiss Federal Institute of Sports Magglingen (EHSM) that he founded in 1967. He was head of the Medical Commission of the FIFA from 1968 until 1972. Hans HOWALD, "Prof. Dr. med. Gottfried Schönholzer," *Schweizerische Zeitschrift für Sportmedizin* 27, no.4 (1979), 148ff.

[199] HOBERMAN, *Mortal,* 261.

[200] Dr. Bernhard Segesser (born 1942), sport medicine specialists, was team doctor of the Swiss Olympic team for several Olympic Games. From 1974 until 1988, he was chief medical officer of the Swiss athletics team. In the late 1980s and early 1990s, he supported the usage of anabolic steroids for therapeutic reasons. Andreas SINGLER and Gerhard TREUTLEIN, *Doping im Spitzensport,* 6th edition (Aachen: Meyer & Meyer Verlag, 2012), 292.

[201] Professor Dr. Armin Klümper (born 1935) is a German sport medicine specialist, who had worked at the University of Freiburg. He became head of the Department of Sports Traumatology in 1977 and received a professorship. He was the team doctor for numerous FRG sport federations and involved in various doping controversies. This also accounts for most recent (March 2015) accusations that he provided the German football clubs SC Freiburg and VfB Stuttgart with doping substances. However, no official report was published until the finalisation of this book.

[202] Report, "Dopingkontrolle Bericht der Gesamtleitung, Prof. G. Schönholzer and Dr. B. Segesser, n.d.," archive collection "Olympische Spiele 1972," folder "9.10. Doping," CuLDA, Cologne, 6.

[203] Note, "Comments to the Report by Prof. G. Schönholzer," archive collection "Olympische Spiele 1972," folder "9.10. Doping," CuLDA, Cologne, 3.

having been drunk during the doping controls.[204] The staffing of the anti-doping laboratory was entirely left to Manfred Donike who presented a list of fourteen chemical experts (who were employed by the University of Cologne, the DSHS, directly by the OK and private chemical companies). Importantly, the NOC of the GDR requested from Manfred Donike to include four GDR doctors to work in the laboratory.[205] During the first meeting of the IOC Medical Commission in Munich, Manfred Donike voiced his discontent with the proposal.[206] The IOC Medical Commission agreed that the GDR´s demand was out of place. However, the request initiated the opening of the laboratory on August 25, 1972, so the team doctors and the press could observe the laboratory equipment.[207] The attempt by the East Germans was not the only approach by self-declared experts to work for Manfred Donike in the laboratory. The medical doctor and German cycling official Dr. Wolfgang Gronen also offered his assistance to Manfred Donike.[208] Interestingly, Wolfgang Gronen reasoned that he had previous experience in the field of doping sampling because he had been appointed doping inspector by the Chelsea College during cycling events in England.[209] However, Manfred Donike probably rejected this proposal, since Wolfgang Gronen´s name does not appear in the official documentation, which only lists names of trained chemists.

Second, the personnel preparations entailed mainly the assembly and training of 20 doping teams, who were responsible for the collection of the doping samples. Each team consisted of a doping official, a doping doctor, a technical assistant and at least one helper from the military services from the

---

[204] Gottfried Schönholzer describes in his report how he arrived in the doping control commission offices one day to find Armin Klümper drunk on the phone trying to speak with Alexandre de Mérode. Note, "Comments to the Report by Prof. G. Schönholzer," 7.

[205] Minutes, "Meeting of the Medical Commission of the International Olympic Committee, August 21, 1972," archive collection "IOC Medical Commission," folder "Meeting in Sapporo 1972, in Munich on 1972, in Moscow on 1973 and in Innsbruck on 1974," IOC Archive, Lausanne, 2.

[206] Ibid.

[207] Ibid.

[208] Letter, "Wolfgang Gronen to Manfred Donike, July 15, 1972," archive collection "Internationales Radsportachiv Wolfgang Gronen," folder "Medizin (22)b," Central Library for Sport Sciences, Cologne.

[209] Ibid.

FRG.[210] The fact that at the 1972 Winter Olympic Games in Sapporo the only doping case came from the FRG also affected the preparations of FRG team doctors. KRÜGER et al. argue that despite the publication of "General Guidelines for Doping Control" in autumn 1970, sport associations in the FRG were not interested in the implementation of the anti-doping regulations,[211] and that this attitude also had an effect on the doctors involved in the medical support of FRG athletes. Due to the Sapporo incident with Franz Schlickenrieder, FRG team doctors were under strict surveillance by the IFs during the Olympic Games. Furthermore, insecurity was detected amongst those doctors, "who thought of themselves as doping experts."[212] Due to the necessity of conducting the doping controls and handling the issue as discretely as possible, Armin Klümper recommended that all doctors should participate in workshops held in conjunction with Manfred Donike´s anti-doping laboratory in Cologne.[213] By holding the workshop in Cologne, not only could a general introduction into the problems with doping, but also information about doping analysis be provided. However, the OK rejected this proposal, and later decided to hold the workshops in conjunction with the two testing weeks for the laboratory staff and equipment in June and July 1972, with the main objective being to educate them about the

---

[210] Minutes, "Sitzung der Dopingkontrollkommission des Organisationskomitees, May 12, 1972," 3. There were very distinctive responsibilities between the doping official and the doping doctor. The official was responsible for the transmission of the information from the Organising Committee on which athletes were to be tested. His task was also to accompany the respective athletes to the doping control station and to assure that the athlete was present within one hour after receiving the information. "Dienststellenbeschreibung für Dopingoffizielle, July 4, 1972," archive collection "Olympische Spiele 1972," folder "9.10. Doping," CuLDA, Cologne. In contrast to this, the doping doctor was in charge of the correct collection of the doping sample as outlined in the *Doping* brochure. It was also he who signed the doping control sheet together with the athlete, the accompanying person, the (medical) representative of the IF and the secretary at the doping control station. Details are listed in: "Arbeitsfolge für Dopingärzte, n.d.," archive collection "Olympische Spiele 1972," folder "9.10. Doping," CuLDA, Cologne.

[211] In fact, according to KRÜGER et al., only four associations, the FRG´s Association of, the FRG´s Athletic Association, the FRG´s Federation of Equestrian Sports and the FRG´s Association of Table Tennis had accepted the anti-doping regulations until 1977. KRÜGER et al., "The Munich Olympics 1972," 539.

[212] Note, "Willing to General Secretary Kunze, Ernst Knoesel, Wolfgang Hegels and Kurt Käfer, March 22, 1972," archive collection "Olympische Spiele 1972," folder "9.10. Doping," CuLDA, Cologne.

[213] Minutes, "Sitzung der Dopingkontrollkommission des Organisationskomitees, May 12, 1972."

processes during the Olympic Games.[214] Nevertheless, one can regard Armin Klümper´s proposal as a move towards a more applicable doping education of sport medicine specialists and a close connection to the working practices of the anti-doping laboratory. Both of these emphasise the increasing awareness for doping analysis issues: medical experts should become more informed about the procedures whereas laboratory staff should become more educated in order to increase the scientific reliability of the tests. The latter initiative was the first educational measure of its kind.

Third, in terms of the technical and organisational preparations, it is necessary again to distinguish between the different sections of responsibilities. While Manfred Donike organised the laboratory equipment and staff in Cologne from a very early stage, the organisation of the overall doping control along with the sampling procedure was more complex. This was a result of the many different involved people in the process. As reported by Gottfried Schönholzer, the laboratory had been in perfect working order during the testing phase.[215] This also indicates that the transportation of the laboratory equipment from Cologne to Munich went without incident, although there is no detailed documentation on this part of the preparations available. The two organisational questions in the months leading up to the Olympic Games that the doping control commission dealt with, were the possibility to install doping tests for horses competing in the equestrian events and – as in Mexico City 1968 – the alcohol controls in the modern pentathlon events. The IOC Medical Commission discussed these during its meetings in Munich ahead of start of the competitions. Whereas all issues concerning personnel were already planned by the organisers in Munich, actual testing matters had to be agreed in conjunction with the IOC Medical Commission.

To summarise, the investigation of the immediate preparation of the doping controls for the 1972 Munich Olympic Games confirms that the anti-doping laboratory was well prepared, especially due to Manfred Donike´s efforts. This gives additional evidence for the new approaching era of anti-doping laboratories.

Role of the Members of the IOC Medical Commission

The vast amount of historical documents on the work of the Munich doping control committee prompts the need for a closer analysis with specific focus on

---

[214] Ibid.

[215] Report, "Dopingkontrolle Bericht der Gesamtleitung, Prof. G. Schönholzer and Dr. B. Segesser, n.d.," 3.

the different individual roles of IOC members, especially since national and international archival material is being used, thus allowing comparisons. Curiously, the arrival of the members in Munich marked a new phase of the doping control preparations and the start of the actual doping controls. This was accompanied by many problems, which Gottfried Schönholzer attributed to the poor communication and performance of Dr. Kurt Käfer, who was the link between the OK and the IOC Medical Commission. Already by June 1972 Schönholzer was criticising such poor communication in a letter.[216]

HUNT contends that the "complex regulatory system of the Olympics," where the Organising Committee, the IFs and the IOC Medical Commission all occupied important roles for the conduction of the doping controls caused confusion because of the list of banned substances.[217] Interestingly, Gottfried Schönholzer similarly argued that the list was not specific enough, and was particularly provoked by the supplementary statement "and related compounds."[218] Whereas the IOC Medical Commission had originally planned to conduct doping tests on horses also,[219] a matter already discussed in Sapporo,[220] the International Federation for Equestrian Sports (FEI) asserted that it did not receive any information on doping controls in their sport during the Munich Games. This was in contrast to Kurt Käfer's position that he had sent them a report by Arnold Beckett containing the list of banned substances.[221] However, because there were no controls for horses mentioned in the rules and it was only a report (which apparently was not received), the IOC Medical Commission decided that the federation should deal with the matter independently, and as a result, the FEI resolved not to have doping tests conducted. This caused consequences for the plans of the doping sampling and the work in the anti-

---

[216] Letter, "Prof. Dr. G. Schönholzer to Dr. med. Käfer, June, 1972," archive collection "Olympische Spiele 1972," folder "9.10. Doping," CuLDA, Cologne.

[217] HUNT, *Drug Games*, 44.

[218] Report, "Dopingkontrolle Bericht der Gesamtleitung, Prof. G. Schönholzer and Dr. B. Segesser, n.d.," 3.

[219] From the available files of the doping control commission of the Munich Organising Committee, it transpires that controls were planned for the military dressage, military show jumping, military cross-country, individual show jumping, dressage and the team show jumping competitions. Also see: Dirk CLASING, Manfred DONIKE and Armin KLÜMPER, "Dopingkontrolle bei den Spielen der XX. Olympiade, München 1972 (III)," *Leistungssport* 4 (1975), 305.

[220] Minutes, "Meetings of the IOC Medical Commission, January 30 and February 3, 1972."

[221] Minutes, "Meeting of the Medical Commission of the International Olympic Committee, August 21, 1972."

doping laboratory, although in this case it resulted in fewer tests and was considerably easier to handle.

Furthermore, the IFs strongly influenced the IOC Medical Commission. Just as ahead of the 1968 Mexico City Olympic Games, the UIPM in the form of its general secretary Willie Grut had asked the IOC Medical Commission to test for tranquillisers, despite them not being included in the official list of banned substances.[222] When asked by Willie Grut, Arnold Beckett confirmed that they could detect probably around 95.0% of all tranquillisers. Even though the UIPM only asked for blood tests, the IOC Medical Commission proposed to conduct urine tests also. Consequently, they took samples of all participating athletes: 59 blood/alcohol tests and 59 urine tests. Again, this influenced the work of the anti-doping laboratory that spontaneously had to deal with 59 additional samples. However, it still had capacity to undertake additional analyses on the day in question. The strong influence of the UIPM was again shown after the doping analysis led to fourteen positive tests, all for tranquillisers.[223] In contrast to his account of the meeting on August 23, Willie Grut, during a second appearance in front of the IOC Medical Commission, denied requesting tests for tranquillisers. He claimed that an assembly of team captains had forced him to make an enquiry about the possibility of taking urine tests. Nevertheless, as HUNT explains, Willie Grut had informed the FRG member of the Organising Committee for the doping controls in the modern pentathlon.[224] Arnold Beckett agreed with Willie Grut that he had stated that some competitors might be able to beat the testing system, however, reporting, "the test carried out in Munich would be regarded sufficiently foolproof anywhere in the world" and "it was possible to detect 99.9% of likely

---

[222] This was because the usage of a sedation to improve performance was only used in the shooting events of the pentathlon. Minutes, "Meeting of the Medical Commission of the International Olympic Committee, August 23, 1972," archive collection "IOC Medical Commission," folder "Meeting in Sapporo 1972, in Munich on 1972, in Moscow on 1973 and in Innsbruck on 1974," IOC Archive, Lausanne, 5.

[223] HUNT states that the German tabloid newspaper *BILD* identified sixteen positive test results and named the countries of origin. However, from the final report of the doping control commission, and Manfred Donike's laboratory team it transpires that there were only fourteen positive test results for tranquilisers. The found substances were: nitrazepam (three cases), glutethimid (one case) and chlordiazepoxid (ten cases). CLASING et al., "Dopingkontrolle," 306.

[224] HUNT, *Drug Games*, 47.

tranquillisers to be misused."[225] The attempt to blame the misunderstanding on the lack of scientific techniques available did not work in this case. In fact, CLASING et al. write in their report that the concentration of the substances was in some cases so high that detection with gas- and mass spectrometer was possible, although hydrolysis products have bad gas-chromatographic characteristics.[226] Consequently, it arose during the meeting that despite the attempt to blame the analytical procedure, the mistake was of a communicative nature. The IOC Medical Commission members were unanimous that the addition of tranquillisers to the list of banned substances was the official request of the federation.[227] However, since there appeared to be no compromise, and no admission of guilt from either side, it did not disqualify the athletes, but ruled that the UIPM should take the blame for not informing its competitors about the rule change.[228] Whereas there was obviously some consternation amongst IOC officials, such as Avery Brundage, who sent a letter to Alexandre de Mérode in October enquiring about the issue,[229] the incident also highlights the problems concerning the different responsibilities of IFs, IOC Medical Commission and doping control team of the OK. Following the Munich Games, there were plenty of written exchanges between the UIPM and Alexandre de Mérode on the matter. The

---

[225] Minutes, "Meeting of the Medical Commission of the International Olympic Committee, September 1, 1972," archive collection "IOC Medical Commission," folder "Meeting in Sapporo 1972, in Munich on 1972, in Moscow on 1973 and in Innsbruck on 1974," IOC Archive, Lausanne, 16.

[226] CLASING et al., "Dopingkontrolle," 306.

[227] Alexandre de Mérode even read out the protocol during the meeting in order to emphasise that the miscommunication was caused by Colonol Willie Grut and not the IOC Medical Commission. Minutes, "Meeting of the Medical Commission of the International Olympic Committee, September 1, 1972," 17.

[228] On the next general assembly of the UIPM in London in 1973, it was decided to eliminate tranquillisers entirely from the federations' list of banned substances. This decision faced a lot of criticism, especially by the representatives from the FRG and the USA. The reason for this was scientific proof that tranquillisers can improve the performance of shooting athletes. CLASING et al. also mention this in their final report, arguing that if the IOC is following this process and excluding tranquillisers from its list, it will be permitted to use a performance-enhancing substance at the subsequent Olympic Games, and thereby manipulate the result. CLASING et al., "Dopingkontrolle," 305.

[229] Letter, "Avery Brundage to Alexandre de Mérode, October 5, 1972," archive collection "Avery Brundage Collection, 1908-1975," film 54, folder 0006 "Medical Commission IOC 1970-1973," IOC Archive, Lausanne, 43.

IOC's technical director, Arthur Takac[230], eventually confirmed the correct response of the IOC Medical Commission, enforcing the prohibition of amendments to the list of banned substances less than one year ahead of the Games.[231] This confirmation was as late as February 1973, and assured that the anti-doping laboratories of the next Olympic Games could prepare even more meticulously.

Finally, it is important to briefly mention further controversies surrounding positive tests. In contradiction to the decision made at the 1972 Winter Olympic Games in Sapporo not to exclude teams that included a positive tested athlete the IOC Medical Commission applied this rule in Munich. The Puerto Rican basketball player Miguel Coll had already tested positive for ephedrine on August 29 during the first round game against Yugoslavia.[232] However, because the Medical Commission only discussed the issue on September 2, Puerto Rico continued to participate in the tournament.[233] The Dutch cycling team had to return its bronze medal due to a positive doping test for coramine by Aad van der

---

[230] Arthur Takac (1918-2004) from Hungary was chosen by Dr. Francis Messerli to serve as his assistant at the Olympic Institute in Lausanne during the Second World War. In 1964, he was appointed IOC president Avery Brundage's assistant for the competition program of the Mexico City 1968 Olympic Games. He served as technical director for the 1972 and 1976 Olympic Games. During his time at the IOC, Artur Takac's main concern was a regular update of the competition programme as well as the participation of women. After the 1984 Winter Olympic Games in Sarajevo, where he served as vice-president of the Organising Committee, he was given the Olympic Order by IOC president Juan Antonio Samaranch. He also made him his personal advisor for all issues concerning the organisation of the Olympic Games. Marié-Hélène ROUKHADZÉ, "Artur Takac, the Stadium as Field of Experience," *Olympic Review* 233 (1987), 106-110.

[231] Letter, "Artur Takac to Lord Killanin, February 15, 1973," archive collection "IOC Medical Commission," folder "Medical Commission: Correspondence 1973," IOC Archive, Lausanne.

[232] Minutes, "Meeting of the Medical Commission of the International Olympic Committee, September 2, 1972," archive collection "IOC Medical Commission," folder "Meeting in Sapporo 1972, in Munich on 1972, in Moscow on 1973 and in Innsbruck on 1974," IOC Archive, Lausanne, 21.

[233] HUNT argues that the decision was taken as late due the duration of the doping analysis. However, this statement is in contrast to the report by the Organising Committee and the publications by the doping laboratory team, who both argue that all doping analysis procedures were finished 24 hours after the receipt of the urine sample. HUNT, *Drug Games*, 48.

Hoek following the 100km team race.[234] The disqualification of the swimmer Rick DeMont (USA) due a positive doping test for ephedrine caused the biggest controversy. Rick DeMont, an asthmatic, had noted the medical product "Marax" on his entry form; however, the American team doctors had not forwarded the information to the IOC Medical Commission. This cast a poor light on the American member Daniel Hanley, who denied all responsibility in front of the IOC Executive Board.[235] The IOC Medical Commission – arguably due to the high profile of the athlete – eventually left it entirely to the IOC Executive Board to make a decision. There was no consensus within the IOC Medical Commission because Daniel Hanley asked for clemency, whereas Alexandre de Mérode first recommended that Rick DeMont could keep his medal, but then argued for his disqualification in order to prevent protests of other competitors. [236] The laboratory reports strongly supported Alexandre de Mérode because the analysis revealed that the concentration of ephedrine was much higher than Rick DeMont claimed to have taken. This highlights how the anti-doping laboratories could offer significant scientific results. The IOC Executive Board followed these arguments, stripped Rick DeMont of his gold medal, and disqualified him from the 1500m race.[237] REINOLD clarifies that the controversial disqualification of Rick DeMont was the prompt for more discussions in the IOC Medical Commission regarding the therapeutic use of medicine.[238] In 1973, it published a list of approved drugs for therapies but again one year later Alexandre de Mérode questioned this initiative. He considered that such a list could never be

---

[234] The president of the Dutch National Olympic Committee Cornelis Lambert Kerdel argued during the meeting of the Executive Committee that this was a particular unfortunate case because Aad Van den Hoek has had to leave the race after the first part of the race due to a bicycle breakdown. Furthermore, it was stated in his defence that codamine was not listed on the banned substance list of the UCI. Minutes, "Executive Board, September 8, 1972," archive collection "IOC Executive Board Meetings 1921-1982," IOC Archive, Lausanne, 42.

[235] Ibid., 46.

[236] Ibid.

[237] However, the International Swimming Federation (FINA) banned Rick DeMont, because he competed at the 1973 World Championships and won the gold medal ahead of the Australian Bradford Cooper, who had been awarded the Olympic gold medal in Munich after Rick DeMont's disqualification. KLUGE, *Olympische Sommerspiele*, 415n468.

[238] REINOLD, "Arguing," 20ff.

conclusive.[239] However, Arnold Beckett, who insisted that such a list was to give the team doctors guidelines for medical treatment, opposed Alexandre de Mérode.[240] As a result, the IOC Medical Commission adopted the following statement:

> The Medical Commission realizes that there are sometimes problems regarding the therapeutic treatment of competitors during the Olympic Games. They emphasise that they are prepared to accept requests for the use of medication in these circumstances and will rule whether in fact the drug in the medication comes within the classes of banned drugs or not.[241]

Furthermore, as REINOLD outlines, the IOC Medical Commission held a meeting with the team doctors prior to the 1976 Winter Olympic Games in Innsbruck, in order to clarify that they had to present written requests for the usage of medicine for therapeutic reasons. For the 1976 Montreal Olympic Games, the IOC Medical Commission permitted beta-2 bronchospasmolytics such as salbutamol for asthma.[242] It categorically forbade ephedrine and related substances.[243]

The other athletes who tested positive in Munich were Mongolian judoist and silver medallist Bakhaavaa Buidaa (ephedrine), Spanish cyclist and bronze medallist Jaime Huelamo (coramine), Austrian weightlifter Walter Legel (amphetamine) and Iranian weightlifter Mohammadreza Nasehi (ephedrine).[244] 2079 urine and 65 blood samples were analysed in total at the 1972 Munich

---

[239] Minutes, "Meeting of the IOC Medical Commission in Innsbruck, April 5-7, 1974," archive collection "IOC Medical Commission," folder "Meeting in Sapporo 1972, in Munich on 1972, in Moscow on 1973 and in Innsbruck on 1974," IOC Archive, Lausanne, 16.

[240] Ibid.

[241] Ibid.

[242] Lan BARNES, "Olympic Drug Testing: Improvements Without Progress," *Physician and Sportsmedicine* 8 (1980), 22.

[243] REINOLD, "Arguing," 21.

[244] Bill MALLON and Ian BUCHANAN, *Historical Dictionary of the Olympic movement* (Oxford: Scarecrow Press, 2006), 367f.

Olympic Games.[245] Despite the interpersonal and interinstitutional controversies, the positive tests illustrate that the analytical equipment used in Munich was working. This was also a result of the meticulous preparations of the doping analysis. The analytical strategy of having an initial screening procedure, based on GC and detection with a nitrogen phosphorus detector, followed by identification through the mass spectrometer for suspicious samples, was used for the very first time by the laboratory staff at the Munich laboratory. Therefore, they followed the recommendations made by the doping technicians in Rome in 1969. Manfred DONIKE et al. note that the doping analysis could be improved and standardised. [246] The well-elaborated preparations in Cologne further allowed Manfred Donike to teach his staff in a precise manner on the usage of the equipment. Furthermore, in contrast to the experience made by Arnold Beckett in Mexico City, the cooperation between the Arnold Beckett and Manfred Donike during the Olympic Games appears to have been faultless. There are no disagreements recorded, and Arnold Beckett regularly praised the work of the anti-doping laboratory. The establishment of a central doping analysis institution for the FRG in Cologne from 1974 onwards is additional proof for the legacy of

---

[245] Some sources also say that there were only 2070 urine samples. However, the list distributed to the members of the IOC Medical Commission in June 1976 outlines 2079 conducted doping tests. Minutes, Meeting of the Medical Commission of the International Olympic Committee, July, 1976, archive collection "IOC Medical Commission," folder "Meeting in Montreal on July-August 1976 and in Barcelona on October 1976," IOC Archive, Lausanne (Appendix 2). This is the same number as stated by CLASING et al. in their academic publication on the doping controls of the 1972 Munich Olympic Games. CLASING et al., "Dopingkontrolle," 305. Interestingly, a statistic on the number of analysed samples has also been published in the Olympic Review in January/February 1973, stating only 2052 taken samples. "Medical Controls," *Olympic Review*, 1973, no. 62-63: 15. However, this statistic had not been authorised, which concerned Alexandre De Merode: "He [Alexandre De Mérode] said that a brief report was published in the *Olympic Review* without any signature and expressed an opinion that the materials on medical matters should be looked through by the Medical Committee before their publication in that or other IOC editions." Minutes, "Meeting of the Medical Commission of the International Olympic Committee, May 25-27, 1973," archive collection "IOC Medical Commission," folder "Meeting in Sapporo 1972, in Munich on 1972, in Moscow on 1973 and in Innsbruck on 1974," IOC Archive, Lausanne, 3.

[246] Manfred DONIKE, Dirk CLASING and Armin KLÜMPER, "Dopingkontrollen bei den Spielen der XX. Olympiade München 1972 – Teil 2," *Leistungssport* 2 (1974), 192.

the anti-doping laboratory. Manfred Donike successfully reinstalled the equipment used for the Munich Olympic Games.[247]

However, this is not to confirm that the entire doping control system at the 1972 Munich Olympic Games performed flawlessly. This is particularly true for the lack of a test on anabolic steroids, which competitors increasingly used at the time. According to a survey by American discus thrower Jay Silvester, 68.0% of the questioned athletes admitted that they had taken anabolic steroids, and 61.0% even replied that this had been in the six months leading up to the 1972 Munich Olympic Games.[248] KRÜGER et al. explore other revelations of the usage of anabolic steroids, such as by head coach of the FRG athletics team, Hansjörg Kofink.[249] As outlined in this chapter, the IOC Medical Commission was aware about the need for a testing method for anabolic steroids. However, because there was no sophisticated and reliable method for steroid testing available, the sport organisations could not test for them. This circumstance led the doping control team to conclude that the tests were the first ones to set internationally approved standards.[250] Therefore, one can conclude that particularly due to the efforts of anti-doping laboratory expert Manfred Donike, the 1972 Munich Olympic Games left a legacy in this regard, as verified by HEMMERSBACH.[251]

Criticism Indicates Future of the IOC´s Fight against Doping

Even though the doping controls at the 1972 Munich Olympic Games were a success, there is evidence for considerable continuing differences amongst the various stakeholders involved with the controls. Gottfried Schönholzer has voiced these in his final report and a letter accompanying the report. His comments give indications about the work of the IOC Medical Commission and the distinction between sport medical specialists and anti-doping laboratory experts. However, it is important to consider the hostile working relationship between the IOC Medical Commission and Gottfried Schönholzer that resulted from his critical nature. Written exchanges between Gottfried Schönholzer, Alexandre de Mérode

---

[247] KRÜGER et al., find it remarkable that the laboratory was installed by the German Ministry of the Interior and the German Association of Sport Physicians (Sportärztebund) and not by the German National Olympic Committee. They relate this to the lack of interest in doping controls by the German sport system in general. KRÜGER et al., "The Munich Olympics 1972," 543.

[248] TODD, "A History," 330.

[249] KRÜGER et al., "The Munich Olympics 1972," 540.

[250] CLASING et al., "Dopingkontrolle," 306.

[251] HEMMERSBACH, "History," 841.

and Avery Brundage reveal that the members of the IOC Medical Commission felt that Gottfried Schönholzer undermined their responsibilities. According to the official minutes, Gottfried Schönholzer had visited the IFs in order to make other arrangements than previously agreed upon, and he attempted to change protocols.[252] Because of Gottfried Schönholzer's actions, Avery Brundage sent a letter to the President of the OK, Willi Daume, requesting the exclusion of Gottfried Schönholzer from any aspect of the doping controls.[253] However, according to Gottfried Schönholzer, the OK did not oblige. He accused Alexandre de Mérode, Kurt Käfer and Armin Klümper of indiscreetness whilst they blamed him for a doping control refusal.[254] The internal hostilities shall not be under in-depth investigation here, but they display that one has to treat Gottfried Schönholzer's remarks carefully due to personal differences. In general, he identified three main interlinked problematic issues.

First, he argued that there was a lack of clear-cut areas of responsibility amongst the involved stakeholders in the doping controls. This was the result of the rule change for the modern pentathlon event shortly before the start of the competitions. Gottfried Schönholzer criticised that IFs were responsible for the selection procedure. As he reported, this could have become "extremely dangerous," and was only prevented due to the detailed preparations of the anti-doping laboratory, which had enough capacity to conduct further tests.[255] This is a first indication for acknowledgement of Manfred Donike's anti-doping laboratory work. Gottfried Schönholzer credited the problematic communication between the local commission and the IOC Medical Commission to the behaviour of Kurt Käfer, who did not fulfil his role as a link between the commissions.[256] Kurt Käfer had influenced other members of both commissions in order to create a negative atmosphere towards Gottfried Schönholzer and his assistant Bernhard Segesser. He stated, Kurt Käfer acted "often as commissionaire of the IOC Medical Commission and cared for its members submissively" instead.[257] Moreover, the IOC Medical Commission later reiterated the controversial role of

---

[252] Minutes, "Meeting of the Medical Commission of the International Olympic Committee, September 2, 1972," 24.

[253] Letter, "Avery Brundage to Willi Daume, September 4, 1972," "IOC Medical Commission," folder "Meeting in Munich on 1972 - Appendices," IOC Archive, Lausanne.

[254] Report, "Dopingkontrolle Bericht der Gesamtleitung, Prof. G. Schönholzer and Dr. B. Segesser, n.d.," 6.

[255] Ibid.

[256] Note, "Comments to the Report by Prof. G. Schönholzer," 2.

[257] Ibid.

Kurt Käfer because it never received an official report on the gender controls and the technical aspects of the medical organisation.[258] Gottfried Schönholzer listed examples, such as the omission to invite him and his assistant to the meeting with the team doctors and not receiving the official protocols of the IOC Medical Commission meetings.[259] He concluded that all these incidents could have been bypassed if one international body was in charge of the entire doping controls. This would have also avoided the reserved attitude of the members of the IOC Medical Commission towards the FRG in general, and the OK in particular.[260] Interestingly, CLASING et al. argue along the same lines. They suggest that there should only be "*one* authority, *one* department, *one* committee or *one* personality [emphasis in the original]" dealing with the doping controls. [261] During international competitions, CLASING et al. write, this body should be of an international nature in order to guarantee all participating nations the implementation of the predetermined conditions. This is interesting, because the IOC Medical Commission had declined the proposal of the NOC of the GDR to include some of their laboratory staff. Furthermore, CLASING et al. argue that running all decisions through several committees slowed down the preparation of the technical aspects of the control. Although the concept for the research, preparation and conduction of the doping analysis procedures had already been suggested in May 1969, the process could only be started in April 1971 – in a very restricted way.[262] Evidently, those not directly involved in the IOC Medical Commission doubted the structure of the Olympic anti-doping system considerably already in its formative years.

Second, Gottfried Schönholzer criticised the structure and membership of the IOC Medical Commission. He knew many of the members through his involvement in the FIMS, as he mentioned in his report. [263] He especially identified the Russian and the French member of the IOC Medical Commission, who must have been Nina Grashinskaya and Jacques Thiebault. According to his report, the two members attempted to demonstrate that the doping controls had a

---

[258] Minutes, "Meeting of the Medical Commission of the International Olympic Committee, April 5-7, 1974," archive collection "IOC Medical Commission," folder "Meeting in Sapporo 1972, in Munich on 1972, in Moscow on 1973 and in Innsbruck on 1974," IOC Archive, Lausanne, 4.

[259] Note, "Comments to the Report by Prof. G. Schönholzer," 2.

[260] Ibid., 8.

[261] CLASING et al., "Dopingkontrolle," 306.

[262] Ibid., 303.

[263] Note, "Comments to the Report by Prof. G. Schönholzer," 8.

leak by stealing a doping protocol.[264] These confrontations and problems with individual members made Gottfried Schönholzer conclude that the IOC Medical Commission was too big and not adequately staffed. He suggested that only one representative of the IOC Medical Commission should be present at the Olympic Games. This person should have competencies in doping analysis. He thought that only Arnold Beckett had such abilities.[265] Furthermore, the set-up should consist solely of "capable and practicing scientists,"[266] who could be trained at the Olympic Academy. Amongst this group of experts, a much smaller working panel, consisting of three members, should only deal with the doping and gender controls. This panel could then act as the highest agency without getting involved in the running of the doping controls by the respective Organising Committee.

Third, Gottfried Schönholzer clearly differentiated between medical and anti-doping laboratory experts in the IOC Medical Commission in a way that no other such early historical account had. He thought that its members only consisted of "doping and sex-administrators," who "are immaterial within their scientific areas and are not professionally qualified."[267] Gottfried Schönholzer highlighted that Arnold Beckett was an exception, attributing him to be the only member subject-specific abilities and fairness. In contrast to the other members, Gottfried Schönholzer wrote, Arnold Beckett had the experience and the expertise in pharmaceutical chemistry.[268] Similarly, he made a differentiation between Manfred Donike and the other members of the German doping control commission, and related his exceptional competencies in doping analysis matters. He noted that in retrospect, he would have taken his own colleagues from within sports medicine to support him during the doping controls in Munich; however, he would have liked to work with Manfred Donike due to his eminent knowledge in doping analysis.[269]

Gottfried Schönholzer's critique identified some key problems that the IOC Medical Commission faced in its early years. With his suggestion to install a specialised working panel on doping controls, he was clearly advanced of his time, because in later years the IOC Medical Committee would implement such measures (see Chapter 6). For Gottfried Schönholzer, the only skilled doping

---

[264] Report, "Dopingkontrolle Bericht der Gesamtleitung, Prof. G. Schönholzer and Dr. B. Segesser, n.d.," 4.
[265] Ibid.
[266] Ibid., 6.
[267] Note, "Comments to the Report by Prof. G. Schönholzer," 3.
[268] Ibid.
[269] Ibid., 9.

experts to deal with the problem were anti-doping laboratory experts with experience in doping analysis, above all Manfred Donike and Arnold Beckett. Clearly, this was an exclusive attitude at the time, especially considering Gottfried Schönholzer himself was a medical professor.

INTERIM RESULTS FOR THE PERIOD 1967-1972: INDIVIDUAL CONSULTANCY ROLES FOR PIONEERS IN ANTI-DOPING LABORATORY EXPERTISE

The reconstruction of the IOC´s fight against doping due to the installation of the IOC Medical Commission brought with it some important changes for the working practices in the practical implementation of doping controls. In contrast to the IOC`s first doping subcommittee, the IOC Medical Commission included external medical experts and one anti-doping laboratory expert. This was Arnold Beckett. From the foundation onwards, he played a central role within international anti-doping efforts because of his professional competencies in the domain of doping analysis. He appeared to be in charge of the compilation of the list of banned substances, was the only member to have technical knowledge on testing mechanisms and coordinated the set-up of the anti-doping laboratory at the Olympic Games. All of these processes were of the highest priority so that Arnold Beckett, because of his professional expertise, became a key consultant for Alexandre de Mérode´s anti-doping policy. However, this does not mean that all his initiatives ran smoothly. The example of the miscommunication, before and during the installation of the doping controls at the 1968 Mexico City Olympic Games prove that there were considerable limits to his influence. In fact, more positive doping tests could have been reported.

The detailed historical review on the preparations for the 1972 Munich Olympic Games by Manfred Donike display that it was an entirely different story in 1972. Whereas the laboratories and its staff in Grenoble, Mexico City and Sapporo all relied heavily on the guidance of Arnold Beckett, Manfred Donike became extremely proactive in the preparation and implementation of the analytical procedures. His expertise in the domain of doping analysis proved to be highly valuable for the OK. Consequently, the anti-doping laboratory work at the 1972 Munich Olympic Games became a turning point in the involvement of anti-doping laboratory expert´s role in the IOC´s fight against doping. In fact, the perceived success of these controls were a result of the initiatives of the local doping control committee, rather than the IOC Medical Commission, whose majority of members appear to have been a disrupting factor. One significant consequence of the detailed preparations was the increasing number of positive doping tests at the Olympic Games, although the actual number of doped athletes must have been much higher.

Yet, despite the involvement of Arnold Beckett and medical doctors with firsthand experience in doping controls, Alexandre de Mérode did not chose members of the IOC Medical Commission by their scientific knowledge and experience in anti-doping matters, but rather for their nationality and sport political lobbying. This was in contrast to Alexandre de Mérode´s original plan of keeping the IOC Medical Commission as small and specific as possible, and shows that he was also subject to adapting his strategy according to the situation of the Olympic Movement. The enlargement is one of the main points of criticism raised by Gottfried Schönholzer following the doping controls in Munich in 1972. A careful read of the minutes of the IOC Medical Commission meetings during and between the Olympic Games reveals that the size of the body influenced the decision-making processes and produced controversial rulings.

Additionally, transformation processes characterise the period between 1967 and 1972. These took place not just within the IOC Medical Commission, but also through the first attempts of a network creation amongst experts on doping analysis. The anti-doping laboratory experts´ professional competencies in doping analysis are acknowledged for the first time. An exchange of knowledge occurred between anti-doping laboratory experts Manfred Donike and Arnold Beckett, but also on the meeting of "Doping Technicians" in Rome in October 1969. Due to the demonstrated lack of exchange forum for experts involved in doping analysis before 1969, the meeting was a first attempt to establish a global network of laboratories and experts. The *Doping* brochure summarised the agreed guidelines on doping analysis, although the booklet was not published as proceedings of the symposium. The consistent procedures eventually led to the first standardised doping controls in Sapporo and Munich, even though the preparations in the FRG, due to the involvement of Manfred Donike, were far more sophisticated than in Japan.

The period under investigation in this chapter also brings to light the necessity in making a distinction between the medical and the anti-doping laboratory experts at the time. This can be noticed in the organisation of the doping controls at the 1972 Munich Olympic Games, which the OK separated between the sampling procedure and the anti-doping laboratory. Whereas national and international sport medicine specialists were in charge of the doping sample, Manfred Donike was solely responsible for the laboratory. For this reason, he also implemented an educational workshop for laboratory staff members. Gottfried Schönholzer, in his final report, also argued in this direction: he stressed Manfred

Donike´s perfect anti-doping laboratory preparations and singled out Arnold Beckett as the only doping control expert on the IOC Medical Commission. There is no doubt that Gottfried Schönholzer recognised their competencies and significance for the doping control system.

In conclusion, the investigations of the period from 1967 until 1972 reveal that the period from the establishment of the IOC Medical Commission to the implementation of the first standardised doping controls at the 1972 Munich Olympic Games, were the first international incorporation of anti-doping laboratory experts into the IOC´s anti-doping activities. This inclusion was based on their professional expertise in the field of doping analysis, which was needed to advance the doping control system. Notwithstanding, Arnold Beckett, despite his influential role in the IOC Medical Commission, along with Manfred Donike, still only occupied individual consultancy roles, and no coordinated procedures to develop testing techniques existed, yet. The majority of the IOC Medical Commission members could still overruled Arnold Beckett, especially since sport medical specialists outnumbered him. Manfred Donike´s role on the international level was clearly less influential. However, he became a role model for future organisers of the doping analysis at the Olympic Games through his sophisticated preparations and execution of the doping analysis. Hence, in this period, the two leading figures of the anti-doping laboratory experts´ evolving network became highly relevant consultants for the IOC in anti-doping questions for the very first time. However, whilst their involvement is notable, they also had to deal with counteracting forces that they could not control, such as the behaviour of Armin Klümper and Kurt Käfer during the 1972 Munich Olympic Games.

CHAPTER 4

Expansion of Consultancy (1973-1977)

ADDRESSING STRUCTURAL PROBLEMS IN THE IOC MEDICAL COMMISSION WITHOUT CONSEQUENCES

As demonstrated in the previous chapter, Gottfried Schönholzer had criticised the size and efficiency of the IOC Medical Commission in the aftermath of the doping controls for the 1972 Munich Olympic Games. After these Games, the Irishman Lord Killanin[1] replaced Avery Brundage as IOC president. Importantly, he suggested ways to improve the working efficiency of the IOC commissions. Similar to Gottfried Schönholzer's concern, he wrote to Alexandre de Mérode in October 1972, enquiring whether the IOC Medical Commission was too large, if it was working rapidly enough and whether there should be a division between doping and medicaments.[2] Lord Killanin considered these two to be separate issues, which Alexandre de Mérode did not. One can attribute Lord Killanin's enquiry to the controversies surrounding the positive test of Rick DeMont (see Chapter 3), that caused extensive public concern. In line with his previous policy, Alexandre de Mérode's reply is characterised by the attempt to strengthen the position of the IOC Medical Commission and it is necessary to emphasise that he relied on the input of Arnold Beckett, attaching a motion drawn up by him.[3] Thus, once again Alexandre de Mérode shifted responsibility to Arnold Beckett, stressing his important consultancy value. Besides more specific tasks, which

---

[1] Michael Morris, 3rd Baron Killanin (1914-1999) (referred to as Lord Killanin) inherited the title of his uncle when he was 13 years old. He was elected as 6th IOC president on the 73rd IOC Session in Munich on August 21, 1972. Lord Killanin studied at Eton and was a passionate sports man, playing several sports such as rugby, boxing, rowing and horse riding. In 1950, he became president of the Irish National Olympic Committee. He was elected onto the IOC Executive Board in 1967. Volker KLUGE, *Olympische Sommerspiele. Die Chronik 1*, 590n1.

[2] Letter, "Lord Killanin to Alexandre de Mérode, October 12, 1972," archive collection "IOC Medical Commission," folder "Medical Commission: Correspondence 1971-1972," IOC Archive, Lausanne.

[3] Letter, "Alexandre de Mérode to Lord Killanin, December 17, 1972," archive collection "IOC Medical Commission," folder "Medical Commission: Correspondence 1971-1972," IOC Archive, Lausanne, 2.

mainly focused on the compilation of the list of banned substances, Arnold Beckett saw the need for a more harmonised approach towards doping controls.[4] The IOC Medical Commission should support the establishment of national anti-doping laboratories of whom only very few existed, because there were no coordinated doping regulations in place yet at sporting events other than the Olympic Games. This pointed towards the realisation of a more scientific approach, which Arnold Beckett clearly favoured. Moreover, it is a move towards the establishment of a bigger institutional network, which would result in more testing and an increased need for competencies in doping analysis. In an accompanying note of his letter to Lord Killanin, Alexandre de Mérode linked the problems that occurred at the 1972 Munich Olympic Games to the lack of regular meetings between the 1968 and 1972 Olympic Games. Thus, he agreed with Arnold Beckett's motion that the IOC Medical Commission should meet annually, by emphasising that "this [the Medical Commission] should stay permanent and that its action should be intensified."[5]

At the first IOC Executive Board meeting after the 1972 Munich Olympic Games in February 1973, Alexandre de Mérode again urged for changes in the IOC's doping rules, but did not agree upon any structural changes. Specifically, he asked to clarify the IOC Executive Board's strategy, in terms of the list of banned substances and the policies in case of a positive test.[6] Lord Killanin again argued that the IOC Medical Commission was too large and that the high number of members was hindering its productivity.[7] He suggested a more pragmatic approach, proposing a standing committee, which could meet much more regularly, so that the full body would only have to meet annually. However, Alexandre de Mérode opposed this by arguing that all members were specialists in their respective fields and that it would not be possible to meet with only a few of them. This appears to be incorrect, since most of the members were medical doctors with very similar backgrounds. Furthermore, from a practical point of view, Alexandre de Mérode's argument was illogical, because it would have been much easier to arrange meetings with only a few members. He clearly did not take into account the lack of experts on doping analysis on the IOC Medical Commission at the time. The IOC Executive Board was also concerned about the long time between the announcements of a positive doping control and the

---

[4] Ibid.

[5] Ibid.

[6] Minutes, "Executive Board, February 2-5, 1973," archive collection "IOC Executive Board Meetings 1921-1982," IOC Archive, Lausanne, 12.

[7] Ibid.

awarding of the medal.[8] In this case, Alexandre de Mérode defended the work of the laboratory, arguing that it worked as fast as possible, whilst also being accurate.[9] Thus, he *did* value the contribution and competencies of the anti-doping laboratory experts, if only during the Olympic Games and not in the IOC Medical Commission, in which Arnold Beckett's presence was sufficient to Alexandre de Mérode.

However, the IOC Medical Commission members themselves also felt the need for a more distinct approach to its anti-doping efforts and voiced such concerns in May 1973. One indication for this is Nina Grashinskaya's request to clearly define the functions and composition of the IOC Medical Commission. She demanded that Alexandre de Mérode draft statutes that included the number of members, the order of work and the regularity of the meetings.[10] It remains unclear, however, if Alexandre de Mérode attempted to create statues of the IOC Medical Commission. He only reported about the wish of the members to make it a more permanent body at the following IOC Executive Board meeting in June 1973.[11] In addition to this, Pieter van Dijk asked for a retirement age for members on the IOC Medical Commission, suggesting that this age limit should be 70 years.[12] His proposal was motivated by his own wish to retire. However, Alexandre de Mérode thought this to be an extraordinary approach because he regarded the membership a privilege. Consequently, he did not agree with Pieter van Dijk, arguing that he had made important contributions and should therefore remain a member.[13] Certainly, the wish for resignation did not come at a good time for Alexandre de Mérode, as his attempt was to keep the IOC Medical Commission's present constitution. However, Pieter van Dijk was not to be convinced and eventually resigned. Both contributions point towards the need for a clearly defined role of the IOC Medical Commission. But because Nina Grashinskaya and Pieter van Dijk were medical doctors, they - unlike Gottfried Schönholzer had in the aftermath of the Munich Olympic Games - did not raise

---

[8] Ibid.

[9] Ibid., 13.

[10] Minutes, "Meeting of the Medical Commission of the International Olympic Committee, May 25-26, 1973," archive collection "IOC Medical Commission," folder "Meeting in Sapporo 1972, in Munich on 1972, in Moscow on 1973 and in Innsbruck on 1974," IOC Archive, Lausanne, 9.

[11] Minutes, "Executive Board, June 22-24, 1973," archive collection "IOC Executive Board Meetings 1921-1982," IOC Archive, Lausanne, 5.

[12] Ibid.

[13] Ibid.

the necessity to include anti-doping laboratory and their suggestions instead addressed the general, structural problems.

Moreover, there were changes in the IOC Medical Commission's membership, demonstrating that Alexandre de Mérode still favoured sport medical specialists. This becomes more obvious in the decision to replace Pieter van Dijk after his resignation. The decision fell on Yoshio Kuroda, and not a representative of Munich's OK such as Herbert Reindell or Manfred Donike, who had been extensively praised for their work (see Chapter 3). Alexandre de Mérode did not explain his discussion, but only suggested the adoption of Yoshio Kuroda to the IOC Executive Board in June 1973.[14] Whatever the reason, the verdict did not reflect the need for more expertise in doping controls or doping analysis. Yoshio Kuroda had no first-hand experience in these fields.

Further personnel changes also point towards the adoption of members without taking into consideration their expertise in anti-doping. When in 1975 Jacques Thiebault needed to be replaced – he could not maintain his membership due to other professional commitments – it was still not regarded necessary to include more anti-doping laboratory experts, even though the work of the Medical Commission focused entirely on the intensification of the doping controls at the time. In fact, Professor Dr. Iba Mar Diop[15], vice-president of the Senegalese National Olympic Committee, replaced Jacques Thiebault.[16] Iba Mar Diop's inclusion was linked to Alexandre de Mérode's increasing efforts to work with the Olympic Solidarity Commission.[17] He had raised this issue for the first time in

---

[14] Ibid.

[15] Iba Mar Diop (1921-2008) was dean of the Faculty of Medicine and Pharmacy of Dakar when he was appointed to the IOC Medical Commission. He specialised in infectious and tropical diseases and had a degree in special studies in biology applied to physical education and sport. INTERNATIONAL OLYMPIC COMMITTEE, *Commission Médicale*, 28.

[16] Minutes, "Executive Board, May 14-16, May 19 and May 23, 1975," archive collection "IOC Executive Board Meetings 1921-1982," IOC Archive, Lausanne, 24.

[17] Due to the large number of NOCs, which were becoming independent from the beginning of the 1960s onwards, the IOC established on initiative of Comte Jean de Beaumont the Committee for International Olympic Aid in 1962. Task of the Committee was to provide the new NOCs with financial and organisational assistance. In 1972, it transformed into the Committee for Olympic Solidarity. In 1981, at the Olympic Congress in Baden-Baden, the IOC set up the Olympic Solidarity Commission, with a strategy to address the needs of the NOCs. Today, it assists them in gaining access to financial, technical and administrative assistance, particularly through the distribution of the broadcasting revenues. HENRY and AL TAUQI, "The Development," 355.

May 1973 and reported to the Executive Board a month later.[18] However, it took until 1979 before efforts were undertaken in this regard.[19] Despite these notable efforts, Iba Mar Diop did not have any experience in anti-doping, but through the connection with other commissions, the IOC Medical Commission gained influence and reputation within the IOC. Again, this pattern fitted Alexandre de Mérode´s strategy. For the same reason, orthopaedic surgeon Dr. Miroslav Slavik [20] from Czechoslovakia joined the IOC Medical Commission. Representatives of the NOCs and the IOC Executive Board agreed on closer cooperation between NOCs and the IOC in May 1975.[21] One of the conclusions was to include NOC representatives on the individual IOC Commissions and the NOCs selected Miroslav Slavik to represent the NOCs in the IOC Medical Commission.[22] This process illustrates that Alexandre de Mérode and the entire IOC Medical Commission were also susceptible to decisions made by the IOC Executive Board.

Consequently, there was no fundamental change in the set-up of the IOC Medical Commission, neither in terms of sizing the number of members down, nor in terms of recruitment criteria. However, as addressed by Gottfried Schönholzer, strengthening would have meant downsizing the membership, but also integrating more experts on doping analysis, and giving Arnold Beckett more power. However, having addressed the personnel changes in the IOC Medical Commission between 1972 and 1976, Alexandre de Mérode regarded it sufficient to rely on Arnold Beckett, whom he considered as the leading expert in the field of doping analysis during this phase. From the minutes of the meetings, it also remains unclear whether Arnold Beckett himself saw the necessity of having more anti-doping laboratory experts as members, because the situation allowed him to occupy a dominant role. Notwithstanding these personal attitudes, the need

[18] Minutes, "Executive Board, June 22-24, 1973," archive collection "IOC Executive Board Meetings 1921-1982," IOC Archive, Lausanne, 4.

[19] "Medical Commission," *Olympic Review* 145 (1979), 648.

[20] At time of his adoption onto the IOC Medical Commission Dr. Miroslav Slavik (1933-) was working as an orthopaedic at the *Orthopaedic Hospital* in Prague. Because of his research in orthopaedy and in traumatology, he was awarded a professorship in 1983. Besides his involvement in the IOC Medical Commission, Miroslav Slavik was also a member of the UCI. Jan BARTONÍČEK, "K 80. narozeninám prof. MUDr. Miroslava Slavíka, CSc," *Ortopedie* 7, no. 5 (2013), 202.

[21] Minutes, "Executive Board, May 14-16, May 19 and May 23, 1975," 10.

[22] Letter, "Lord Killanin to Miroslav Slavik, October 21, 1975," archive collection "IOC Medical Commission," folder "Medical Commission: Correspondence 1975," IOC Archive, Lausanne.

for their advice and more active involvement became most apparent in the ongoing debate about the necessity to introduce a doping test for anabolic steroids, addressed in the following chapter.

ANTI-DOPING LABORATORY EXPERTISE NEEDED FOR THE INSTALLATION OF TESTS FOR ANABOLIC STEROIDS

Two aspects emphasise the need for more expertise in doping analysis following the 1972 Munich Olympic Games. First, Arnold Beckett continued to occupy a leading role in the IOC Medical Commission's work. He was responsible to search for appropriate laboratory facilities for the 1976 Montreal Olympic Games.[23] This clearly demonstrates that the IOC Medical Commission wanted to maintain a high laboratory standard. Importantly, Arnold Beckett outlined that the main issue would be to find experts for conducting the analytical part of the doping controls since he had already been in talks with the University of Montreal, who would provide the laboratory equipment.[24] Arnold Beckett made a distinction between the laboratory equipment and the personnel in charge, therefore emphasising that it was crucial to have experienced laboratory staff. This can be related to both the very good Munich and very bad Mexico City experiences.

Even more so, the development of a doping test for anabolic steroids displays the need for more anti-doping laboratory expertise. The IOC Medical Commission decided in May 1973 not to include anabolic steroids on the list of banned substances, "because of impracticability to prove its misuse if an athlete ceased to have it several days before the control test."[25] Hence it upheld its policy to include only detectable drugs. Moreover, although there were people such as the chairman of the British Sports Council, Roger Bannister[26], who were calling

---

[23] Minutes, "Meeting of the Medical Commission of the International Olympic Committee, May 25-26, 1973," 3.

[24] Ibid.

[25] Ibid., 5.

[26] Sir Dr. Roger G. Bannister (born 1929) was the first runner to run a mile faster than four minutes. After his sporting career, he became a neurologist and was chairman of the British Sports Council from 1971 until 1974. For several historical and cultural essays on his achievement to break the four-minute mile, see: John BALE and P. David HOWE, eds., *The Four-Minute Mile* (London: Routledge, 2008).

for "snap checks" to control athletes during training periods, [27] the IOC maintained its stance to test only during the Olympic Games, contradictory to its from time to time voiced self-understanding to lead the global fight against doping. At the meeting, Arnold Beckett also briefly commented on research conducted in the field of steroid detection at his institution for the first time, while explaining that some methods might prove to be effective. [28] It took over half a year before more information became available on the research project. Similar to the approach of including Arnold Beckett into the IOC Medical Commission, the British Sports Council informed the IOC about the developments in anabolic steroid testing. [29] Walter Winterbottom reported that Professor Dr. Raymond Brooks of the Department of Pathology at the St. Thomas Hospital in London had successfully conducted research on a method to analyse urine samples for anabolic steroids. He, like Arnold Beckett, was an expert in clinical chemistry, and had, since 1968, focused on the development of a test for anabolic steroids. DIMEO claims that Professor F.T.G. Prunty, who also worked at the St. Thomas Hospital and received financial support through the British Sports Council from 1972, conducted this research. [30] However, a document reveals that Roger Bannister had already made an enquiry at the St. Thomas Hospital about the possibility to undertake research on the issue as early as 1968. [31] In October 1969 eventually, Ph.D. student Richard Firth received a three-year grant, to focus on the study of the metabolism of orally active anabolic steroids, and the possibility of detecting them by using gas-liquid chromatography. After two years, it appeared that the approach with gas-liquid chromatography was unlikely to be successful and the focus shifted onto radioimmunoassay (RI). This decision was based on the first published application of RI for the measurement of steroids in

---

[27] HUNT, *Drug Games*, 55. Besides the comment by HUNT on the issue, further proof for the suggestion to install unannounced out-of competition testing could be found in a letter by the director of the British Sports Council Walter Winterbottom to the new technical director of the IOC, Henry Richard Banks. Letter, "Walter Winterbottom to Henry Richard Banks, February 22, 1974," archive collection "IOC Medical Commission," folder "Medical Commission: Correspondence 1974," IOC Archive, Lausanne.

[28] Minutes, "Meeting of the Medical Commission of the International Olympic Committee, May 25-26, 1973," 5.

[29] Letter, "Walter Winterbottom to Henry Richard Banks, February 22, 1974."

[30] DIMEO, *A History*, 112.

[31] Overview, "Chronology of St. Thomas Hospital involvement with the Sports Council," archive collection "CDPM/FPA2 Beckett," King's College London Archives, London.

biological fluids.[32] Once Richard Firth's grant ended in 1972, Nigel Sumner continued with the research project and received a two-year post-doctoral fellowship for his research. His work aimed to find a way to screen the 14 orally active anabolic steroids at the time. This was eventually achieved through an increase of immunoglobins that could target two alkyl substituents, which all of the known steroids had in common. Any potentially positive sample could then be analysed with GC-MS in the full-scan mode for identification.[33] This second part dealing with the confirmation of the result was nothing new to doping analysis and Manfred Donike had refined it regularly. However, as a journal on doping analysis did not exist, the advancements were all published in biochemical papers.[34] It remains unclear if, and how, F.T.G. Puntry and Raymond Brooks' team linked up in their research. As DIMEO points out, the two worked at the same hospital.[35] Nevertheless, there is reason to doubt an intensive involvement by F.T.G. Puntry because the published academic papers do not mention his name.[36] Consequently, one has to attribute the scientific success to Raymond BROOKS et al., who eventually published the results of their work in 1975.[37] The anabolic steroid testing method was used prior to publication for the first time at the 1974 Commonwealth Games in Christchurch, New Zealand, in February 1974. The laboratory confirmed the effectiveness of the method as nine out of 55 taken samples failed the immunoassay screen and the anabolic steroids could be identified by GC-MS.[38]

---

[32] Andrew T. KICMAN and DB GOWER, "Anabolic steroids in sport: biochemical, clinical and analytical perspectives," *Annals of Clinical Biochemistry* 40 (2003), 323.

[33] Ibid.

[34] In fact, between 1973 and 1975 Manfred Donike published numerous articles on new ways to improve gas chromatography for sports drug testing. Amongst them the following: Manfred DONIKE, "Acylierung mit Bis(Acylamiden): N-Methyl-bis-(trifluoracetamid) und Bis(trifluoracetamid), zwei neue Reagenzien zur Triflouracetylierung," *Journal of Chromatography* 78 (1973), 273-279. Manfred DONIKE, "Der gas-chromatographische Nachweis von Catecholaminen im Femtomol-Bereich durch massenspezifische Detektion," *Chromatographia* 7 (1974), 651-654. Manfred DONIKE, "N-Trifluoracetyl-O-trimethylsilyl-phenolalkylamine: Darstellung und massenspezifischer gaschromatographischer Nachweis," *Journal of Chromatography* 103 (1973), 91-112.

[35] DIMEO, *A History*, 112.

[36] BECKETT, "Problems."

[37] Raymond V. BROOKS, Richard G. FIRTH, and Nigel T. SUMNER, "Detection of Anabolic Steroids by Radioimmunoassay," *British Journal of Sports Medicine* 9, no. 2 (1975), 89-92.

[38] KICMAN and GOWER, "Anabolic steroids," 323.

Importantly, whilst BROOKS et al. published their research results only in 1975, the close working relationship between Arnold Beckett and Raymond Brooks enabled the IOC Medical Commission to act instantly with the installation of a test for anabolic steroids. This can also be attributed to the information given by Walter Winterbottom to Henry Banks in the above-mentioned letter. Despite the late introduction of the test considering the widespread usage of steroids at the time, it was an advancement from the implementation of the previous testing methods. The IOC Medical Commission strongly depended on Raymond Brooks' research. However, at the beginning of 1974 there still appeared to be confusion on whether Raymond Brooks' research was actually dealing with anabolic steroids or amphetamines. Walter Winterbottom reports that Joseph Keul and even Manfred Donike associated it with the latter.[39] Consequently, a frequent exchange between anti-doping laboratory experts outside of their respective countries and on an international level did still not exist.

Because of his scientific success, the IOC Medical Commission invited Raymond Brooks to its meeting in April 1974.[40] At the same meeting, Manfred Donike presented his report about the doping controls in Munich. Thus, for the first time Arnold Beckett had support by other experts with professional competencies in doping analysis during an IOC Medical Commission meeting. During Raymond Brooks' remarks on the new testing technique, this became rather obvious. He explained the scientific aspects of the test in general, admitting that a urine test did not allow for the detection of stanozolol, but it could be found in blood.[41] However, the IOC Medical Commission had strong objections against a blood test and eventually decided to work only with the urine test.[42] Furthermore, Raymond Brooks had to acknowledge that anabolic steroids were still only detectable in the human organism for up to eight days if used in large doses. The significance of the attendance of Manfred Donike at the meeting becomes obvious when he enquired about the production of the antisera, which was necessary to detect the steroids.[43] Raymond Brooks had to admit that this was not an easy task, however, once scientists had produced a good antiserum, it could be used in very high delusions.[44] This could enable other laboratories –

---

[39] Letter, "Walter Winterbottom to Henry Richard Banks, February 22, 1974."

[40] Minutes, "Meeting of the Medical Commission of the International Olympic Committee, April 5-7, 1974," 1.

[41] Ibid., 7.

[42] Ibid.

[43] Ibid., 8.

[44] Ibid.

such as Manfred Donike's in Cologne – to be supplied with the antiserum without having to develop their own. This points towards an anticipated closer relationship between leading institutions in doping analysis.

The official IOC Medical Commission statement on anabolic steroid testing reads as follows:

> A positive result will be defined as failure to pass a test for the absence of anabolic steroids in urine as measured by a radio-immunoassay based upon the use of a number of antisera with selectivity for structures in anabolic-steroid molecules.
>
> At present Gas-Liquid Chromatography / Mass Spectrometry definitive methods are also available for particular anabolic steroids taken in normal doses and theses and other techniques maybe used in the identification procedures.[45]

Therefore, it considered a remark by Manfred Donike to allow for other types of analysis, as well, because future developments could lead to new methods.[46] As will be discussed later, he already anticipated further technical advancements in all aspects of the doping controls and consequently wanted to make sure that the rules did not have to change constantly. This was a very pragmatic approach, and in contrast to the usual IOC Medical Commission's strategy of only naming already existing methods.

In addition to this, a specific press release explained the IOC's policy:

> The Medical Commission realizes that a competitor could misuse anabolic steroids for a long periods [sic] and then discontinue their use a week or two before the Games so that a negative result in the doping test at the Games would occur despite the drug misuse.
>
> However, the Medical Commission hopes that the International Federations will follow their lead on banning the misuse of anabolic steroids and will introduce testing at various events held under their rules. Thus it would then be difficult for a competitor to misuse anabolic steroids for prolonged periods and yet to evade detections.[47]

---

[45] Ibid., 14.

[46] Ibid.

[47] Ibid.

This press release is both an indication for an increasingly strong position of the IOC Medical Commission, which is now making recommendations for the IFs, and also an outlet to get around the discussion on out-of competition testing. Actually, the IOC Medical Commission did not debate this difficulty at all. Rather, the statement reads that through doping controls by the IFs, the possibility of catching offenders would increase considerably. An assumption, which is of course true, but does not pay any attention to the fact that athletes could still use anabolic steroids during the training periods.

Eventually, in May 1976 Alexandre de Mérode reported to the IOC Executive Board that anabolic steroids were now included on the list of banned substances.[48] However, it was also determined that the tests for anabolic steroids were to be made before the Olympic Games actually began, in order to prevent offenders from participating in the Games. This had consequences for the entire doping control regime (see later in this chapter). Finally, the IOC Medical Commission announced that it did not screen for anabolic steroids at the 1976 Winter Olympic Games in Innsbruck. This decision can be traced back to a comment by Manfred Donike. He had already mentioned in April 1974 that anabolic steroids would not provide a major advantage in winter sports, and therefore proposed to drop the screening.[49] This was a controversial statement because positive tests in later years proved that athletes were using anabolic steroids in winter sports.[50]

To summarise, Raymond Brooks' key role for the installation of the test is nothing new to research. Nevertheless, the specific focus on the contribution of anti-doping laboratory experts allowed investigating into his role in more detail. Anti-doping laboratory experts apart from Arnold Beckett were central to the introduction of the test for anabolic steroids at the Olympic Games. The Olympic Movement depended on such scientific advancements, because the anti-doping laboratory experts' professional competencies allowed adding substances to the banned list. Since Alexandre de Mérode was simultaneously aiming to strengthen the position of the IOC Medical Commission within the world of sport, the technical development played an important role for him. Nevertheless, the comparison with the changing membership illustrates that he did not consider

---

[48] TODD and TODD, "Significant Events," 74.

[49] Minutes, "Meeting of the Medical Commission of the International Olympic Committee, April 5-7, 1974," 9.

[50] For example at the 1984 Winter Olympic Games in Sarajevo, the Mongolian cross country skier Batsukh Purevjal was tested positive on the anabolic steroid methandienon (see Chapter 6).

them for a position on the IOC Medical Commission. However, this did not prevent the few anti-doping laboratory experts creating an increasing exchange of knowledge. For example, Manfred Donike invited Dr. Robert Dugal, who was to head the anti-doping laboratory team at the 1976 Montreal Olympic Games, to visit his laboratory in Cologne in order to observe his work.[51] Robert Dugal had earned his doctorate in pharmacology from the University of Wisconsin before he began working at the National Institute of Scientific Research (Institute Nationale de la Recherche Scientifique, INRS), the institution responsible for the doping analysis in Montreal, from 1973.[52] In the following years, he headed the INRS laboratory until 1990, and became an important addition to the inner circle of the anti-doping laboratory experts' network. Evidence for the increasing interest in the scientific aspects of doping controls is also contained in a letter sent to the IOC by Professor Dr. Wang-Kee Jhoo from the Department of Pharmaceutical Sciences of the Gangwon National University in the Republic of Korea. Wang-Kee Jhoo requested to have Raymond Brooks' scientific articles in order to implement a doping control centre.[53] Interestingly, Henry Banks directly forwarded his request to Raymond Brooks without consulting the IOC Medical Commission.[54] Raymond Brooks answered in October 1974, but there is no evidence that Wang-Khee Jhoo set up an anti-doping laboratory in the Republic of Korea at the time.

INITIATION OF THE IAAF'S FIGHT AGAINST DOPING

Role of Anti-doping Laboratory Experts in the Foundation Period

As mentioned in Chapter 1, the IAAF was the first major international sport organisation which addressed the issue of doping and prohibited the usage of

---

[51] Minutes, "Meeting of the Medical Commission of the International Olympic Committee, April 5-7, 1974," 6.

[52] Report, "Games of the XXIst Olympiad – Analytical Doping Control Scientific Report by Robert Dugal and Michel Bertrand, June, 1978," archive collection "Summer and Winter Olympic Games: Medical files," folder "Analysis of drug tests at the 1976 Summer Olympic Games in Montreal," IOC Archive, Lausanne.

[53] Letter, "Wang-Kee Jhoo to Henry Banks, September 14, 1974," archive collection "IOC Medical Commission," folder "Medical Commission: Correspondence 1974," IOC Archive, Lausanne.

[54] Letter, "Raymond Brooks to Henry Banks, October 1, 1974," archive collection "IOC Medical Commission," folder "Medical Commission: Correspondence 1974," IOC Archive, Lausanne.

performance-enhancing drugs in 1928.[55] However, similar to the IOC, the IAAF did not undertake any testing efforts for a period of more than 35 years. Consequently, the IAAF did not consult anti-doping laboratory experts. As within the IOC, sport medicine specialists were supporting the IAAF through their involvement as team doctors and the links to the FIMS. In this way, if questions on doping arose, the medical IAAF members and the IAAF's medical consultants dealt with them. This tendency mirrors the processes within the IOC until the 1960s. It was only in the aftermath of more doping incidents in the 1960s and the increased efforts by governments to combat doping, that the IAAF became active again. The installation of doping tests at the 1968 Mexico City Olympic Games influenced the IAAF's beginning anti-doping activities. In fact, the Polish IAAF member Jerzy Bogobowicz proposed the formation of an IAAF Medical Committee at the IAAF Congress during the Games in October 1968.[56] Notably, he suggested that the new body should consist of experts from outside the IAAF, and that the new members did not necessarily have to be doctors. The IOC Medical Commission served as an example here. Marea Hartman, chair of the IAAF Women's Commission, also proposed to have at least one woman on the Committee.[57]

However, the IAAF eventually refrained from constituting an official Committee but established the IAAF Medical Advisory Panel instead. The IAAF Council argued that it would be easier to call together a meeting of particular members of a panel instead of a full Committee meeting whenever urgent matters arose.[58] Using a panel set-up, a few members could make binding decisions without the need for approval through a full Committee meeting. Furthermore, in a letter to all IAAF members, the IAAF honorary secretary-treasurer Frederick Holder[59] informed that the IAAF Council kept the IAAF Medical Advisory Panel

---

[55] Minutes, "9th Congress of the IAAF in Amsterdam, July 27 and August 6-7," 1928, 55.

[56] Minutes, "26th Congress of the IAAF in Mexico City, October 12 and 21-31, 1968," archive collection "IAAF Congresses," IAAF Archive, Monaco, 17.

[57] Ibid.

[58] Letter, "Frederick W. Holder to the Members of the Medical Advisory Panel, August 25, 1971," archive collection "IAAF Medical Committee," folder "Medical Correspondence 1971-1972," IAAF Archive, Monaco.

[59] Frederick W. Holder (1913-2009) from Great Britain was the IAAF's honorary secretary-treasurer from 1970 until 1984. Afterwards, he became IAAF honorary life vice-president. In 1980, he was awarded the Olympic Order. "Athletics mourns loss of Frederick Holder, IAAF Honorary Life Vice President," *International Association of Athletics Federations*; http://www.iaaf.org/news/news/athletics-mourns-loss-of-frederick-holder-iaa [accessed February 15, 2015].

deliberately as small as possible, "to avoid the valuable time of experts who kindly offered their services being taken up in meetings to discuss matters outside their own specialist fields."[60] In consideration of the opposite approach by the IOC Medical Commission, this statement must be given special significance. In fact, the structure in theory allowed the IAAF to have a more focused approach, which is exactly what Gottfried Schönholzer suggested for the IOC Medical Commission (see Chapter 3).

In reality, the implementation appears not to have been that different at all, because the individual memberships within the IAAF Medical Advisory Panel were very similar to the IOC Medical Commission. Once the body was officially set up by the time of the IAAF Congress in Stockholm in 1970, the members of the IAAF Medical Advisory Panel were its chairman Dr. Max Danz (FRG), Dr. Waldemar Areno (Brazil), Dr. Robert Andrivet (France), Arnold Beckett, Dr. Bilic (Poland), Dr. Manfred Höppner[61] (GDR), Ludwig Prokop, Herbert Reindell, Professor Dr. Jacques van Rossum[62] (Netherlands) and Dr. Grigory Vorobiev[63] (USSR).[64] In contrast to the initial intention, all members were medical doctors with the exception of Arnold Beckett and Jacques van Rossum, who was a pharmacologist. Therefore, Arnold Beckett also occupied, from 1972 onwards, the position as leading expert in the field of doping analysis in the most influential sport federation. As suggested, there was one vacancy held for a female expert. However, the approached Dr. Marshall from Great Britain was not available.[65] Moreover, the Panel did not come together as much as anticipated, as

---

[60] Ibid.

[61] Dr. Manfred Höppner (born 1934) had studied medicine at the Karl-Marx University in Leipzig and became a sport medicine specialist. From 1967 onwards, he was vice-president of the GDR's Sport Medical Services (Sportmedizinischer Dienst, SMD) and played a leading role in the organisation and implementation of the state doping system in the GDR (see Chapter 6). Giselher SPITZER, *Doping in der DDR. Ein historischer Überblick zu einer konspirativen Praxis* (Cologne: Sportverlag Strauß, 1998).

[62] Professor Dr. Jacques van Rossum (born 1930) was awarded a Ph.D. from the University of Nijmegen in 1958. In 1965, he became professor for general pharmacology at the Medical Faculty and the Faculty of Mathematics and Natural Sciences at the University of Nijmegen. In the 1980s, he headed the anti-doping laboratory in Nijmegen/Utrecht.

[63] Dr. Grigory Vorobiev (born 1929) is a sport medical specialist that graduated from Leningrad Medical Institute. He was the Olympic team doctor for the USSR at several Olympic Games

[64] Minutes, "27th Congress of the IAAF in Stockholm, August 30-31, 1970," archive collection "IAAF Congresses," IAAF Archive, Monaco, 36.

[65] Ibid., 36.

reported by Frederick Holder May 1972.[66] Members of the IAAF Medical Advisory Panel also complained about this.[67]

It is important to emphasise that Frederick Holder quickly established an IAAF Doping Working Group – in the official documents sometimes referred to as Subcommittee – to deal with only the issue of doping. This group consisted of Arnold Beckett, Ludwig Prokop and Jacques van Rossum. Max Danz acted as chairman.[68] This clearly reflects a more focused and concentrated approach to the doping problem, since all of the members were experts with first-hand experience in doping controls. Even though Ludwig Prokop was a sport medicine specialist, the group had a strong focus on the analytical aspects of the doping controls. Therefore, the IAAF Doping Working Group was the first international body to discuss only methods and techniques for doping analysis within the framework of an international sport organisation or event. The IAAF Doping Working Group made abundantly clear that all analytical aspects should be dealt with by experts within the scientific field, and not by the IAAF itself.[69] This strengthened the position of anti-doping laboratory experts. Subsequently, in the rules submitted to the IAAF Council it is stated, "for the chemical testing of samples, the Doping Committee shall avail itself to the services of competent experts and scientific Institutes."[70] Obviously, Arnold Beckett and Jacques van Rossum had a strong interest in this because their laboratories were amongst the leading ones in doping analysis.

In addition to the formulation of the IAAF anti-doping rules for the IAAF Council, the IAAF Doping Working Group published a booklet, which contained detailed anti-doping regulations. Due to the involvement of Arnold Beckett and Ludwig Prokop, it is understandable that it was highly similar to the *Doping* brochure, developed during the same period by the IOC Medical Commission. In contrast to the IOC´s brochure, however, the IAAF Doping Working Group again emphasised the standard of the anti-doping laboratory in its booklet:

---

[66] Letter, "Frederick W. Holder to the Members of the Medical Advisory Panel, May 11, 1972," archive collection "IAAF Medical Committee," folder "Medical Correspondence 1971-1972," IAAF Archive, Monaco.

[67] Ibid., 2.

[68] Ibid., 1.

[69] Minutes, "27th Congress of the IAAF in Stockholm, August 30-31, 1970," 61.

[70] Ibid.

> Only laboratories accredited and approved by the IAAF on the advice of
> the Medical Advisory Panel should be used to carry out the analytical
> work in connection with dope control.[71]

It seems that the IAAF was faster to realise the need for an accreditation scheme
for anti-doping laboratories, meeting certain standards and working according to
uniform principles, than the IOC, which did not include any reference to
institutional requirements in its brochure. Certainly, this has partly to be
attributed to the reason that the IOC Medical Commission had much greater
control over the implementation of the doping controls at the Olympic Games
than the IAAF in its many athletic events. Nevertheless, it cannot be denied that
the experience made by Arnold Beckett and Ludwig Prokop at the first doping
controls at the Olympic Games also contributed to stressing the significance of
high laboratory standards. Importantly, these discussions had already taken place
before the first standardised doping controls at the 1972 Munich Olympic Games.

Despite the efforts of the IAAF Doping Working Group, leading IAAF
officials felt that it needed to increase the efforts to combat doping in its sport.
Since the IAAF Medical Advisory Panel only met once with of all its members,
an IAAF Medical Committee replaced the Panel based on a decision on the IAAF
Congress in Munich in 1972.[72] In contrast to the other IAAF Committees,
however, the members should not be voted onto the Committee by an open vote
during the IAAF Congress, but through recommendations submitted to the IAAF
Council. The IAAF president, David Burghley, argued, "experts at the top of their
profession from all over the world" could become members of the IAAF Medical
Committee.[73] This opened the possibility for anti-doping laboratory experts to
participate more actively. Eventually it was decided that:

1. The Medical Panel should become the I.A.A.F. Medical
   Committee and
2. The Committee members should be nominated by Council on
   the recommendation of the Medical Committee, the numbers of

---

[71] Letter, "Frederick W. Holder to the Members of the Medical Advisory Panel, August 25, 1971," 4.
[72] Minutes, "28th Congress of the IAAF in Munich, August 30 and September 10-11, 1972," archive collection "IAAF Congresses," IAAF Archive, Monaco, 21ff.
[73] Ibid.

members being limited to a maximum of thirteen, to include as far as possible at least one representative from every country.[74]

The maximum number of thirteen members was in contrast to the original recommendation made in 1970 where a maximum of eight members was proposed. Max Danz explained the increase by a need to have a specialist from different branches of medicine on the Committee. In the report to the IAAF Congress, these branches were specified into "doping problems, chemistry and biochemistry, physiology, tropical diseases, the functions of the heart, dietary questions in connection with sport and the determining of sex."[75] The distinction between doping problems to be dealt with by medical doctors and biochemical/chemical aspects was unique for the time. The IOC did not make such a distinction.

Finally, the IAAF Congress discussed creating a "Doping Committee" to deal solely with the legal aspects of positive doping tests in 1972. This proposal can be traced back to a suggestion made by the Danish IAAF member Emanuel Rose in a letter to the IAAF Council members in April 1971.[76] Emanuel Rose explained that only the medical views had been addressed while legal aspects had been completely neglected. His premonition, that legal questions would arise when doping tests were made, was also exceptional at the time. Nevertheless, considering the controversies that the IOC Medical Commission faced in the aftermath of the doping controls at the 1972 Munich Olympic Games, Emanuel Rose's suggestion appears not to be too early at all. Nevertheless, the IAAF Council determined not to establish the "Doping Committee," because it wanted to decide independently about disqualification and re-installation whereas at Area Games[77] it was not always practicable to include a legal expert.[78] This reaction demonstrates that legal aspects were not a priority at the time, and that it was not deemed necessary to include a legal expert in the newly established IAAF Medical Committee.

---

[74] Ibid.

[75] Minutes, "28th Congress of the IAAF in Munich, August 30 and September 10-11, 1972," Appendix M, 71ff.

[76] Letter, "Emanuel Rose to IAAF Council Members, April 25, 1971," archive collection "IAAF Medical Committee," IAAF Archive, Monaco.

[77] In the official minutes of the IAAF, national and regional athletic events such as the Asian or European Athletics Championships are commonly referred to as "Area Games".

[78] Minutes, "28th Congress of the IAAF in Munich, August 30 and September 10-11, 1972," 23.

Increased Focus on Anti-doping Laboratory Experts

The IAAF Medical Committee mainly dealt with the installation of a test for anabolic steroids in the period between 1972 and 1976, even though it took almost two years more before the members met again, showing that the change of status from a panel into a committee did not have the desired effect at all. The first full meeting took place in Frankfurt in June 1974.[79] A close exchange with the IOC Medical Commission becomes apparent here for the first time because Alexandre de Mérode also attended the meeting and reported about its functions. Primarily, the sport organisations decided to forbid anabolic steroids and planned tests for the European Championships in Rome in September 1974. These tests, implemented and organised by the FMSI with the anti-doping laboratory in Rome at the University of Sassari under the guidance of Michele Montanaro, were to become the initial tests for anabolic steroids undertaken under the umbrella of the IAAF.[80]

Significantly, the procedure to inform the IAAF Medical Committee members about the tests was the same one as in the IOC Medical Commission: it invited Raymond Brooks and Manfred Donike to present their research. Interestingly, they were both listed in the official reports as "invited doctors," rather than experts in doping analysis.[81] Furthermore, whereas at the IOC meeting, Manfred Donike had primarily been present to speak about the 1972 doping controls, he was asked to describe the MS method for steroid identification. Clearly, their presence displays that the same anti-doping laboratory experts were influential in the IAAF and in the IOC during this time, and that both organisations needed their advice on the implementation of the tests.

In contrast to the IOC, the IAAF Medical Committee continuously involved anti-doping laboratory experts in its working groups before the 1976 Olympic Games. This becomes obvious in the constitution of the IAAF Working Group on Anabolic Steroids in March 1976.[82] Its members were Arnold Beckett, Max Danz, Manfred Höppner and Jacques van Rossum from within the IAAF Medical

---

[79] Minutes, "29th Congress of the IAAF in Rome, August 30-31, 1974," archive collection "IAAF Congresses," IAAF Archive, Monaco, 53f.

[80] CALIFANO, *Istituto di Medicina*, 34.

[81] Minutes, "Medical Committee/Working Group on Anabolic Steroid Controls in Amsterdam, March, 1976," archive collection "IAAF Medical Committee," IAAF Archive, Monaco.

[82] Ibid.

Committee plus Raymond Brooks, Manfred Donike, Dr. H.C.J. Ketelaars[83] and
Dr. Arne Ljungqvist[84]. The designated IAAF president Adriaan Paulen had set up
the Working Group.[85] According to an unofficial protocol of the meeting by
Manfred Donike, a productive exchange of technical aspects, covering the
experience on working with the anabolic steroid test, occurred during the
meeting.[86] The conclusions and recommendations reveal that the IAAF regarded
the further development of steroid testing as a matter of urgency. The group
decided to extend research in order to allow for more controls and to extend the
range of anabolic steroid substances that could be detected. The competencies of
the anti-doping laboratory experts were necessary for more research and assured
themselves future involvement in the anti-doping body. Furthermore, the IAAF
informed the IOC about future cooperation in light of the planned tests at the
1976 Montreal Olympic Games, whereby samples could be taken from the
athletes before, and during the Olympic Games.

---

[83] HJC Ketelaars was a pharmacologist, working with chromatography at the *Department
of Pharmacology* of the *University of Nijmegen*. It was not possible to get more
information on his biographical data. H.J.C. KETELAARS and J.G.P. PETERS,
"Determination of guaiphenesin and its metabolite, β-(2-methoxyphenoxy) lactic acid, in
plasma by high-performance liquid chromatography," *Journal of Chromatography B:
Biomedical Sciences and Applications* 224, no. 1 (1981), 144-148.

[84] Arne Ljungqvist (born 1931) participated at the 1952 Helsinki Olympic Games in the
high jump. Following his sporting career, he became the president of the Swedish Athletics
Association from 1973 until 1981. He was an IAAF Council member in 1976 and was one
of its vice presidents from 1981 to 1999, and IAAF's senior vice president 1999-2007.
Because Arne Ljungqvist also pursued a medical career, conducting research mainly in the
areas of cardiovascular diseases, he became chairman of the IAAF Medical Committee in
1980 and chairman of the IOC Medical Commission in 2003 (he became a member of the
IOC Medical Commission in 1987). At the 103rd IOC Session in Paris in 1994, he was
voted to become member of the IOC. His own perspective on the history of the
international fight against doping can be found in: Arne LJUNGQVIST, *Doping's Nemesis*
(Cheltenham: Sportsbooks Limited, 2008).

[85] Adriaan Paulen (1902-1985) was a participant in the 1920, 1924 and 1928 Olympic
Games in middle distance running events. After his sporting career and the end of the
Second World War, he played an influential role in the re-building of the IAAF. He was
president of the Dutch Athletic Committee from 1946 until 1964 and from 1965 until 1970
director of the Dutch Olympic Committee. In 1976, he succeeded Lord Killanin as
president of the IAAF. "Obituary," *Olympic Review* 213 (1985), 400.

[86] Minutes, "Sitzung der Arbeitsgruppe Anabole Steroide, March 8, 1976," archive
collection "Nachlass August Kirsch," File 091 "Doping von 1968-1977," CuLDA,
Cologne.

Finally, the IAAF Medical Committee installed an IAAF Anti-Doping Subcommittee to deal with the technical aspects of the doping control permanently in 1977. Max Danz, Arnold Beckett, Manfred Höppner and Manfred Donike, who was co-opted to become a member of the IAAF Medical Committee at the same meeting, became its first members.[87] Undeniably, the establishment of the IAAF Anti-Doping Subcommittee was the most explicit initiative in the IAAF's efforts to shift responsibility away from sport medical specialists and towards anti-doping laboratory experts instead. In fact, from the beginning, there appears to have been a much more pragmatic approach to the doping problem in the IAAF. One can recognise a consistent attempt to keep discussion groups as small as possible, and to integrate external professionals. This allowed anti-doping laboratory experts to exert more influence in making doping analysis a central aspect. The major important outcome of their influence was the increasing attention paid to the standards of the doping laboratories by the IAAF Medical Committee, which is central to the specific focus of this book.

Emphasis on the Anti-doping Laboratories

The emphasis on the standards of the anti-doping laboratories by the IAAF Medical Committee was significantly different to the work of the IOC Medical Commission. In its first guidelines for the conduction of doping controls, the IAAF Medical Advisory Panel stressed the importance of having well-equipped laboratories to conduct the doping analysis by naming the issue in its first paragraph already.[88] It appears that there was a great concern for laboratories being unsuitable for doping analysis, especially during Area Games. Whereas the IOC Medical Commission did not deal with such issues, because it only felt responsible for the doping controls at the Olympic Games, the IAAF Medical Committee had to address the matter in order to guarantee the validity of the testing results for all athletics competitions. Despite the proposal to have accredited laboratories though, there was no discussion on the implementation of an accreditation procedure, yet. It seems that the "accreditation" was given to the laboratories on an individual basis and not through the installation of standardised regulations. During the IAAF Council meeting in 1972, where the anti-doping rules were subject to debate, it was eventually stated that the doping controls

---

[87] Ibid.

[88] Letter, "Frederick W. Holder to the Members of the Medical Advisory Panel, August 25, 1971," 4.

should be conducted "providing always that laboratories were satisfactory and well proven."[89] Again, no specification is made.

Following the transformation into the IAAF Medical Committee, anti-doping laboratory experts were decisive in the process to develop international guidelines for anti-doping laboratories. As both Raymond Brooks and Manfred Donike had made appearances during the meetings of the IAAF Medical Committee, they played a major role in this process. They deemed that it was necessary to have a list of recognised doping laboratories, because of the introduction of doping tests for anabolic steroids. In fact, Raymond Brooks had already compiled a list of existing laboratories in various countries:

> Dr. Brooks of London, the pioneer of the now universally accepted method for steroid testing, had prepared a list of centres in various countries, known to him to be capable of doing the radio-immunoassay tests.

> A principle had been agreed that, wherever possible, a centre should be capable of conducting testing for amphetamines etc. as well as anabolic steroids, as this considerably simplified the testing procedure.

> Letters had been sent to 10 centres capable of doing radio-immunoassay tests in various countries, not all of them in Europe, and it was hoped as soon as possible to draw up a list of accredited centres. [...]

> Professor Brooks had confirmed to the IAAF that he and his laboratory were prepared to make available testing kits with control samples included for centres where radio-immunoassay facilities existed and which were willing to carry out tests for sporting events. The costs of each kit would be £50.00 enabling at least 300 tests to be conducted.[90]

It results from this statement by the IAAF Council that Raymond Brooks had full authority to address testing centres that he considered capable of conducting tests for both amphetamines and for anabolic steroids. Regarding the fact that Raymond Brooks was not even a member of the IAAF Medical Committee, this was surely an extraordinary step, because it meant that every laboratory Raymond

---

[89] Minutes, "28th Congress of the IAAF in Munich, August 30 and September 10-11, 1972," 72.
[90] Minutes, "IAAF Council Meeting in Nairobi, April 18-20, 1975," archive collection "IAAF Council Meetings," IAAF Archive, Monaco, 17.

Brooks had addressed automatically became an IAAF certified laboratory. The reason that the headquarters of the IAAF was in London, must have contributed to the installation of this process. It certainly made the communication between the involved individuals a lot easier. The IAAF Medical Committee also asked Raymond Brooks and Arnold Beckett to occupy a pioneering role in educating other laboratories and equipping them with the necessary testing kits.[91] Moreover, it also shows the significance given to the tests for anabolic steroids because full recognition was only possible if the laboratory could also conduct the analysis for anabolic steroids. In actuality, during all the discussions on the standards of the anti-doping laboratories, there appeared to be no concerns that the testing for stimulants should also take place in accredited laboratories, since all of the debates focused on the test for anabolic steroids.

In October 1975, it was finally revealed which laboratories were amongst those addressed by Raymond Brooks. In addition to the laboratory at the KCL, the anti-doping laboratory in Rome and the testing centre at the University of Ghent, were recognised, although the latter only installed the required analytical equipment at the end of that year.[92] These three laboratories were the only testing centres able to do RI testing. The laboratories in Cologne (headed by Manfred Donike) and Nijmegen (headed by Jacques van Rossum) also tested for steroids, however, using an identification method developed by Manfred Donike based on only MS.[93] The IAAF also officially recognised them. At a meeting with FRG officials, Manfred Donike revealed how the official recognition had automatically led to a more extensive exchange of knowledge between the leading figures in the institutions, which he praised emphatically.[94] Therefore, the establishment of a closer network of anti-doping laboratory experts was a welcome consequence of the emphasis on the laboratories in the IAAF. This is important, because a coordinated network had not yet existed, even though there had been individual efforts as highlighted earlier in this chapter.

The efforts were clearly limited to the European continent due to the lack of a global exchange forum for anti-doping laboratory experts, but also to the

---

[91] Ibid.

[92] Minutes, "IAAF Council Meeting in Rouen, October 10-12, 1975," archive collection "IAAF Council Meetings," IAAF Archive, Monaco, 8.

[93] It is important to mention that similar to the IOC, the IAAF always demanded another test based on MS despite the effectiveness of the radioimmunoassay method. Therefore, the specific type of steroid could be detected. Consequently, it was the combination of both tests that was needed in order to fulfil the demands of the anabolic steroid controls.

[94] Minutes, "Sitzung der Arbeitsgruppe Anabole Steroide, March 8, 1976."

European-dominated make-up of the anti-doping bodies in the IOC and the IAAF. In October 1975, IAAF president Adriaan Paulen even argued that there was not a great deal of attempts made on the American continent to test athletes for doping, and he criticised the IOC for not giving enough support to the IAAF in its anti-doping efforts on the American continent. [95] Frederick Holder approached Eduardo Hay, in his role as member of the IOC Medical Commission about the conduction of tests for anabolic steroids at the 1975 Pan American Games in Mexico City.[96] Despite emphasising the quality of the laboratory chosen for the doping tests, Eduardo Hay replied that the organisers did not plan tests for anabolic steroids. [97] IOC technical director Henry Banks backed this decision because according to him it was difficult to impose the introduction of such a testing procedure, which "may not have the required specialists on hand, and in view of the fact that the testing procedure is still not fully advanced."[98] Moreover, the realisation of having human expertise in doping analysis becomes apparent with this example again. Henry Banks regarded anabolic steroid testing as such a sensitive issue that he would rather not have any tests at all than tests that were not conducted by leading experts in the field. Therewith, he enabled the few already advanced anti-doping laboratory experts from Europe to occupy a monopolistic role.

After having established a first list of recognised laboratories, the newly founded IAAF Working Group on Anabolic Steroids pushed for a fast and broad extension of the laboratory network. At its meeting in March 1976, it put together several recommendations to be presented at the IAAF Council and IAAF Congress. At the meeting, it was mentioned once more that the tests should only be conducted in "convenient designated laboratories." [99] Furthermore, it recommended a procedure for the case of a positive test:

---

[95] Minutes, "IAAF Council Meeting in Rouen, October 10-12, 1975," 8.
[96] Letter, "Frederick W. Holder to Eduardo Hay, June 26, 1975," archive collection "IOC Medical Commission," folder "Medical Commission: Correspondence 1975," IOC Archive, Lausanne.
[97] Letter, "Eduardo Hay to Frederick W. Holder, July 4, 1975," archive collection "IOC Medical Commission," folder "Medical Commission: Correspondence 1975," IOC Archive, Lausanne.
[98] Letter, "Henry Banks to Frederick W. Holder, July 25, 1975," archive collection "IOC Medical Commission," folder "Medical Commission: Correspondence 1975," IOC Archive, Lausanne.
[99] Minutes, "Medical Committee/Working Group on Anabolic Steroid Controls in Amsterdam, March, 1976," 1.

> The procedure for dealing with a recheck when a positive result is challenged by a competitor should be modified, to fall into line with the IOC procedure. Under the revised procedure the recheck of the reserve sample would take place in the SAME LABORATORY as the original analysis but with different persons conducting the tests [emphasis in the original].[100]

The proposed rule demonstrated that by setting strict and harmonised rules for the working procedures in an anti-doping laboratory, the equipment should not be contested. Certainly, this initiative could only be established if accreditation procedures for laboratories became standardised. The newly founded IAAF Anti-Doping Subcommittee should develop these standards.

Finally, it is important to attest that the IAAF Working Group on Anabolic Steroids realised the IAAF's pioneering role in the official recognition of anti-doping laboratories and its lead over the IOC in this regard. In its recommendations, it stated:

> The IOC should also be informed about the IAAF proposal to draw up a list of accredited laboratories and asked to give a lead in helping to establish an approved list on a worldwide basis of laboratories which would be able to provide service for all International Sport Federations.[101]

There was a personnel overlap between the anti-doping efforts of the two sport organisations through Arnold Beckett, which made him a very influential figure within anti-doping politics at that time. Hence, an exchange of information must have taken place. This is despite the fact that he was not as dominant in the IAAF's anti-doping bodies. The more pragmatic approach of leading IAAF figures to install small working groups of specialised experts resulted in an advantage over the IOC. Naturally, it led to an increased involvement of anti-doping laboratory experts, who compiled recommendations on the standards of anti-doping laboratories, and eventually took the lead in the recognition of official institutions for doping analysis. However, the statement also illustrates awareness that the IAAF's possibilities were actually limited, and that the IOC Medical Commission's support was necessary to extend the network of anti-doping laboratories. The statement called the IOC into account and recommended that

---

[100] Ibid.
[101] Ibid.

the IOC Medical Commission should also deal with the standards of anti-doping laboratories beyond the ones at Olympic Games in order to fulfil its responsibility as the leading international sports organisation. This is a first indication for the desire of more involvement of anti-doping laboratory experts in the IOC Medical Commission from within the group itself. Whereas previously, "outsiders" such as Gottfried Schönholzer and Lord Killanin had raised this issue, they now began to realise the opportunities through growing involvement on the political level, which were also for their own advantage. They wanted to increase this influence and were aware that only the IOC Medical Commission could reach a further expansion of doping tests.

INDICATIONS FOR THE SPECIFIC ROLE OF ANTI-DOPING LABORATORY EXPERTS

Doping Controls at the 1976 Winter Olympic Games in Innsbruck

Often omitted in historical reviews on doping, is that the doping controls at the 1976 Winter Olympic Games were characterised by the decision not to install tests for anabolic steroids. Curiously, Árpád Csánadi still claimed that the IOC wanted to carry out anabolic steroid tests in Innsbruck during an IOC Executive Board meeting in October 1975.[102] It remains unclear why he was not up-to-date on this issue.

Ludwig Prokop was responsible to find appropriate laboratory facilities for the 1976 Winter Olympic Games in Innsbruck.[103] However, preparations were extremely slow and the Organising Committee did not pay much attention to the doping controls. As late as mid-1973, there was no representative of the medical services appointed to the IOC Medical Commission. In fact, Ludwig Prokop informed the members at the meeting in June 1973 that the Organising Committee had only discussed the issue so far without making any decisions.[104] This mirrors the attitude that doping at Winter Olympic Games was a minor concern. Importantly, however, it appears from the next IOC Medical Commission meeting in April 1974 that Manfred Donike was involved in the

---

[102] Minutes, "Executive Board, October 4-6, 1975," archive collection "IOC Executive Board Meetings 1921-1982," IOC Archive, Lausanne, 26.
[103] Minutes, "74th Session of the IOC in Varna, October 5-7, 1973," archive collection "IOC Sessions 1894-2009," IOC Archive, Lausanne, 12ff.
[104] Ibid.

preparations of the anti-doping laboratory.[105] This might also explain why Arnold Beckett did not contribute to the preparations, but focused on the 1976 Montreal Olympic Games instead.

The entire medical department was under the leadership of Dr. Ernst Raas, who eventually represented the Organising Committee on the IOC Medical Commission. The official head of the doping controls was Dr. Gottfried Machata of the Chemical Department of the Institute for Forensic Medicine in Innsbruck.[106] According to the official documents of the Organising Committee and the IOC Medical Commission, the official head of the laboratory was the head of the Institute of Analytical Chemistry of the University of Vienna, Professor Dr. Josef Franz Karl Huber[107]. His name also appears on the laboratory reports. Significantly, Manfred Donike was in charge of the conduction of the second sample in case there was a positive test.[108] Manfred Donike selection was instigated by his involvement in the preparation phase, and the Cologne anti-doping laboratory providing parts of the equipment.[109] This is a crucial detail because for the first time a non-IOC Medical Commission member was responsible for this key part of the doping analysis. At previous Olympic Games,

---

[105] Minutes, "Meeting of the Medical Commission of the International Olympic Committee, April 5-7, 1974," 2.

[106] HEMMERSBACH, "History," 840.

[107] Dr. Franz Karl Josef Huber (1925-2000) was a specialist in analytical chemistry and in particular in the separation methods, including gas and liquid chromatograhphy. He contributed much to the exchange between scientists in the East and West in the 1980, especially through the organisation of the "HLPC" meetings, which were entirely devoted to liquid phase seperations. Charles W. GEHRKE, Robert L. WIXON and Ernst BAYER, "Prominent Chromatographers and their Research – Seminal Concepts in Chromatography/Separation Sciences," in: *Chromatography. A Century of Discovery 1900-2000*, eds. Charles W. GEHRKE, Robert L. WIXON and Ernst BAYER (Amsterdam: Elsevier Science, 2001), 248ff.

[108] Report, "Medical Report of the 1976 Innsbruck Winter Olympic Games, o.d.," archive collection "IOC Medical Commission," folder "Correspondence and reports of the medical control during the Olympic Winter Games of Innsbruck 1976," IOC Archive, Lausanne, 29ff. Professor Dr. Erich Schmid, who was also involved in the Innsbruck laboratory, recently claimed that he was in charge of the doping analysis. However, after a statement by Gottfried Machata, Erich Schmid had to admit that Gottfried Machata was the head of the doping controls but confirmed that he was also involved in the analytical procedures. See: Karl ZOJER, "Eindeutige Aussagen zu komplexen Fragestellungen," *Chemiereport* 5 (2010), 36. Also see: "Wer war für die Doping-Kontrolle 1976 verantwortlich?" *Chemiereport* 8 (2010), 51.

[109] Report, "Medical Report of the 1976 Innsbruck Winter Olympic Games, o.d.," 29.

this responsibility had been delegated to Arnold Beckett. Certainly, this underlines Manfred Donike´s increasing influence and reputation.

In contrast to the proposal made following the 1972 Munich Olympic Games, local doctors, and not international teams, again undertook the sample collection of the 390 urine samples.[110] A detailed list of the individual responsibilities in Innsbruck can be found in the medical report.[111] Similar to the doping controls at previous Games, problems arose in Innsbruck. These illustrate that even though the IOC Medical Commission had now dealt with the conduction of doping tests for almost ten years, there was still an obvious degree of inexperience. However, the difficulties were mainly linked to the organisational issues connected with the collection of the urine samples, and not with the doping analysis. For example, the IOC Medical Commission decided that a car had to be permanently available to drive an athlete to the Olympic Village if he/she was not able to provide a urine sample.[112] Furthermore, it is stated in the minutes, "the athlete is allowed to drink beer if he pays it."[113] As the IOC Medical Commission determined this after the competitions had already started, the incidents point toward problems in the collection procedures. Moreover, for the first time at the Olympic Games, the controllers kept the two doping samples (A-sample and B-sample) in different boxes to avoid confusion.[114] Whereas the laboratory staff instantly reopened the A-sample to conduct the doping analysis, the IOC Medical Commission stored the B-sample in the safe of the major of the Olympic Village. Consequently, the urine samples were leaving the supervision of the IOC Medical Commission for the first time.

In accordance with previous attempts to have more pharmaceutical expertise available during the Olympic Games, Arnold Beckett suggested employing a pharmacist supporting the team doctors in questions regarding medical products. The team doctors had requested the same in a meeting with the IOC Medical Commission ahead of the Olympic Games.[115] REINOLD claims that this concern

---

[110] ORGANISING COMMITTEE OF THE GAMES OF THE XIIITH OLYMPIC WINTER GAMES, *Official Report of the XIIth Olympic Winter Games, Innsbruck 1976*, Part 2 (Innsbruck: Organising Committee of the Games of the XIIth Olympic Winter Games, 1976), 366.

[111] Report, "Medical Report of the 1976 Innsbruck Winter Olympic Games, o.d.," 29ff.

[112] Individual Minutes, "Meetings of the IOC Medical Commission in Innsbruck, February 2-13, 1976," archive collection "Summer and Winter Olympic Games: Medical files," folder "Correspondence and reports of the medical control during the Olympic Winter Games of Innsbruck 1976," IOC Archive, Lausanne, 30.

[113] Ibid., 8.

[114] Ibid., 14.

[115] Ibid., 3.

was a result of the even more differentiated rules of the IOC about the usage of medicaments, following the controversies surrounding Rick DeMont in Munich in 1972.[116] Similar to previous Olympic Games, Arnold Beckett also wanted to add more substances to the banned list. However, the other IOC Medical Commission members rejected this proposal in order to avoid difficulties in case of a positive test result. Also, his suggestion to have a pharmacist available was deemed too difficult to implement.[117] Nevertheless, it shows that Arnold Beckett wanted to have more support for the team doctors. He considered this the main weakness of the doping control system. In addition, it would have released pressure from the anti-doping laboratory.

In light of the only two positive doping tests, Arnold Beckett´s concerns appeared justifiable because in both cases, the team doctors played a central role. First, in the positive test for ephedrine of cross-country skier Galina Kulakova (USSR), the IOC ruled a doping offense, although her positive test was not the result of "wilful doping."[118] The IOC Medical Commission estimated that the case was very unfortunate and that one had to consider the "extenuating circumstances."[119] This attitude resulted from a report on the case compiled by Arnold Beckett, where he had highlighted the validity of the positive test from the laboratory´s point of view, but also included the positions of the USSR delegation. According to the athlete and the officials, Galina Kulakova had not known about the ban of the substance. Consequently, the IOC Executive Committee decided to withdraw her bronze medal from the 5km race but it allowed her to participate in the remainder of the Olympic Games.[120] Second, the positive doping test of codeine of ice hockey player František Pospíšil (Czechoslovakia) also illustrates the significance of the team doctors and their knowledge about pharmacological products. The player had been given a medical product, containing codeine, by the Czechoslovak team doctor Dr. Otto Trefny to cure the influenza. Several team members of the ice hockey team had suffered from it during the entire tournament. Otto Trefny was, according to his own

---

[116] REINOLD, "Arguing," 54.

[117] Minutes, "IOC Medical Commission, February 9, 1976," archive collection "Summer and Winter Olympic Games: Medical files," folder "Correspondence and reports of the medical control during the Olympic Winter Games of Innsbruck 1976," IOC Archive, Lausanne.

[118] Minutes, "Executive Board, January 30 and 31, February 5-15, 1976," archive collection "IOC Executive Board Meetings 1921-1982," IOC Archive, Lausanne, 30.

[119] Individual Minutes, "Meetings of the IOC Medical Commission in Innsbruck, February 2-13, 1976," 17.

[120] She won the gold medal in the 4x5km relay. KLUGE, *Olympische Winterspiele*, 302.

account, unaware that codeine had been included as a related compound on the list of banned substances.[121] In a desperate attempt to undo his actions, he eventually submitted a medical form for the athlete: but he did this after the IOC Medical Commission had already announced the result of the doping test.[122] Consequently, the IOC banned Otto Trefny for life.[123] REINOLD maintains that the resulting ban on the team doctor was an exception, because the IOC's testing regime was catered to penalise the athletes and not the doctors. It did not have the "organisational capabilities to establish the responsibility of other persons and groups potentially involved."[124] In addition, the IOC annulled Czechoslovakia's 7-1 win over Poland and assigned a 1-0 defeat instead.[125]

The two positive test results show that Arnold Beckett's proposal to have more pharmaceutical support was justified. Moreover, the episode surrounding František Pospíšil emphasises the significance of the laboratory work. Josef Franz Karl Huber, the head of the anti-doping laboratory, confirmed to the IOC Medical Commission that both urine samples of František Pospíšil had contained codeine.[126] He also mentioned that besides codeine, the first analysis had displayed further foreign constituents in the urine but he was not yet able to determine these on the day following the sample collection. Two days later, he sent another note, explaining that the sample also showed the presence of morphine.[127] The additional conducted tests are important when regarded in conjunction with a letter sent by Ludwig Prokop to Alexandre de Mérode. In the letter, Ludwig Prokop outlined that in a conversation with Günther Sabetzki, president of the IIHF, he had argued that codeine should not be regarded a related

---

[121] Minutes, "Executive Board, January 30 and 31, February 5-15, 1976," 33.

[122] Ibid.

[123] Letter, "Lord Killanin to Chef de mission of the Czechoslavak delegation to the XIth Olympic Winter Games, February 12, 1976."

[124] REINOLD, "Arguing," 54.

[125] ORGANISING COMMITTEE OF THE GAMES OF THE XIIITH OLYMPIC WINTER GAMES, *Official Report*, 141.

[126] Note, "Josef Franz Karl Huber, February 11, 1976," archive collection "Summer and Winter Olympic Games: Medical files," folder "Correspondence and reports of the medical control during the Olympic Winter Games of Innsbruck 1976," IOC Archive, Lausanne.

[127] Note, "Josef Franz Karl Huber, February 13, 1976," archive collection "Summer and Winter Olympic Games: Medical files," folder "Correspondence and reports of the medical control during the Olympic Winter Games of Innsbruck 1976," IOC Archive, Lausanne.

compound to morphine, due to its different pharmacological effect.[128] In contrast
to this, Arnold Beckett reported to the IOC Executive Committee, that codeine
was a related compound scientifically. According to Arnold Beckett, "any doctor
who did not know that codeine changed to morphine in the body was not
competent."[129] Therefore, he accused Ludwig Prokop of not having sufficient
qualified knowledge to make such a statement. Arnold Beckett saw himself
confirmed in his accusations by the presence of morphine in the second sample.
Consequently, Ludwig Prokop had to backpedal, admitting, "about 20% of the
dose of codeine is changed into morphine in man and that a small part of the dose
appears of morphine appears in the urine."[130] Clearly, whereas Arnold Beckett
seemed to support his statements through scientific evidence, sport medical
specialists such as Ludwig Prokop often had close contacts to IFs and supported
their positions. KRÜGER et al. state that the IFs did not have a great interest in the
rigorous handling of doping offenders and potential positive doping cases had a
negative impact on the public perception of the sport.[131] Thus, it would have been
better to situate doping controls, analysis and penalisation outside sport. Bearing
this in mind, more involvement of *external* anti-doping laboratory experts could
have also helped to avoid certain difficulties and controversies.

To summarise, Arnold Beckett, but also Manfred Donike, again occupied key
roles at the 1976 Winter Olympic Games. Similar to 1972 Munich Olympic
Games, the latter's influence was reduced to anti-doping laboratory work. In
contrast to this, Arnold Beckett was crucial for the controversies surrounding the
two positive findings. In terms of their involvement in the Olympic Games, they
both continued in their consultancy roles, which they had already occupied during
the 1972 Munich Olympic Games. It enabled them to continue with their attempts
to base the usage of doping solely on scientific evidence.

Doping Controls at the 1976 Montreal Olympic Games

Chemical Aspects Dominate Preparation

The emphasis and increasingly apparent distinction between medical and doping
issues at the Olympic Games, and within the IOC Medical Commission, becomes

---

[128] Letter, "Ludwig Prokop to Alexandre de Mérode, February 13, 1976," archive
collection "Summer and Winter Olympic Games: Medical files," folder "Correspondence
and reports of the medical control during the Olympic Winter Games of Innsbruck 1976,"
IOC Archive, Lausanne.

[129] Minutes, "Executive Board, January 30 and 31, February 5-15, 1976", 36.

[130] Letter, Ludwig Prokop to Alexandre de Mérode, February 13, 1976."

[131] KRÜGER et al., *Doping und Anti-Doping*, 86.

obvious in an innovative decision by the Organising Committee of the 1976 Montreal Olympic Games (COJO). COJO proposed a change of the official term from "medical controls" to "doping controls" to emphasise clearly what was related to doping matters and which issues were of a medical nature.[132] The IOC Medical Commission agreed to the new term, which shows a distinction between the two fields becoming increasingly necessary.

Through the involvement of Carroll Laurin[133], who COJO appointed as medical representative, the IOC Medical Commission was regularly informed about all ongoing preparation processes of the doping controls for the 1976 Montreal Olympic Games. This was also the case for the doping analysis procedures and the anti-doping laboratory. In total, COJO and the IOC Medical Commission held four major meetings ahead of the Olympic Games. During the first meeting in October 1974, COJO informed the IOC Medical Commission that it had signed a contract on the logistics and organisation of the doping controls with the INRS in May 1974.[134] Robert Dugal and Dr. Michel Bertrand led this section. Whereas the latter was mainly responsible for running the laboratory and the doping analysis during the Games, Robert Dugal coordinated the organisational tasks and cooperated closely with the IOC Medical Commission, especially Arnold Beckett.

The decision to use the INRS is significant when compared to the anti-doping laboratory at the 1972 Munich Olympic Games. As addressed in Chapter 3, the OK chose Manfred Donike and his laboratory team due to their specialisation in sports drug testing. In contrast to this, the INRS was involved in various areas of chemical research: toxicology, toxicomania, clinical pharmacology, psychological/neurological pharmacology and biopharmaceutics, psycholinguistic psychiatry as well as methodology and mathematics applied to clinical research.[135] Dr. Léon Tétreault, director of the INRS, explained to the members of the IOC Medical Commission during their meeting in April 1975 that the INRS had integrated the anti-doping programme into the field of biopharmaceutics and

[132] Minutes, "Minutes of the Special Meeting of the Health Department, October 20, 1974," archive collection "IOC Medical Commission," folder "Medical Commission: Meeting in Montreal on April 23-15, 1975," IOC Archive, Lausanne, 1.
[133] Professor Dr. Carroll Laurin (born 1928), an orthopaedic surgeon, graduated from McGill University in 1952 and joined the University of Montreal after. In 1982, he became the director of the Orthopaedics Department of McGill University.
[134] Minutes, "Minutes of the Special Meeting of the Health Department, October 20, 1974," 12.
[135] Report, "Games of the XXIst Olympiad – Analytical Doping Control Scientific Report by Robert Dugal and Michel Bertrand, June, 1978," 27ff.

clinical toxicology/toxicomania. [136] Awarding the conduction of the doping controls to a scientific institution brought a major advantage to COJO: the INRS received financial support from the federal and regional governments because sport's efforts to eliminate drugs were in line with the policy of the Canadian Ministry of Health and Welfare.[137] Against the background of the huge financial losses of the 1976 Montreal Olympic Games, this has to be regarded important.[138]

Similarly, Robert Dugal also illustrated that the integration into regular scientific research areas resulted in a restriction in terms of developing the already existing tools for doping analysis. According to Robert Dugal, this posed no difficulties as since 1967, the methods had been in place. He remarked, "it was done in Munich, and I see no reason why we could not do it here." [139] Nevertheless, one has to retain that the INRS did not have any prior experience in sports drug testing until the preparations for the doping controls at the 1976 Olympic Games began. However, in his final report on the doping controls, Robert Dugal emphasised that the cooperation between several scientists contributed to the success of the doping controls. He thought that the increased number of substances used by athletes and the growing multiplicity of the physical, chemical and biological sciences made it necessary to consult experts from analytical chemistry, physico-chemistry, organic chemistry and biochemistry in order to detect and identify the substances.[140] Furthermore, the interpretation of the results could only be done with knowledge in pharmacokinetics, pharmacology and physiology. He felt the involvement of the different sciences could best be achieved by including the organisation of the doping controls into a well-positioned scientific institution:

> The dynamic exchange between scientists in different branches made it possible not only to change tactics rapidly, when these proved

---

[136] Report, "Medical report on the meeting of the IOC Medical Commission in Montreal, April 23-25, 1975," archive collection "IOC Medical Commission," folder "Medical Commission: Meeting in Montreal on April 23-25, 1975 – working papers," IOC Archive, Lausanne, 16.

[137] Ibid., 18.

[138] Originally, COJO estimated that the Olympic Games would cost around $310 million. However, because of cost overruns on the building of the Montreal Olympic stadium, the City of Montreal was left with debts of more than $2 billion. It only paid of its debts in 2006. Michael PAYNE, *Olympic Turnaround* (Oxford: Infinite Ideas, 2005), 9.

[139] Report, "Medical report on the meeting of the IOC Medical Commission in Montreal, April 23-25, 1975," 17.

[140] Robert DUGAL, "Doping Tests in Montreal," *Olympic Review* 116 (1977), 383.

unpromising, but also to follow up and swiftly implement an interesting idea.[141]

Additionally, an institution specialised in pharmacological aspects brought a clear focus on the technical matters of the doping tests. Primarily, this can be seen at the installation of a "Doping Control Consultative Committee" with the mandate to act as advisors to the IOC Medical Commission and to the anti-doping laboratory. [142] COJO identified the following areas of support: MS, pharmaceutical chemistry, clinical pharmacology and pharmacokinetics. This was decided upon on during a meeting with Robert Dugal and the IOC Medical Commission in February 1976.[143] The "Doping Control Consultative Committee" was composed of five specialists from Canadian universities and headed by Professor Dr. Albert Nantel, the director of the Québec Center for Toxicology at Laval University.[144] The Committee's main task was to consult the team doctors about pharmaceutical questions on medical products, and scientific questions that arose during the Games. [145] Therefore, it dealt with the specific tasks, which Arnold Beckett had in mind when he proposed pharmacological support to team doctors during the 1976 Winter Olympic Games. After the Olympic Games, the IOC Medical Commission reasoned that the Doping Control Consultative Committee was crucial because of the lack of knowledge on compounds from the side of the team doctors.[146] This again shows the necessity to have specialists with specific professional competencies to support the doping controls.

The preparations for the doping controls and in particular the involvement of the INRS point towards the continuation of the increasingly more intensive focus on anti-doping laboratory expertise. In Robert Dugal, a specialist in chemical analysis was in charge of the organisation of the doping controls, from which an even more intensive focus on doping analysis resulted. In addition, one can attribute this to the introduction of the anabolic steroid tests and the resulting sophisticated doping analysis. Hence, a continuation of the processes triggered through Manfred Donike at the 1972 Munich Olympic Games took place. Finally,

[141] Ibid.
[142] Ibid., 385.
[143] Individual Minutes, "Meetings of the IOC Medical Commission in Innsbruck, February 2-13, 1976," 22.
[144] Ibid.
[145] DUGAL, "Doping Tests," 385.
[146] Minutes, "Meeting Medical Commission Scientific Committee, March 19-20, 1977," achive collection "IOC Medical Commission," folder "Meeting in Lausanne on mai 7-8," IOC Archive, Lausanne, 3.

the introduction of a double protection system to seal the urine samples, [147] demonstrates an increasing anxiety within COJO and the IOC Medical Commission about the doping controls and all its technical aspects. In particular, they wanted to be prepared for potential complaints in the case of positive testing results. Certainly, this was linked to the installation of the tests for anabolic steroids and all its elaborate technical set-up.

Installing the First Olympic Doping Tests for Anabolic Steroids

When Robert Dugal first explained the organisation of the doping controls in October 1974, he noted that he had not yet received an official request for anabolic steroid control. [148] Nevertheless, his team was still preparing all the necessary steps to install the controls. Thus, all technical aspects for the conduction of the tests were prepared to be in place from a very early stage. The IOC Executive Board estimated the costs for the tests too high in spring 1975, mainly because Alexandre de Mérode did not attend the meeting. [149] However, the IOC Medical Commission had decided that the tests were going to take place, but left it to the IFs to make the final decision. Eight sports decided to have tests conducted: athletics, basketball, canoe-kayak, judo, rowing, swimming, weightlifting and wrestling. [150] Importantly, due to the long duration of the doping analysis, the samples had to be taken before the start of the Olympic Games.

In February 1976, the IOC Medical Commission asked Arnold Beckett and Robert Dugal to prepare a draft document on the system of the anabolic steroid tests. [151] However, because the two had already cooperated with each other, and Arnold Beckett had provided the laboratory team with "moral and scientific

---

[147] Report, "Medical report on the occasion of the meeting of the IOC Medical Commission in Montreal, April 23-25, 1975, 15."

[148] Minutes, "Minutes of the Special Meeting of the Health Department, October 20, 1974," 13.

[149] Minutes, "Executive Board, May 14-16, 19 and 23, 1975," archive collection "IOC Executive Board Meetings 1921-1982," IOC Archive, Lausanne, 26.

[150] Minutes, "Minutes of the Meeting of the IOC Medical Commission, April 23-15, 1975," archive collection "IOC Medical Commission," folder "Medical Commission: Meeting in Montreal on April 23-15, 1975," IOC Archive, Lausanne, 2.

[151] Minutes, "Meeting of the IOC Medical Commission, January 15 – February 30, 1976," archive collection "Summer and Winter Olympic Games: Medical files," folder "Correspondence and reports of the medical control during the Olympic Winter Games of Innsbruck 1976," IOC Archive, Lausanne, 2.

support"[152] from the initial preparation phase, they could already address the technical aspects at the meeting. As one would expect, their draft focused on the analytical procedures, and essentially reproduced the official statement made by the IOC Medical Commission in October 1974 following the adoption of anabolic steroids on the list of banned substances.[153] The applied method was the method developed by Raymond Brooks: the screening procedure was based on RI as explained in BROOKS et al., confirmation was done by GC and MS after hydrolysis, purification, concentration and trymethylsilyl derivatisation as developed by DONIKE.[154]

However, due to technical advancements, Robert Dugal and his team were also able to use improved methods for the stimulant controls. Previous historical scholarship has overlooked this development. By fitting a new detector possessing a selective sensitivity to the doping agents onto the new appliances, the methods became more accurate. [155] This advancement was the result of systematic research done at the INRS laboratory to improve the testing techniques.[156] The chromatographs were connected to computers that contained software, which numerically standardised the results. Hence, the result of each sample was presented simultaneously in the form of a graph and in the form of an analytical report.[157] It also offered the possibility to draw a direct comparison between the characteristics of the samples already present in the computer's memory. For the detection of the volatile and non-volatile doping agents, the laboratory staff used six Hewlett-Packard 5730 gas chromatographs equipped with temperature programme facilities. When it was necessary to establish the identity of a chromatographic peak, or to verify peak homogeneity, the laboratory staff submitted the samples the GC-MS analysis and the mass spectra recorded on one of two Hewlett-Packard 5982A integrated GC-MS systems.[158] Therefore, as it

---

[152] Carroll A. LAURIN and Georges LÉTOURNEAU, "Medical Report of the Montreal Olympic Games," *The American Journal of Sports Medicine* 6, no. 2 (1978), 60.

[153] Minutes, "Meeting of the IOC Medical Commission, January 15 – February 30, 1976," 2.

[154] DONIKE, "Zum Problem."

[155] DUGAL, "Doping Tests," 386.

[156] Michel BERTRAND, Robert DUGAL, Cyrus VAZIRI, Gabriel SANCHEZ and S.F. COOPER, "A special dimension of the nonmedical use of drugs. II. Systematic approach to the analytical control of doping]," *Union Med Can.* 104, no. 6 (1975), 952-960.

[157] Alexandre DE MERODE, "Doping Tests at the Olympic Games in 1976," *Olympic Review* 135 (1979), 14.

[158] Report, "Games of the XXIst Olympiad – Analytical Doping Control Scientific Report by Robert Dugal and Michel Bertrand, June, 1978," 27ff.

happened in Munich, the anti-doping laboratory staff was able to develop the doping analysis considerably further.

In retrospect, it was essential to have the testing equipment in place and the laboratory staff educated on anabolic steroid testing. Only a couple of days before the beginning of the Olympic Games the IOC Medical Commission created a subcommittee to investigate into the implementation of the tests.[159] By this time, the sampling procedures had begun. Importantly, this small group consisted of very few experts in the field: Arnold Beckett, Iba Mar Diop, Robert Dugal, Michel Bertrand and Albert Nantel.[160] When considering the previous policy of Alexandre de Mérode to refrain from appointing small working groups, this committee was a new approach. Moreover, the group members had different organisational affiliations, coming from COJO and the IOC Medical Commission, which was also unusual. In fact, Alexandre de Mérode referred to the members of the group during the IOC Session in Montreal as "a commission of five pharmacologists."[161] The subcommittee mainly investigated into the duration of the doping analysis for anabolic steroids. Such was the primary IOC concern that it did not announce the testing results ahead of the athletes participating in the competition. Moreover, the IOC Medical Commission expected most of the test results only after the end of the Olympic Games.[162] An acceleration of this process was not possible because the IOC Medical Committee wanted to be certain about the scientific proof of the presence of an anabolic steroid.

Importantly however, the subcommittee and the IOC Session did not address two important aspects. First, the elusiveness of many athletes because they were living outside the Olympic Village with some of them training in Mexico. Robert Dugal had already addressed this problem at the beginning of the year.[163] Second, the difficulties that arose during the US Olympic track and field trials where 23 athletes were tested positive on anabolic steroids but not sanctioned.[164] This gives

---

[159] Statement, "Anabolic Steroid Controls, July 13-19, 1976," archive collection "Summer and Winter Olympic Games: Medical files," folder "Minutes of the IOC Medical Commission of the 1976 Summer Olympic Games in Montreal: 24 meetings between 10 July and 1 August," IOC Archive, Lausanne.

[160] Ibid.

[161] Minutes, "78th Session of the IOC in Montreal, October 5-7, 1973," archive collection "IOC Sessions 1894-2009," IOC Archive, Lausanne, 41.

[162] Statement, "Anabolic Steroid Controls, July 13-19, 1976."

[163] Individual Minutes, "Meetings of the IOC Medical Commission in Innsbruck, February 2-13, 1976," 28.

[164] HUNT, *Drug Games*, 57.

rise to the impression that the IOC was initially satisfied with the installation of the anabolic steroid tests, especially due to the organisational difficulties that came with it, but did not want to create any additional problems. Notwithstanding, the set-up of the subcommittee, and the technically challenging task to install controls for anabolic steroids, confirm the ongoing process of increasingly necessary competencies in doping analysis.

Significance of Anti-doping Laboratory Work

In total, the IOC collected 1786 urine samples ahead of, and during the 1976 Montreal Olympic Games, then analysed for the "traditional" doping substances according to the discussed methods.[165] The laboratory team screened 275 samples for anabolic steroids, since the duration of the analysis did not allow conducting more tests.[166] Three athletes were tested positive for stimulants: Paul Cerotti (Monaco, shooting), Dragomir Ciorosian (Romania, weightlifting) and Lorne Liebel (Canada, sailing).[167] The low figure of positive tests related to stimulants, led Carroll Laurin and Georges Létourneau to summarize, "the lowest incidence yet reported in Olympic Games, [suggests] that this battle at least appears to have been won."[168] Obviously, this statement was far too optimistic, even though their briefing of the data on the anabolic steroids was a different one. They made eight adverse findings in the 275 urine samples, leading them to conclude, "this battle would seem to have just begun." [169] The positive tested athletes were the weightlifters Blagoi Blagoev (Bulgaria), Mark Cameron (USA), Phil Grippaldi (USA), Zbigniew Kaczmarek (Poland), Valentin Khristov (Bulgaria), Arne Norrback (Sweden), Petr Pavlasek (Czechoslovakia), and discus thrower Danuta Rosani (Poland).[170] Not drawing on the positive cases, Robert Dugal summarised that the controls were successful from a technical point of view and the applied techniques effective:

---

[165] HEMMERSBACH, "History," 840.

[166] DUGAL, "Doping Tests," 387.

[167] Individual Minutes, "Meetings of the IOC Medical Commission in Montreal, July 6 – August 1, 1976," archive collection "Summer and Winter Olympic Games: Medical files," folder "Minutes of the IOC Medical Commission of the 1976 Olympic Games in Montreal: 24 meetings between 10 July and 1 August," IOC Archive, Lausanne.

[168] LAURIN and LÉTOURNEAU, "Medical Report," 60.

[169] Ibid.

[170] Individual Minutes, "Meetings of the IOC Medical Commission in Montreal, July 6 – August 1, 1976."

> The gas chromatographic/mass spectrometric technique has proved particularly useful in the confirmation of anabolic steroids. As a result of the techniques developed in our laboratories, it was possible during the Games to identify the nature of the steroid administered, which enabled the sanctions, with which you are all familiar, to be taken subsequently.[171]

Several authors have already illustrated the positive doping cases and HUNT has discussed the legacy of the (positive) tests in light of the political situation in which the Olympic Movement found itself in the 1970s.[172] However, as at previous Olympic Games, the historical documents also provide insights into the work and significance of the anti-doping laboratory experts in these cases.

The laboratory reported the first three positive tests on anabolic steroids by Mark Cameron, Peter Pavlasek and Danuta Rosani to the IOC Medical Commission on July 28.[173] The analyses of the B-sample took place the following day and Arnold Beckett, who, together with Robert Dugal, was in charge of the analysis of the B-sample, confirmed all positive results. Curiously, neither a representative from the IAAF nor a representative from the International Weightlifting Federation (IWF) was present. The reactions of the attending NOC officials were quite indifferent. Whereas the American delegation opposed the decision and appeared dissatisfied with the selection of the athletes for doping controls ahead of the Games, the Czechoslovak team doctor approved the result and received applause for his confession from the IOC Medical Commission members.[174]

In addition, two major issues arose from the announcement of the second set of positive tests on anabolic steroids, made following the end of the Olympic Games. First, the Bulgarian NOC, represented by its general secretary Christo Marazanov, and the Polish team doctor Dr. Michal Firsowicz complained about the sealing procedure of the urine bottles. Christo Marazanov argued that the Finnish weightlifter Juhani Avellan could not give his urine sample at the competition site and had to provide it on the bus to the anti-doping laboratory. Consequently, the box, in which the doping control officers had also stored the doping samples of six other athletes, had to be unsealed and the two control

---

[171] DUGAL, "Doping Tests," 386.
[172] HUNT, *Drug Games*, 58ff.
[173] Individual Minutes, "Meetings of the IOC Medical Commission in Montreal, July 6 – August 1, 1976," 99.
[174] Ibid., 107.

bottles added. As reported by the Bulgarian delegation, the labelling with a code number and placing the sample in the plastic cylinder (which had to be sealed again) was not done on the bus.[175] Therefore, Christo Marazanov concluded that it could have been opened in any other place as well, which was a clear violation of the IOC's rules. Furthermore, he claimed that once the box with the samples was taking out of the fridge for the recheck, it was visible that the lead seal of the outer container was crushed.[176] Arnold Beckett confirmed this in a short note to Christo Marazanov after the recheck, but stated that all code numbers were intact and under the correct plastic seals of the bottles. Similarly, Michael Firsowicz reasoned that technicians could remove the coded band with an air blower and reapply it onto the bottle afterwards.[177] He demonstrated this also to the laboratory staff, including Arnold Beckett, who again confirmed that this was possible. Notwithstanding, the IOC Medical Commission based its final decision to recommend disqualification to the IOC Executive Board on the positive analysis of the B-samples of Bulgarian athlete Blagoi Blagoev and Polish athlete Zbigniew Kaczmarek. This procedure took place on August 22, 1976. Besides the representatives of the IFs, Robert Dugal, Michel Bertrand, Léon Tétreault, Carroll Laurin, Daniel Hanley and Arnold Beckett were present during these procedures. They claimed that the urine samples were all stored in a fridge unlocked by Robert Dugal, all seals of the urine bottles were intact and that none of the competitors had made any complaints during the sampling and transportation procedures.[178] A paragraph was included into the official statement, where the group admitted that the sealing of the outer container was crushed but still intact. Furthermore, the group stated that the container was not part of the identification procedure and only an additional safeguard.[179] Even more importantly, the doping control officer in charge at the weightlifting competitions reported that he did not

---

[175] Ibid.

[176] Letter, "Declaration of the Bulgarian Weightlifting Federation, n.d.," archive collection "Summer and Winter Olympic Games: Medical files," folder "Doping in weightlifting at the 1976 Summer Olympic Games in Montreal," IOC Archive, Lausanne.

[177] Letter, "Dr. Med Michal Firsowicz to Arnold Beckett, August, 1976," archive collection "Summer and Winter Olympic Games: Medical files," folder "Doping in weightlifting at the 1976 Summer Olympic Games in Montreal," IOC Archive, Lausanne.

[178] Statement, "Arnold Beckett, September 22, 1976," archive collection "Summer and Winter Olympic Games: Medical files," folder "Doping in weightlifting at the 1976 Summer Olympic Games in Montreal," IOC Archive, Lausanne.

[179] Report, "Arnold Beckett, Daniel Hanley and Caroll Laurin, August 23, 1976," archive collection "Summer and Winter Olympic Games: Medical files," folder "Doping in weightlifting at the 1976 Summer Olympic Games in Montreal," IOC Archive, Lausanne.

transport the box with the samples of the six athletes together with Juhani Avellan. Instead, he had sent it directly to the laboratory, where the laboratory staff added the final urine after arrival.[180] Thus, it appears from the official reports, but also from the exchange of letters, that the sealing of the bottles was only a minor issue to the IOC Medical Commission. Rather, it stressed that the analysis of the urine samples was "first class," and that it had no doubt about the identity of the material found in the urine.[181] Georges Létourneau also confirmed this in a letter to Arnold Beckett.[182] Consequently, they dismissed the problems as less important than the fact that the laboratory had produced positive results for anabolic steroids and was able to confirm them in the second check. Because he did not regard the sampling and sealing part of the responsibility of the anti-doping laboratory experts but rather procedure problems, Arnold Beckett affirmed, "the laboratory on the technical side was at the height of the situation." [183] HENNE is therefore correct to conclude that despite likely irregularities in the sampling procedures, the IOC Medical Commission's decisions stood up to scrutiny. According to the data presented here, this was mainly due to the conviction that the laboratory results in the newly introduced processes for anabolic steroid testing were correct.[184] It transpires that by that time, this was all that mattered and gives further proof for the ongoing tendencies within the IOC Medical Commission. There was an apparent need for even more standardised procedures and an increasing number of laboratory experts to be involved. The introduction of the anabolic steroid test brought with it the necessity to have entirely ironclad techniques, for which only anti-doping laboratory experts could give insurance.

---

[180] Telegram, "Duncan Thorpe to Department of Pharmacy Chelsea College of Science and Technology, September 7, 1976," archive collection "Summer and Winter Olympic Games: Medical files," folder "Doping in weightlifting at the 1976 Summer Olympic Games in Montreal," IOC Archive, Lausanne.

[181] Letter, "Arnold Beckett to Monique Berlioux, August 26, 1976," archive collection "Summer and Winter Olympic Games: Medical files," folder "Doping in weightlifting at the 1976 Summer Olympic Games in Montreal," IOC Archive, Lausanne.

[182] Letter, "Georges Létourneau, August 26, 1976," archive collection "Summer and Winter Olympic Games: Medical files," folder "Doping in weightlifting at the 1976 Summer Olympic Games in Montreal," IOC Archive, Lausanne.

[183] Individual Minutes, "Meetings of the IOC Medical Commission in Montreal, July 6 – August 1, 1976," 18.

[184] Kathryn HENNE, "The Emergence of Moral Technopreneurialism in Sport: Techniques in Anti-Doping Regulation, 1966–1976," *International Journal for the History of Sport* 31, no. 8 (2014), 895.

Second, communication problems and confidentiality matters arose, again pointing towards insufficient information management within the IOC Medical Commission. Hence, the two American shot put athletes Al Feuerbach and George Woods were apparently not informed that they had to give samples for anabolic steroid tests, and left Montreal without a doping control. The IOC Medical Commission stated that this was out of their control and as a result, the athletes were not ordered to return to Montreal.[185] Besides this regularly omitted episode, a more prominent issue had been the early announcement of five positive doping tests on anabolic steroids that the IOC Medical Commission confirmed officially on August 22, 1976. As HENNE illustrates, the former IWF general secretary Oscar State had already known about the positive A-sample on August 10, when he called IWF president Gottfried Schödl.[186] He claimed that he had read about the names of the athletes in a German newspaper before Albert Dirix had officially informed him.[187] Written exchanges display controversies about the disclosure of information. Eventually the IOC Medical Commission announced that it condemned the publication of the results before the confirmation through the B-sample, but argued that the information did not come from the IOC Medical Commission itself.[188] Importantly, Lord Killanin was also concerned by this issue and was very interested in discovering who had been the IOC spokesperson to whom is referred in the press publications.[189] It appears that he felt vindicated in his belief that too many individuals were involved in doping matters through the size of the IOC Medical Commission. Thus, in light of the previously discussed set-up, the doping controls at the Montreal Games are a confirmation of the ongoing developments. Moreover, importantly, the members requested more compact and shorter meetings for the first time during the Games.[190]

---

[185] Individual Minutes, "Meetings of the IOC Medical Commission in Innsbruck, February 2-13, 1976," 41.

[186] HENNE, "The Emergence," 895.

[187] Letter, "Gottfried Schödl to Alexandre de Mérode, August 31, 1976," archive collection "Summer and Winter Olympic Games: Medical files," folder "Doping in weightlifting at the 1976 Summer Olympic Games in Montreal," IOC Archive, Lausanne.

[188] Individual Minutes, "Meetings of the IOC Medical Commission in Montreal, July 6 – August 1, 1976," 118.

[189] HUNT, *Drug Games*, 58.

[190] Individual Minutes, "Meetings of the IOC Medical Commission in Montreal, July 6 – August 1, 1976," 118.

The Role of Arnold Beckett

Besides the apparent need for higher technical standards and more anti-doping laboratory expertise in doping controls in general, the decisive role of Arnold Beckett is revealed when closely examining the documents on the controls at the 1976 Olympic Games. Thus, previous historical scholarship has overlooked his important role during the early phase of doping controls at Olympic Games. This becomes evident at four interrelated examples.

First, Arnold Beckett appears to be the primary contact for the complaints about the flaws in the doping control. One would expect these to be directed to Alexandre de Mérode but this was not the case. The perception of the team doctors and representatives of the federations reveals Arnold Beckett´s standing within the Olympic Movement´s anti-doping activities. Going through the official channel would have meant going through Alexandre de Mérode. Certainly, as most of the issues to be dealt with were of technical nature, there is no doubt that Arnold Beckett was the correct contact. In any case, Alexandre de Mérode had always delegated all technical matters to Arnold Beckett anyway. After his return to the Great Britain, Arnold Beckett gave indeed many detailed technical explanations concerning the complaints, despite considering them as sampling and not laboratory issues. Throughout his explanations, he emphasised the extraordinary work of the INRS laboratory team while clarifying that each of the positive doping controls had been verified with methods of the highest technical level. He concluded, "the evidence on the cases in question, in my opinion, will stand up any degree of cross examination in any court of law."[191]

Second, Arnold Beckett was in charge of the all-important analysis of the B-samples. Especially after the leak of the information to the press prior to the recheck, this analysis had to be conducted under special circumstances. Alexandre de Mérode was not present during this procedure. Hence, Arnold Beckett did not only run the technical parts of the controls, but also the organisational and communication operations. Already ahead of the controversial cases, he had maintained that the urine sampling procedure for steroid testing should only be controlled by members of the IOC Medical Commission.[192] These should be present at the doping control station so that they would be taken under

---

[191] Statement, "Implications of the Declarations from Poland and Bulgaria, September 22, 1976," archive collection "Summer and Winter Olympic Games: Medical files," folder "Doping in weightlifting at the 1976 Summer Olympic Games in Montreal," IOC Archive, Lausanne.

[192] Individual Minutes, "Meetings of the IOC Medical Commission in Montreal, July 6 – August 1, 1976," 82.

the supervision of the highest order. It appears that he already anticipated complaints in cases of positive tests. Whereas Arnold Beckett discussed with the complaining delegations on a technical level, Alexandre de Mérode´s lack of understanding for such as issues becomes apparent at this stage. He had argued that it would be completely natural to make mistakes because it had been the first tests for anabolic steroids.[193] In addition, he reasoned in the IOC Executive Board that he was the "sole guardian of the key to the safe where the samples were stored."[194] This statement is in stark contrast to the documents found in the IOC archive in which Robert Dugal provided confirmation in writing that he had been the only person in possession of the key, which Arnold Beckett also affirmed.[195]

Third, Arnold Beckett signed and made all announcements on the positive doping tests, demonstrated through the analysis of the B-sample after the Olympic Games. Of course, this is linked to the fact that he was in charge of the analysis and apart from Daniel Hanley (who was believed to be biased because an American athlete was amongst the positive tests), the only IOC Medical Commission member present at the re-check. Moreover, Arnold Beckett informed Lord Killanin about the positive cases and warned him that more countries might make a political issue out of positive doping controls if reliable scientific evidence was not given.[196] In order to get ahead of further complaints, Lord Killanin suggested publishing an article on the problems of steroid controls, to be written by Arnold Beckett and not Alexandre de Mérode. Just two months later, the article appeared in the *Olympic Review*.[197] It was very similar to the publication Arnold Beckett had written for the *Sunday Times* a couple of years before. The only publication on the doping controls of the 1976 Montreal Olympic Games by Alexandre de Mérode was published in the *Olympic Review* in January 1979.[198] However, this was a copy of an article by Robert Dugal, which had already appeared in the same publication in its June/July 1977

---

[193] Ibid., 119.

[194] Minutes, "Executive Board, October 13-17, 1976," archive collection "IOC Executive Board Meetings 1921-1982," IOC Archive, Lausanne, 32.

[195] Statement, "Arnold Beckett, September 22, 1976," archive collection "Summer and Winter Olympic Games: Medical files," folder "Doping in weightlifting at the 1976 Summer Olympic Games in Montreal," IOC Archive, Lausanne.

[196] Letter, "Lord Killanin to Harry Banks, September 1, 1976," achive collection "IOC Medical Commission," folder "Medical Commission: Correspondence: 1976," IOC Archive, Lausanne.

[197] BECKETT, "Problems," 591-598.

[198] DE MÉRODE, "Doping Tests at the Olympic Games in 1976."

edition. [199] Furthermore, the appreciation of Arnold Beckett's commitment through Lord Killanin is also evidenced in a letter, sent to him by the IOC president in January 1977. In the letter, Lord Killanin praised Arnold Beckett for the article and stated, "I do appreciate so much your contribution, as probably the world's leading pharmacologist, to the problem of doping, with special reference to the anabolic steroids." [200] Lord Killanin appeared not know, however, that Arnold Beckett was not an expert in anabolic steroids but only dealt with the issue so intensively because he was still the exclusive anti-doping laboratory expert on the IOC Medical Commission.

Fourth, Professor Dr. Victor Rogozkin[201] (see Chapter 5), a new member of the IOC Medical Commission, stated during the meetings of the IOC Medical Commission, "in certain decisions relating more particularly to the level of the laboratory are taken by only one person." [202] Although Victor Rogozkin does not specifically name him, the person referred to must be Arnold Beckett. Hence, the fact that he had so much influence was not only perceived positively. Moreover, Victor Rogozkin suggested that a subcommittee should be formed to deal with laboratory issues and the development of the analytical procedures. According to the minutes, Alexandre de Mérode approved this suggestion. Without directly opposing Victor Rogozkin's point of view, Arnold Beckett reasoned that the analytical procedures were regularly making progress anyway and that a close cooperation with the laboratory had been in place so that all of the decisions were made jointly. [203] In any case, this appears to be the first time he faced opposition to his dominant role from other members of the IOC Medical Commission.

The above information about Arnold Beckett's role during the 1976 Olympic Games offers an extension of previous research. In her article on the emergence of the "moral technopreneuralism" in sport, HENNE concludes that by the end of the 1976 Montreal Olympic Games, the IOC Medical Commission had a more secure place within the Olympic Movement, mainly because of Alexandre de Mérode's lobbying efforts and the influence of doping testing. [204] This assumption

---

[199] DUGAL, "Doping Tests."

[200] Letter, "Lord Killanin to Arnold Beckett, January 18, 1977," archive collection "IOC Medical Commission," folder "Medical Commission: Correspondence: 1977 – June, 29, 1978," IOC Archive, Lausanne.

[201] Vladimir I. MOROZOV, "Professor Victor Alekseevich Rogozkin," *European Journal of Applied Physiology* 103 (2008), 379-380.

[202] Individual Minutes, "Meetings of the IOC Medical Commission in Montreal, July 6 – August 1, 1976," 118f.

[203] Ibid.

[204] HENNE, "The Emergence," 896.

is certainly correct as has been highlighted in this chapter. However, the focus on the work of the anti-doping laboratory experts shows that they were not only influential but crucial for the IOC′s fight against doping and that they occupied a strong advisory role within the Olympic Movement towards the end of 1976. The leading role of Arnold Beckett is certainly an obvious indication for this. Many resolutions were solely made by him. Hence, there was more to the IOC′s anti-doping efforts than lobbying through Alexandre de Mérode to strengthen the position of the IOC Medical Commission. One could quickly arrive at the conclusion that Alexandre de Mérode also realised the significance of analytical aspects, when reading this paragraph of the article published under his name in 1979:

> One often tends to forget, to underestimate or even simply to realise the technical and scientific complexities of the analytical doping controls, especially when they have to be carried out during Olympic Games. We would remind you that it is the IOC's policy to prohibit only those potentially doping substances for which there exist one or more scientifically reliable analytical techniques of detection and identification. To accuse an athlete of doping merely on the basis of clinical impressions – no matter how justified they may be – is not sufficient motive for intervention. it is essential to prove the presence of the medicine (or a metabolite) in the samples of urine taken, under clearly defined conditions laid down in regulations drawn up not only for the protection of athletes, but also for the integrity of the whole testing system.[205]

The significance of the analytical procedures and individuals with professional competencies in doping analysis is clearly emphasised here. However, with the knowledge that an almost identical article had been published under the name of Robert Dugal, it remains unclear whether this was actually Alexandre de Mérode′s opinion. It mirrors the view of an increasingly important anti-doping laboratory expert in Robert Dugal and must be classified an attempt to show the relevance of his work.

---

[205] DE MÉRODE, "Doping Tests," 12.

Flaws in the Doping Controls

It is important to mention that even though anabolic steroid tests were installed and perceived as successful, there was still considerable doubt about the efficiency of the tests. There were also other flaws.

First, problems occurred with the anabolic steroid tests. Members of the IOC Medical Commission criticised heavily the long amount of time required for the doping analysis. Robert Dugal and Michel Bertrand also expressed the need for more sophisticated methods to speed up the analytical procedure:

> It therefore seemed desirable that a fast and specific method for the detection of these substances should be developed, in order to achieve the overwhelming task of doping control of anabolic steroids, particularly in the context of the Olympic Games. In circumstances such as these, a large number of analyses have to be performed within a rigid time schedule.[206]

In actuality, the anti-doping laboratory could test considerably less than the originally planned number of 2279 samples for stimulants because the analysis for anabolic steroids absorbed a big amount of the laboratory's capacity.[207] Besides the duration of the analytical procedure, sport officials also raised concerns about the reliability and effectiveness of the tests. Amongst them was the Canadian IOC Member James Worrall, who had previously explained his resistance against the implementation of tests, arguing that athletes could simply discontinue the use of the substance for a period prior to the competition.[208] Whereas the medical experts on the IOC Medical Commission along with Alexandre de Mérode appeared to be satisfied with the installation, anti-doping laboratory experts Manfred Donike (in his scientific publication on the problems of the anabolic steroid controls from the year 1975)[209] and Robert Dugal strongly supported this view, suggesting the introduction of out-of competition tests.[210] Certainly, the support for the idea was not without a degree of self-interest,

---

[206] Report, "Games of the XXIst Olympiad – Analytical Doping Control Scientific Report by Robert Dugal and Michel Bertrand, June, 1978," 52.

[207] Minutes, "Meeting Medical Commission Scientific Committee, March 19-20, 1977," 4.

[208] Letter, "James Worrall to Alexandre de Mérode, January 3, 1975," "IOC Medical Commission," folder "Medical Commission: Correspondence: 1975," IOC Archive, Lausanne.

[209] DONIKE, "Zum Problem," 5.

[210] DUGAL, "Doping," 387.

because it would have provided their institutions with a considerable increase in work and financial income.

Second, there was no test for exogenous testosterone introduced yet. The usage of testosterone was an increasing problem for the anti-doping laboratory experts at the end of the 1970s because its application was not detectable: men and women naturally produce testosterone in small quantities and therefore its misuse could only be obtained through a quantitative determination. This allowed the athletes to cease the steroid usage and change to testosterone prior to the Olympic Games. Arnold Beckett presented the progress on a testing method for testosterone – of which he appeared to be very well versed – at the concluding meeting of the IOC Medical Commission in Montreal.[211] At the meeting, he asserted that ascertaining the normal or abnormal level on woman was the main problem, which was very complicated from a scientific point of view.[212] As a result, he encouraged the laboratory in Montreal to conduct further research on testosterone in urine with the samples from the Olympic Games. He even suggested that if there were a positive test, there would be no sanction.[213] The investigation should only serve scientific goals. Such research projects changed the work of the anti-doping laboratory because their tasks were not done after the end of the Olympic Games but instead integrated into the developing network of doping research and analysis.

Third, the anti-doping laboratory experts were also involved in controversies. Henk Erik MEIER and Marcel REINOLD describe the discussions in the FRG to apply the "air clyster" method to improve the hydrodynamics of swimmers,[214] which occurred in the broader context of doping scandals in the country at the end of the 1970s.[215] The "air clyster" method included pumping air into the bowels of the competitors. When offered the method for one million D-Mark, the German

---

[211] Ibid.

[212] Individual Minutes, "Meetings of the IOC Medical Commission in Montreal, July 6 – August 1, 1976," 123.

[213] Ibid.

[214] Henk E. MEIER and Marcel REINOLD, "Performance Enhancement and Politicisation of High Performance Sport: The West German 'air clyster' Affair of 1976," *The International Journal for the History of Sport* 30, no. 12 (2013), 1361.

[215] The most controversial incident was the so-called "Kolbe injection". The FRG rower Peter-Michael Kolbe had been given a compound of cocarboxylase and thioctacid by Joseph Keul ahead of his final run for which he was the clear favourite. However, he lost the race to Pertti Karppinen from Finland, which was attributed to the usage of the substance. According to KRÜGER et al., Joseph Keul had been given athletes "vitamin injections" for many years. KRÜGER et al., *Doping und Anti-Doping*, 87.

Swimming Association and the German Ministry of the Interior felt obliged to accept the offer. However, both organisations emphasised that the method could only be used if it was not a violation of the IOC's anti-doping regulations, not health damaging, not an impediment to performance nor endangering the participation of athletes at the Olympic Games.[216] Thus, the BMI asked Manfred Donike whether the method would violate Olympic or FINA doping regulations. Since the method was not on the banned list, Manfred Donike confirmed that the method did not violate any rules and the Germans tested the "air clyster" in the pre-Olympic training camp in Calgary.[217] Nevertheless, they eventually decided against the usage due to a lack of technical requirements.[218] Evidently, sport organisations used the knowledge of anti-doping laboratory experts and scientists to bypass doping regulations. Although not officially a member of the IOC Medical Commission, the FRG institutions turned to Manfred Donike when they required detailed knowledge about the doping regulations.

INTERIM RESULTS FOR THE PERIOD 1973-1977: MORE INFLUENCE FOR THE ANTI-DOPING LABORATORY EXPERTS IN ADVISORY ROLE

The IOC's anti-doping efforts between the 1972 Munich Olympic Games and the 1976 Montreal Olympic Games were highly influenced by the attempt to install a reliable analytical procedure to detect anabolic steroids. This is nothing new to research. However, the undertaken investigations reveal that several processes concerning the work of the anti-doping laboratory experts, commencing with the foundation of the IOC Medical Commission in 1967, were intensified because of the introduction of the test.

First, the focus on the significance of the work of anti-doping laboratory experts becomes apparent in the preparation phase for anabolic steroid testing. Once Alexandre de Mérode realised that anabolic steroids presented the most severe problem, he and other sport administrators began to rely more intensively on individuals with professional competencies in the field of doping analysis. In fact, the scientific breakthrough of the research by Raymond Brooks and his colleagues finally enabled the IOC to install such a test for the 1976 Montreal Olympic Games. Thus, anti-doping laboratory experts triggered a key turning point in the installation of the global doping control system. The scientific orientation of the INRS added enhanced focus on chemical aspects. Robert Dugal

---

[216] MEIER and REINOLD, "Performance Enhancement," 1362.
[217] Ibid.
[218] KRÜGER et al., *Doping und Anti-Doping*, 90.

and Michel Bertrand emphasised this in their extensive final report, where they referred to the "scientific multidisciplinary character of an organised doping control programme."[219] In retrospect, this proved an extremely useful decision because the initiation of the anabolic steroid tests required a very high degree of understanding of such issues. The introduction enabled highly specialised scientists from various scientific disciplines to work together, thus ensuring a high technical standard. The decision to change the term from "medical controls" to "doping controls" also displays awareness that the nature of problem was now more than a medical one. The medical justification for doping tests had been given until the mid-1970s, but there is evidence that this period ended by 1976, because the doping control system demanded more experts in doping analysis.

Second, the implementation of the anabolic steroid tests allowed Arnold Beckett playing an even more central role within the IOC Medical Commission and the supervision of the anti-doping laboratory at the Olympic Games. He became the main reference person for the IFs, even though he did not personally conduct research on anabolic steroids. Whereas Alexandre de Mérode kept pushing for a better standing of the IOC Medical Commission on the political level, Arnold Beckett dealt with the development of the testing procedures in an extended advisory role. In his publication on the misuse of anabolic steroids following the Montreal Olympic Games, Arnold Beckett´s rigorous attitude towards doping offenders becomes clear. He stressed:

> the administrators in sport and the scientists and physicians in dope control bear a heavy responsibility to ensure that sport is cleansed from the cancerous growth of misuse of anabolic steroids in sport.[220]

Not only does he highlight the necessary distinction between sport officials, sport medical specialists and anti-doping laboratory experts, but demonstrates his willingness to invest heavily into the matter. One can find the same attitude in a letter written previously in 1975 where he confirmed his stance that science would always find a way to detect doping substances:

> The introduction of doping control by the IOC Medical Commission and by the International Sports Federations has led to a substantial reduction of drug misuse of those drugs which were included in the banned

---

[219] Report, "Games of the XXIst Olympiad – Analytical Doping Control Scientific Report by Robert Dugal and Michel Bertrand, June, 1978," 1.
[220] BECKETT, "Problems," 598.

classes. When testing has been carried out in various events the small percentage of positive results found indicates that the deterent [sic] aspects of the tests are in operation (...). New drugs are becoming available and there may be a temptation to use the new drugs to defeat doping control; nevertheless at the same time detection methods are continuing to improve rapidly both in sensitivity and specificity and thus attempt to circumvent doping controls are not likely to succeed.[221]

Later revelations show this was an overly enthusiastic and optimistic standpoint, but it provides researchers with another argument that those responsible actually believed that they would win the fight against doping in the 1970s. This appears to be true for sport administrators and sport medicine specialists, but also for Arnold Beckett.

Third, despite the increased focus on doping analysis and the expertise of anti-doping laboratory experts in this field, this was not yet reflected in the membership of the IOC Medical Commission. Instead, Alexandre de Mérode appeared unconcerned that the majority of the members had their strengths in medical fields. This hindered the IOC Medical Commission's effectiveness. Notwithstanding, as a result of the ongoing consultation with Raymond Brooks and Manfred Donike, a few more anti-doping laboratory experts adopted external consultancy roles, if not as members of the IOC Medical Commission. The leading people in the execution of the doping controls in Montreal, Robert Dugal and Michel Bertrand, who were after all two educated pharmacists, confirm this assumption. They interpreted their role similar to Manfred Donike in Munich in 1972.

Fourth, even though there was a more intensified exchange, no significant extension of the network of anti-doping laboratory experts appears to have taken place. They did not hold any meetings such as the one in Rome in 1969. Nevertheless, the distinction between medical and anti-doping laboratory experts definitely still widened. This also becomes important when considering the foundation of the International Association of Olympic Medical Officers (IAOMO), who mainly dealt with the practical care of the athletes from the perspective of the team doctors. It was not the objective of IAOMO to conduct research, or to be a rival body for the IOC Medical Commission, but rather

---

[221] Letter, "Arnold Beckett to Harry Banks, September 24, 1975," archive collection "IOC Medical Commission," folder "Medical Commission: Correspondence 1975," IOC Archive, Lausanne.

concentrate on "different problems."[222] Furthermore, the foundation of IAOMO provides additional evidence for the well-established network of sport medicine specialists in the 1960s and 1970s,[223] which anti-doping laboratory experts still lacked.

Fifth, the in-depth analysis of the establishment and the first working years of the IAAF Medical Committee proved to be enlightening for the subject under research. This international anti-doping body concentrated more extensively on the technical aspects of the doping controls. The responsible individuals achieved this through the establishment of a small working group of anti-doping laboratory experts, who dealt only with doping tests and the analytical aspects of the controls. Its efforts resulted in the first list of officially recognised laboratories in 1975, showing that their roles in the IAAF went beyond consultancy and led to the implementation of actual procedures. Moreover, the inclusion of Arnold Beckett, Raymond Brooks, Manfred Donike and Jacques van Rossum allowed the leading figures in the research on doping analysis to exchange information more frequently. The link between the IOC and IAAF was Arnold Beckett, who was a member on both bodies. Indeed, the UCI had previously listed three appointed laboratories in its doping regulations from 1968,[224] but had not selected them based on their scientific suitability. Rather, three members of the UCI Medical Commission simply appointed their own institutions.

In conclusion, one can recognise that Alexandre de Mérode himself provided a suitable summary of the period between 1972 and 1976. During of the IOC Executive Board meeting in October 1976, he remarked "the trial period for steroid testing was over, the testing procedure well practiced by the IAAF and this knowledge passed on to the Medical Commission through Professor Beckett and Dr. Brooks."[225] Thereby, he does not only acknowledge the contribution of the IAAF Medical Committee with its earlier initiatives in terms of anabolic steroid testing, but also the input of the two individual anti-doping laboratory experts as consultants of the IOC in anti-doping affairs. Thus, although Alexandre de Mérode did not yet see the need for more inclusion of anti-doping laboratory experts in the IOC Medical Commission, he certainly highly valued their expertise in the field of doping analysis.

---

[222] Raymond J. OWEN, "The Organisation of the International Association of Olympic Medical Officers," *Olympic Review* 105 (1976), 372.

[223] DIMEO, *A History,* 93, 101 and 128. KRÜGER et al., *Doping und Anti-Doping,* 46.

[224] Minutes, "IOC Medical Commission, July 13 and 14, 1968."

[225] Minutes, "Executive Board, October 13-17, 1976," 29.

CHAPTER 5

Transition Phase (1977-1980)

SIGNS OF A CHANGING FOCUS WITHIN THE IOC MEDICAL COMMISSION

Expansion of the IOC Medical Commission's Expertise

It has already been discussed in the previous chapter that at its very first meeting following the 1976 Montreal Olympic Games in October 1976, the IOC Medical Commission dealt primarily with the disqualification of the five athletes who tested positive for anabolic steroids. By that time, Victor Rogozkin had joined the IOC Medical Commission to replace Nina Grashinskaya.[1] On first view, this decision appears obvious because Victor Rogozkin replaced another Soviet expert. However, in an important contrast to other previously added members, Victor Rogozkin also had professional competencies in doping analysis. In 1958, he had obtained a Ph.D. from the Biochemistry Department of Leningrad State University. From 1966, he was deputy director of the Research Institute of Physical Culture, and from 1975 its director. Besides conducting research on the molecular mechanisms underlying the physiological and biochemical adaptations of exercise, he also headed the Doping Control Department of the Research Institute of Physical Culture.[2] Ahead of the 1980 Moscow Olympic Games, he became chair of the Doping Control Committee,[3] which appears to be an obvious decision because his department was the only Soviet institution dealing with doping controls at the time.[4] However, despite his expertise in biochemistry, Alexandre de Mérode did not recruit Victor Rogozkin based on his scientific

---

[1] Letter, "Lord Killanin to Victor Rogozkin, June 4, 1976," archive collection "IOC Medical Commission," folder "Medical Commission: Correspondence January-June 1976," IOC Archive, Lausanne.

[2] MOROZOV, "Professor Victor Alekseevich Rogozkin" 379f.

[3] As in Montreal, the Organising Committee decided to install a Doping Commission for the organisation of the doping controls, headed by Victor Rogozkin, and a Medical Committee, responsible for all other medical matters.

[4] ORGANISING COMMITTEE OF THE GAMES OF THE XXIITH OLYMPIAD, *Official Report of the 1980 Olympic Games in Moscow*, Volume 1, Part 3 (Moscow: Organising Committee of the Games of the XXIIth Olympiad, 1981), 193.

knowledge. Rather, Lord Killanin accepted a suggestion of Soviet IOC member Nikolay Andrianov to replace Nina Grashinskaya with Victor Rogozkin. [5] Consequently, he was the choice of Soviet sport officials over an adoption based on the expertise that the IOC Medical Commission required. Nevertheless, his experience in doping analysis became instantly recognisable, when he challenged Arnold Beckett's "monopoly" on the conduction of the doping analysis during the 1976 Montreal Olympic Games along with his suggestion to install a scientific committee (see Chapter 4). In fact, Victor Rogozkin eventually fulfilled a double role on the IOC Medical Commission, because it did not adopt any additional representative from the Organising Committee of the 1980 Moscow Olympic Games (OCOG-80). He presented the initial draft of OCOG-80's doping control plan to the IOC Medical Commission in 1977. [6]

Besides Victor Rogozkin, two key members of the 1976 doping control team became permanently involved in the IOC Medical Commission. Carroll Laurin became its advisor to future Organising Committees. Alexandre de Mérode acknowledged that the IOC Medical Commission had "to establish not only the anti-doping control but a complete medical infrastructure." [7] Consequently, he was now beginning to distinguish actively between doping controls and other *medical* tasks. Further evidence for this is the addition of Robert Dugal to the IOC Medical Commission. He did not become a full member or advisor, but a member on a new Scientific Committee, [8] which the IOC Medical Commission officially decided to install in October 1976. [9] It was agreed that Alexandre de Mérode, Arnold Beckett, Robert Dugal, Victor Rogozkin and Albert Dirix (he was not regarded as a full member but he occupied the role of the secretary) should be on the new body. The selection of Robert Dugal was significant because he was not

---

[5] Letter, "Lord Killanin to Alexandre de Mérode, June 4, 1976," archive collection "IOC Medical Commission," folder "Correspondence January-July 1976," IOC Archive, Lausanne.

[6] Note, "Proposals on organisation of anabolic control at the Games of XXII Olympiad in Moscow, 1977," archive collection "IOC Medical Commission," folder "Correspondence 1977 – june 26, 1978," IOC Archive, Lausanne.

[7] Minutes, "Meeting of the Medical Commission of the International Olympic Committee, May 7-8, 1977," archive collection "IOC Medical Commission," folder "Meeting in Lausanne on mai 7-8," IOC Archive, Lausanne, 9.

[8] In the official documents, the body is sometimes referred to as "subcommission" and on other occasions as "committee". In order to stick with a constant approach, the term "Scientific Committee" is used in this book.

[9] Minutes, "Meeting of the Medical Commission of the International Olympic Committee, May 7-8, 1977," 10.

an official member of the IOC Medical Commission. However, the focus on doping analysis made it necessary to have more anti-doping laboratory experts on the Scientific Committee. Hence, the IOC Medical Commission adopted a former head of an Olympic anti-doping laboratory for the first time. Curiously, this was neither Manfred Donike nor Raymond Brooks, who had contributed so much to the introduction of the anabolic steroid tests. Nevertheless, the installation of the Scientific Committee definitely stands for a changed approach by Alexandre de Mérode, who started to recognise that the IOC's anti-doping initiatives needed an increased focus on technical aspects of doping analysis in order to keep up with the consumed substances.

Focus of the New Scientific Committee

The Scientific Committee met for the first time in March 1977. Because Robert Dugal and Victor Rogozkin were members, they could exchange information on the conduction of the doping controls at Olympic Games directly. This had not been the case between previous heads of laboratories. Thus, the main issues discussed at the meeting were the doping controls in Montreal, along with suggestions for the approach in Moscow. The Scientific Committee briefly discussed the problems with the sealing procedure and the members decided to put in place a new procedure at least one year ahead of the next Olympic Games. The members did not make any concrete proposal, but insisted that only one person should be responsible for the storage device of the samples.[10] Furthermore, the members discussed the problem of blood transfusion for the first time and decided to contact haematologists at the Harvard Medical School, who were studying the issue.[11] This is an interesting aspect, because the inclusion of additional substances and the introduction of testing methods was still an issue the IOC Medical Commission as a whole needed to deal with.[12] By May 1977, Robert Dugal had compiled an extensive report on the issue, where he mentioned studies on the positive effects of blood transfusion on physical work capacity,

---

[10] Minutes, "Meeting Medical Commission Scientific Committee, March 19-20, 1977," 1.

[11] Minutes, "Meeting Medical Commission Scientific Committee, March 19-20, 1977," 6.

[12] It also explains why John GLEAVES concludes that the issue of blood doping was not discussed amongst the members of the IOC Medical Commission from 1976 until 1985. John GLEAVES, "Manufactured Dope: How the 1984 US Olympic cycling team rewrote the rules on drugs in sport," *International Journal for the History of Sport* 32, no. 1 (2015), 94.

going back to the 1960s.[13] However, he concluded that there were major issues with the collection of blood samples, since athletes would oppose such a measure. Thus, he recommended a) an examination of the moral issue of blood auto-transfusion in order to find out whether it actually opposed the doping definition b) an examination of the detrimental effects of blood doping c) research to establish reliable scientific methods to detect blood doping.[14] It shows how early the IOC Medical Commission discussed blood doping although it remained unsolved for more than twenty years (see Chapter 7).

Furthermore, the Scientific Committee also made plans for two symposia on the problem of the scientific aspects of anabolic steroids. The members planned that these would take place in London in 1978 and in Moscow in 1979.[15] The intention to hold such meetings gives further proof to the increased awareness about the necessity of having more dialogue on technical anti-doping matters. Certainly, the intended topic of the symposia illustrates that these were mainly linked with the problem of anabolic steroid testing.[16] Considering the composition of the Scientific Committee, and the contributions made at the meeting, the anti-doping laboratory experts intended to use these symposia primarily to exchange information on laboratory issues and technical matters.

With doping being the predominant topic, it is unsurprising that the IOC Medical Commission mainly discussed similar issues at its meeting in May 1977. It also focused on the possible addition of several compounds to the banned list. In the cases of beta-blockers and exogenous testosterone, medical doctor Ludwig Prokop advocated not adding them to the list. He claimed to refrain from adding beta-blockers because he was of the opinion that, like tranquilisers and anti-depressants, they had no effect on performance.[17] The other members of the IOC Medical Commission partly agreed with his argument, but also asked for more studies on the issue, including the development of possible analytical methods to detect beta-blockers. In the case of exogenous testosterone, Ludwig Prokop

---

[13] In particular, Robert Dugal refers to the following study: B. GULLBRING, A. HOLMGREN, T. SJÖSTRAND and T. STRANDELL, "The Effect of Blood Volume Variations on the Pulse Rate in Supine and Upright Positions and During Exercise," *Acta Physiologica Scandinavica* 50, no. 1 (1960), 62-71.

[14] Report, "A Status Report on Blood Doping, April, 1977," archive collection "IOC Medical Commission," folder "Correspondence 1977 – june 26, 1978," IOC Archive, Lausanne, 4.

[15] Minutes, "Meeting Medical Commission Scientific Committee, March 19-20, 1977," 7.

[16] Ibid.

[17] Minutes, "Meeting of the Medical Commission of the International Olympic Committee, May 7-8, 1977," 5.

argued that it was hard to distinguish between artificial and natural testosterone.[18] Despite these reservations, Arnold Beckett reported of several studies dealing with the issue, some of them from his own institution.[19] However, because the research was expensive, he urged other laboratories to conduct studies, too. The IOC Medical Commission followed both suggestions; it did not add beta-blockers and testosterone but asked for more research.[20] Thereby it continued its strategy to only ban detectable substances.

Moreover, the influence of the anti-doping laboratory experts developed from the debates about the organisation and quality of the doping laboratories. The IOC Medical Commission discussed this issue for the first time in May 1977. It decided to test every anti-doping laboratory six months before the Olympic Games to give the laboratory staff members a feeling of security about the applied methods.[21] In addition, the members hotly debated the laboratories in the context of tests for anabolic steroids at Regional Games. Arnold Beckett was in favour of sending an observer to Regional Games to supervise the doping controls and consider establishing more laboratories worldwide.[22] He justified this with the additional sports performed at the Regional Games and the insufficient laboratory facilities. Iba Mar Diop and Eduardo Hay suggested asking Olympic Solidarity for financial support for the local organising committees. The IOC Medical Commission did not make a final decision on the issue because it wanted to await the outcome of the 79th IOC Session, of whether the IOC gave patronage to Regional Games at all. Eventually, this was the case,[23] and the IOC Medical Commission adopted the suggestion of Arnold Beckett and the Scientific Committee to have an observer at Regional Games.[24] Hence, Arnold Beckett appeared again as advocate for standardised doping controls and thereby reiterated the IAAF´s approach for IOC support in order to extend the anti-doping laboratory network.

---

[18] Ibid.

[19] Ibid., 6.

[20] Ibid.

[21] Minutes, "Meeting of the Medical Commission of the International Olympic Committee, May 7-8, 1977," 4.

[22] Ibid., 8.

[23] Minutes, "79th Session of the IOC in Prague, June 15-18, 1977," archive collection "IOC Sessions 1894-2009," IOC Archive, Lausanne, 38.

[24] Ibid., 112.

Critique on the Scientific Committee by Sport Medicine Specialists

The discussions demonstrate an inevitable need to enhance anti-doping laboratory expertise within the anti-doping efforts of the IOC Medical Commission from the 1972 Munich Olympic Games onwards. The installation of the Scientific Committee appears to be the first direct reaction to this. However, those members of the IOC Medical Commission, who were not included, did not perceive the Scientific Committee as positive and linked their critique to its focus on doping analysis.

Both Giuseppe La Cava and Ludwig Prokop raised concerns about the role of the Scientific Committee on the meeting of the IOC Medical Commission. Giuseppe La Cava criticised the composition of the Scientific Committee in particular. He believed that it should not be only composed of "pharmacologists," because the scope of the work undertaken was far more general.[25] Similarly, Ludwig Prokop showed his discontent with the fact that Arnold Beckett, on behalf of the Scientific Committee, proposed a new list of banned substances. Ludwig Prokop especially opposed the decision to include codeine, because he thought that codeine had no effect on performance.[26] Moreover, he stressed that the Scientific Committee should not make such decisions alone. This is interesting, because the IOC Medical Commission had already added codeine to the list before the 1976 Winter Olympic Games. Furthermore, Arnold Beckett had stated clearly that the drugs to be added were only proposals.[27] Finally, towards the end of the meeting, Ludwig Prokop, still dissatisfied with the dominating role of the Scientific Committee members, maintained that the Scientific Committee should be named differently, "since the Medical Commission itself was scientific."[28] Similarly, Giuseppe La Cava argued that the problems existed not only in the fields of biology and chemistry, but also in other areas. Giuseppe La Cava proposed three possible names: "Technical Commission," "Technological Commission" and "Subcommittee for Bio-analytical aspects of doping control."[29]

The proposals by the two medical doctors reveal that they felt overlooked in an area where they clearly saw their responsibility and competencies. The complaints are an interesting development because they prove the different

---

[25] Minutes, "Meeting of the Medical Commission of the International Olympic Committee, May 7-8, 1977," 4.
[26] Ibid.
[27] Ibid.
[28] Ibid., 10.
[29] Ibid., 12.

approaches to anti-doping. Anti-doping laboratory experts had lobbied for more influenced before, but now representatives of the medical profession felt ignored. The fact that the Scientific Committee was regarded important enough to discuss major issues of doping controls, but did not have discretionary competence, did aggravate the situation. It meant that issues had to be discussed twice and could only be decided through the incorporation of both medical and anti-doping laboratory experts. One example for this is the debate on blood transfusion. Whilst the IOC Medical Commission received Robert Dugal's report positively, Ludwig Prokop, in his capacity as medical doctor, was asked to compile more information on whether blood transfusions actually had a positive effect on performance.[30] Moreover, the different opinions of Arnold Beckett and Ludwig Prokop illustrate that the two individuals had different approaches to the addition of doping methods to the banned list. Whereas Ludwig Prokop regularly stated reservations about the performance-enhancing effects of certain substances and their detectability, Arnold Beckett constantly encouraged research to develop analytical methods, no matter whether the IOC Medical Commission was supportive or not. This resulted in an acceleration of many processes and was also a consequence of his involvement in many scientific fields outside sport.

In contrast to the medical experts on the IOC Medical Commission, it seems that Alexandre de Mérode began to value the additional anti-doping laboratory knowledge. He supported the Scientific Committee in his report to the IOC Session in Prague in 1977:

> Since Barcelona, two meetings have been held. The first in Brussels, attended by members of our sub-committee, consisting of Professors Beckett, Rogozkin, Dugal and Dirix. This meeting discussed a certain number of scientific problems and paved the way for the Medical Commission meeting in Lausanne. *The Brussels meeting showed how a specialized group of this kind was necessary in order to be able to cope successfully with the complexity of the problems we currently face.* Several very detailed studies are in the course of being carried out, in particular with regard to blood transfusions, blocking betas, A.C.T.H., and testosterone as well as with regard to the new methods of detection

---

[30] Minutes, "Meeting of the Medical Commission of the International Olympic Committee, May 7-8, 1977," 11.

required owing to the increasingly sophisticated nature of the substances and techniques used [emphasis added].[31]

Therefore, he acknowledged the contribution of smaller working groups for the first time. He clearly stated that the Scientific Committee was crucial in the preparation of the IOC Medical Commission meeting, and also referred to the increasing scientific nature of the doping problem. It is the beginning of a transition in Alexandre de Mérode´s attitude from considering doping controls a medical matter to seeing them more as a technical matter.

In addition, Arnold Beckett continued to push for more initiatives and changes. For example, he challenged Henry Banks in November 1977 about the delayed release of the updated list of banned substances, which the IOC Medical Commission had approved in its meeting.[32] He was concerned that the Organising Committee of the 1978 Commonwealth Games could not update its regulations. Similarly, he approached Alexandre de Mérode about the distribution of prepared urine samples to several laboratories worldwide to discover whether they could get the right testing results. He argued that it was "imperative that we have information on the matter of the ability of the laboratories to carry out the work,"[33] and wanted to send samples to the laboratory of the University of Edmonton, responsible for the tests at the Commonwealth Games. Thus, Arnold Beckett again appeared as an advocate of universal standards and regulations.

Therefore, one has to conclude that the foundation of the Scientific Committee was a turning point in the IOC´s approach to address the doping problem. Although the outcome of its meeting was in fact very limited, the acknowledgement of the need for more advice on technical matters was a new strategy. Arnold Beckett´s efforts, which he also continued in the IAAF, are one reason for this.

---

[31] Minutes, "79th Session of the IOC in Prague, June 15-18, 1977," Annex 43.

[32] Letter, "Arnold Beckett to Henry Banks, November 28, 1977," archive collection "IOC Medical Commission," folder "Correspondence 1977 – june 26, 1978," IOC Archive, Lausanne.

[33] Letter, "Arnold Beckett to Alexandre de Mérode, January 11, 1978," archive collection "IOC Medical Commission," folder "Correspondence 1977 – june 26, 1978," IOC Archive, Lausanne.

IAAF PROVIDES FRAMEWORK FOR ADVANCEMENTS OF DOPING ANALYSIS

More Involvement of Anti-doping Laboratory Experts

A detailed analysis of the IAAF Medical Committee's work between 1976 and 1980 reveals that it maintained its scientific focus. In January 1977, John Holt sent out a letter to all members of the IAAF Medical Committee and members of the IAAF Council where he included new doping regulations.[34] Although there was no official accreditation procedure in place yet, the first point under the topic "doping analysis" stated, "only accredited and by the IAAF on recommendation of the Medical Committee recognised laboratories should be used for the analysis of the samples of the doping controls."[35] Thus, the IAAF certainly considered the laboratories it recognised in 1975 (see Chapter 4) as officially "accredited."

In addition, there was a continuous strong desire within the IAAF Medical Committee to enhance its efforts in guaranteeing the reliability of doping analysis results. A key tactical move in this regard was to include Manfred Donike as official member in the IAAF Medical Commission.[36] The need to have more permanent anti-doping laboratory expertise available becomes evident with this decision, and it is an indication of the appreciation of Manfred Donike's experience in anti-doping laboratory work. Moreover, similar to the IOC, the IAAF Council decided in March 1977 to install a working group to deal with only the issue of doping controls. This new body was the IAAF Doping Subcommittee.[37] The IAAF Council envisaged two main tasks for it: sample taking and its analysis. Importantly, the decision to establish the IAAF Doping Subcommittee came on the back of a discussion within the IAAF Council about the introduction of blood sample taking. The IAAF Council members were convinced that only anti-doping laboratory experts could deal with this problem appropriately, which was not the case (see Chapter 7).[38]

---

[34] Letter, "John Holt to all Members of the IAAF Medical Committee and IAAF Council Members, January 20, 1977," archive collection "Nachlass August Kirsch," File 007 "DLV Doping 1977," CuLDA, Cologne, 5.

[35] Ibid.

[36] Letter, "John Holt to Manfred Donike "New Doping Regulations, October 26, 1976," archive collection "Nachlass August Kirsch," File 007 "DLV Doping 1977," CuLDA, Cologne.

[37] Minutes, "IAAF Council Meeting in Düsseldorf, March 18-20, 1977," archive collection "IAAF Council Meetings," IAAF Archive, Monaco, 19f.

[38] Ibid.

The IAAF Doping Subcommittee was the successor of the IAAF Working Group on Anabolic Steroids (see Chapter 4). The members on the IAAF Doping Subcommittee were Arnold Beckett, Manfred Donike, Manfred Höppner, Arne Ljungqvist and Grigory Vorobiev.[39] Similar to the Scientific Committee of the IOC Medical Commission there was consequently an insistence on having anti-doping laboratory experts on the IAAF Doping Subcommittee. However, the IAAF Doping Subcommittee did not restrict itself in dealing only with technical aspects as it had originally intended either. For example, it strongly recommended allowing codeine for therapeutic usage, while it removed exogenous testosterone and its esters from the list of banned substances. This is an extraordinary case because the IAAF Medical Committee had never decided to ban exogenous testosterone in the first place. Nevertheless, the *1977-1978 Handbook of the IAAF* included the substance, a fact that Manfred Donike pointed out.[40] He claimed that the main reason why exogenous testosterone could not be added was that it was a natural hormone, and therefore far more difficult to detect. As in the case of Arnold Beckett within the IOC, Manfred Donike appears to be well aware of the anti-doping regulations. He did not only stress that the addition of exogenous testosterone was an administrative mistake, but also outlined the scientific complications.[41] Similar to Arnold Beckett, he referred to the policy that sport organisations should only ban detectable substances.

The anti-doping bodies of the IAAF also continued to deal with the standard of the doping laboratories because of the increasing number of regional events. At the IAAF Council Meeting in March 1977, Adriaan Paulen reported about the ongoing debates in the IOC along with an agreement with Alexandre de Mérode, which foresaw doping tests at all Regional Games.[42] It triggered a debate about the need to establish more laboratories all over the world. The IAAF members Amadeo Francis (Puerto Rico) and Charles Mukora (Kenya) raised concerns over the feasibility of the agreement, and said that their respective countries could not host any athletics meeting if providing a suitable laboratory was made obligatory.[43] However, Max Danz reassured them that if there were no laboratories in the host country, a member of the IAAF Medical Committee

---

[39] Ibid.

[40] Letter, "Manfred Donike to Dr. Danz."IAAF Handbuch 1977-1978, Regel 144, March 8, 1977," archive collection "Nachlass August Kirsch," File 007 "DLV Doping 1977," CuLDA, Cologne.

[41] Ibid.

[42] Minutes, "IAAF Council Meeting in Düsseldorf, March 18-20, 1977," 18.

[43] Ibid., 20.

would collect the sample in order to take it to a recognised laboratory. IAAF general secretary John Holt also appeared concerned about the quality of the anti-doping laboratories, and noted that to his knowledge only the laboratories in Cologne, London and Rome were able to test on both stimulants and anabolic steroids. [44] Decision-making officials in the IAAF were clearly far more concerned about the laboratory issue than the IOC. Of course, this was favourable to the anti-doping laboratory experts, who could then exert influence and strengthen their position more easily.

The IAAF Doping Subcommittee, under the growing influence of Manfred Donike, adopted a pragmatic approach and came up with a concrete set of recommendations that it had made following initial meetings in 1977 and 1978. In the recommendations, it becomes obvious that the IAAF Doping Subcommittee had two priorities: a) to assure that testing would only occur to standardised analytical methods by experts within the field b) to establish testing centres in different parts of the world to ensure testing for all major sporting events.[45] Moreover, it recommended that doping controls should take place at all IAAF events. Certainly, this is unsurprising considering the set-up of the group: its members ensured that an increasing number of doping tests would be analysed in their institutions. In order to guarantee that this was possible, the IAAF Doping Subcommittee formulated the aim to install at least one anti-doping laboratory per continent.[46] Until this was achieved, a medical officer should attend the event, collect samples and submit them to one of the few approved laboratories. [47] Obviously, this meant that athletes and the public had to wait for a very long time for the results of the doping tests. However, the procedure allowed assurance that the analysis of the sample was made according to approved methods.[48] Hence, in contrast to the IOC Medical Commission, the validity of the testing results was more important than a fast publication of the results. Furthermore, the members foresaw educational activities for laboratory staff through the shipping of sample testing packs and specialist courses on doping controls. The IAAF Doping Subcommittee intended that these courses take place in London at Arnold Beckett's anti-doping laboratory.[49]

---

[44] Ibid., 21.

[45] Report, "Doping Regulations Working Group, March 13, 1978," archive collection "IAAF Medical Committee," IAAF Archive, Monaco.

[46] Ibid.

[47] Ibid.

[48] Ibid.

[49] Ibid.

The processes within the IAAF highlight the striving for more doping laboratories around the world to conduct doping tests at regional events. Without a doubt, the IAAF demanded high-quality laboratories more than the IOC at the time. Regional events such as continental athletics championships posed a challenge for the federation. The IAAF committed itself to a strict testing policy, where reliable doping tests were essential. The installation of an IAAF Doping Subcommittee on doping controls, composed of experts with experience in the conduction of doping controls, is further proof for this development. Although not directly involved in the final decision-making process, the anti-doping laboratory experts began to extend their role beyond the advisory level.

Introduction of the Official Accreditation System by the IAAF

The IAAF Council agreed to all proposals of the IAAF Doping Subcommittee unanimously in April 1978, which is additional proof that the laboratory issue was of the highest priority. Arne Ljungqvist, who eventually became the successor of Max Danz as head of the IAAF Medical Committee,[50] claimed that from the perspective of the IAAF Medical Committee, the "scarcity of laboratories" was the real problem of doping controls.[51] The IAAF even suggested that:

> Any Organising Committee, which could not provide doping control or at least arrange satisfactorily for it to be conducted in an acceptable laboratory, should not stage the Games or Championships.[52]

However, the IAAF Council regarded this proposal too unrealistic because it would have excluded a large number of countries from hosting athletics events, and the IAAF Council did not want to make themselves dependent on the pre-conditions for doping controls. Parallel, anti-doping laboratory experts thought that the IOC's efforts were too slow and preferred to take more concrete steps by themselves. In September 1978, Manfred Donike noted in a document to all members of the IAAF Doping Subcommittee, that he expected no support from the IOC Medical Commission over the installation of an accreditation system:

---

[50] Minutes, "IAAF Council Meeting in Moscow, July 19-20, 1980," archive collection "IAAF Council Meetings," IAAF Archive, Monaco, 12.

[51] Minutes, "IAAF Council Meeting in Seoul, April 14-16, 1978," archive collection "IAAF Council Meetings," IAAF Archive, Monaco, 46.

[52] Ibid.

Ausgehend von der Prämisse, daß auf internationaler Ebene es unbedingt erforderlich ist, die Arbeitsweise von Doping-Kontroll-Laboratorien zu überprüfen, erscheint es mir wesentlich, zumindest für den Bereich der IAAF, verbindliche Vorschriften über die anzuwendenden analytischen Verfahren und die Durchführung von Qualitätstests – zur Akkreditierung und zur intermittierenden Überprüfung der Arbeitsweise der Labors – auszuarbeiten. General wäre dies eine Aufgabe, die die Medizinische Kommission des IOC für alle olympischen Sportarten übernehmen könnte bzw. sollte. Da von dieser Seite zur Zeit jedenfalls, keine Hilfe auf diesem Gebiet zu erwarten ist, sollte die Subkommission Doping der Medizinischen Kommission der IAAF bis zur Frühjahrstagung in Berlin eine beschlußreife Vorlage erarbeiten (…).

[Based on the premise that it is absolutely necessary to check the quality of the doping control laboratories on the international level, it appears essential to me to develop compulsory regulations – at least within the IAAF – about the analytical procedures and the conduction of quality test for the purpose of accreditation and the intermittent check on the operating principles of the laboratories. Generally, the IOC Medical Commission can and should take over this task for all Olympic sports. However, one cannot expect support in this area from it now and therefore the doping subcommittee of the IAAF Medical Committee should work on decision-making recommendations until its meeting in Berlin in spring (…).][53]

Manfred Donike clearly was a strong advocate of the introduction for an accreditation system for anti-doping laboratories. He was aware that this would bring financial and reputational advantages to the leading institutions such as his own. However, he did not expect support from the IOC Medical Commission, of which he was not a member. This clearly points to the difficulties in the system but also to the intention to achieve more inclusion of anti-doping laboratory experts in the anti-doping bodies of international sports organisations.

In his note, Manfred Donike presented the individual technical standards a laboratory was required to have.[54] This must be considered the first attempt to

---

[53] Note, "Manfred Donike - Standardisierung von Qualitätstests und von den analytischen Verfahren für Doping-Kontroll-Laboratorien," archive collection "Nachlass August Kirsch," File 101 "Doping (1)," CuLDA, Cologne.
[54] Ibid.

draft a concrete proposal of an accreditation process for anti-doping laboratories. Significantly, the IAAF Doping Subcommittee discussed his proposed guidelines at a subsequent meeting in Cologne in 1979.[55] Despite some minor amendments, the proposal was accepted and put forward to the meeting of the IAAF Medical Committee in East Berlin in March 1979.[56] There, it unanimously accepted the "Requirements for Accreditation – Standardization of Analytical Procedures and Quality-Test for Doping Control Laboratories".[57] The requirements contained four main aspects: (1) Essential Equipment (2) Analytical Procedures (3) Accreditation of Analytical Laboratories (4) Cost of Accreditation.[58] Despite the obvious requirement to do GC, TLC and MS, it is important to mention that the first accreditation scheme also included a reaccreditation process. Therein, laboratories were required to analyse six control samples every two years in order to prove a consistency in the quality of its testing.[59] However, the original analytical method to detect anabolic steroids with RI was not made compulsory, because the IAAF Doping Subcommittee members believed it to be unreliable. One can link this to the influence of Manfred Donike, for whom MS was the preferred screening method. In addition to fulfilling the requirements, the laboratories also had to complete a questionnaire for the IAAF headquarters in London.[60] This was necessary so laboratories could officially apply for IAAF accreditation. Clearly, the accreditation process reflects the institutional influence of the IAAF Doping Subcommittee and the personal influence of Manfred Donike.

From this stage onwards, it was the task of the IAAF Doping Subcommittee, and not the IAAF Medical Committee, to handle all organisational and scientific issues. This is evidence for the significance of the body and a considerable

---

[55] Letter, "Manfred Donike to August Kirsch, Ausstattung von analytischen Laboratorien für Doping-Kontrollen, Anforderung für die Akkreditierung durch die IAAF, February 9, 1979," archive collection "Nachlass August Kirsch," File 101 "Doping (1)," CuLDA, Cologne.

[56] Letter, "Manfred Donike to August Kirsch, Aktennotiz Donike bzgl. Tagung der Medizinischen Kommission, Ost-Berlin, March 29, 1979," archive collection "Nachlass August Kirsch," File 101 "Doping (1)," CuLDA, Cologne.

[57] Minutes, "IAAF Council Meeting in Dakar, April 26-28, 1979," archive collection "IAAF Council Meetings," IAAF Archive, Monaco, 26.

[58] Circular Note, "IAAF Medical Commission, Anti Doping Control. The Standardization of Analytical Procedures and Quality Tests for Doping Control Laboratories," archive collection "IAAF Medical Committee," IAAF Archive, Monaco.

[59] Ibid.

[60] Ibid.

expansion of the administrative tasks for its members. From a practical and organisational point of view, it is necessary to emphasise that to obtain official accreditation, the laboratory teams of Manfred Donike and/or Arnold Beckett prepared urine samples with banned substances, and sent them to the laboratories.[61] Hence, the two occupied a central role in the accreditation process. The samples had then to be correctly analysed in the presence of a member of the IAAF Doping Subcommittee.

The IAAF Council, at its meeting in April 1979, accepted the official accreditation procedure. [62] Interestingly, the acceptance of the official accreditation procedure had an immediate effect on the willingness by different countries to get a laboratory accredited. Kenyan IAAF Council member Charles Mukora, who had expressed that there was no suitable laboratory in his country in a previous meeting, now stated that he wanted to certify an institution in Nairobi immediately.[63] Similarly, Admiral Pedro Galvez from Peru also expressed his desire to get an accreditation for an anti-doping laboratory in Lima.[64] In both cases, the IAAF Medical Committee prepared the accreditation process.[65]

The IAAF granted only five laboratories official accreditation until the 1980 Moscow Olympic Games. These were the testing centres in Cologne (headed by Manfred Donike), Kreischa (GDR, headed by Dr. Claus Clausnitzer and linked closely to Manfred Höppner, see Chapter 6), Leningrad (USSR, headed by Victor Rogozkin), London (headed by Arnold Beckett) and Montreal (headed by Robert Dugal). The accreditation of these institutions was a result of the representation of their heads in the IOC and the IAAF, and their already existing involvement in international doping controls. Thus, the most influential heads of anti-doping laboratories had essentially created an accreditation procedure for their own category of institutions. Clearly, this brought two advantages. First, with the knowledge that their own anti-doping laboratories would meet the criteria, but others might struggle, they created a monopoly for doping analysis. Second, they legitimised the existence of their institutions and profited from the financial rewards that resulted from it. At the end of the 1970s, the number of doping controls increased. The Cologne laboratory, for example, reported an increase of

---

[61] Ibid.

[62] Minutes, "IAAF Council Meeting in Dakar, April 26-28, 1979," 26.

[63] Ibid.

[64] Ibid.

[65] Ibid.

78.6% from 1977 to 1979.[66] This was an intended benefit for the anti-doping
laboratory experts´ efforts in the IAAF as they evidently encountered more
opposition in the IOC Medical Commission.

The IAAF Congress discussed the need for more laboratories in 1980. Some
IAAF members argued that the few accredited laboratories could not conduct all
the doping analysis for every competition within athletics.[67] New rules and
regulations could only be adopted if the experts could assure that the testing
procedures were reliable, and the laboratories had enough capacity to conduct all
the planned tests. John Holt stressed this, when stating, "with the expansion of the
Laboratory Accreditation Programme the possibility of greater testing became
more likely."[68] Thus, the IAAF Doping Subcommittee and the IAAF Medical
Committee discussed further applications for accreditation in July 1980.
Numerous laboratories had applied for accreditation, but the Committee decided
to focus on the accreditation of laboratories in Australia, Bulgaria,
Czechoslovakia, France, Italy (Rome), Sweden (Stockholm), Switzerland
(Magglingen), USA and Yugoslavia.[69] At the same meeting, it becomes apparent
that the introduction of the accreditation procedure did not have the desired effect
for sport administrators´ trust in the doping controls. Previously in 1978, there
had been five positive doping tests at the Balkan Games, the European Cup Semi-
Final and the European Junior Championships.[70] According to IAAF rules, this
would have normally resulted in an 18-month ban. However, after a lengthy
discussion at the IAAF Council Meeting in March 1980, the IAAF reduced the
ban so the athletes could take part at the 1980 Moscow Olympic Games.[71] The
arguments brought forward by the IAAF Council members focused on flaws in
the sampling procedures along with language problems. The most opposition
against this decision voiced Arne Ljungqvist, who believed that the decision was
a "slap in the face of sporting and scientific experts who are now making a
common effort to solve the problem of doping."[72] He felt that through a reduction
of the ban, the IAAF undermined its own anti-doping regulations. Thereby, he

---

[66] Report, "Jahresstatistik 1988 by Manfred Donike, January 26, 1989," archive collection
"Nachlass August Kirsch," File 89 "Doping (6)," CuLDA, Cologne.

[67] Minutes, 32nd Congress of the IAAF in Moscow, 1980," archive collection "IAAF
Congresses," IAAF Archive, Monaco, 14.

[68] Ibid.

[69] Minutes, "Meeting of the Medical Committee of the IAAF, July 17, 1980," 2.

[70] Ibid.

[71] Minutes, "IAAF Council Meeting in Paris, March 10-12, 1980," archive collection
"IAAF Council Meetings," IAAF Archive, Monaco, 17ff.

[72] Ibid., 20.

reiterated the disapproval by the anti-doping laboratory experts, who thought that the IAAF Council were counteracting their efforts. For example, Manfred Donike hoped, "political discussions in Council could be avoided. If the laboratory confirmed positive cases, that should be accepted without further discussion and the penalty applied automatically". [73] According to him, a positive test was evidence enough for a violation of the anti-doping rules.[74] Arnold Beckett also voiced his concern about the decision,[75] and consequently the IAAF Medical Committee included the following statement into the medical report to the IAAF Congress:

> The Committee extends to the IAAF Council its appreciation of the Council's strong efforts to conduct and increase Doping Controls in the past two years. In the light of the Council's policy to fight against the abuse of drugs in athletics, the Committee finds it all the more regrettable that the Council took a decision in March 1980 to reinstate 5 women athletes from July 1st onwards. This meant a period of only 10 months ineligibility, whereas the Doping Regulations approved by the Puerto Rico Congress call for a minimum Suspension of 18 months. The Committee asks the Council in future not to repeat a deviation from the Doping Regulations, since these form the basis for the Committee's work.[76]

The controversy demonstrates that the belief (that the introduction of an accreditation procedure would reduce the political discussions) was naïve. Although the delegations of the positive tested athletes emphasised that there were no doubts about the validity of the doping analysis,[77] there were loopholes for officials and athletes. With the implementation of a strict doping policy, the anti-doping laboratory experts were still very much dependent on the decision-makers within the IAAF. At the same time, however, the complaint by the IAAF Medical Committee shows that the experts felt undermined by sport

---

[73] Letter, "Manfred Donike to August Kirsch, Aufhebung der Sperren durch die IAAF Resolution der Medizinischen Kommission der IAAF [Resolution der Medizinischen Kommission der IAAF], August 12, 1980," archive collection "Nachlass August Kirsch," File 101 "Doping (1)," CuLDA, Cologne.

[74] Ibid.

[75] Minutes, "Meeting of the Medical Committee of the IAAF, July 17, 1980," 3.

[76] Ibid.

[77] Minutes, "IAAF Council Meeting in Paris, March 10-12, 1980," archive collection "IAAF Council Meetings," IAAF Archive, Monaco, 18.

administrators. The anti-doping laboratory experts in particular were aware about
the reliance of the entire world of sport on their work, and thus attempted to
increase the pressure on the IAAF Council with their statement. In fact, the
testing policy was only feasible when anti-doping laboratories were available.
Arne Ljungqvist highlighted this in his report to the IAAF Council in June 1980:

> Our Doping Control experts from the Medical Committee had been
> upset by the action. He agreed with the President that the chemists were
> not there to decide the punishment, but if their help was not appreciated
> they could withdraw this and devote their time and energy elsewhere.[78]

Thereby, although not an anti-doping laboratory expert himself, Arne Ljungqvist
showed understanding for their importance, and attempted to increase the
pressure on the IAAF Council to apply stricter rules. Moreover, the statement
carries the implicit threat that the anti-doping laboratory experts could refrain
from working with sport organisations, whilst also acknowledging that the
decision-making body was still the IAAF Council. From the subsequent
discussion amongst the IAAF Council members, it evolves that they were clearly
worried about losing cooperation with the anti-doping laboratory experts.[79] The
IAAF Council accepted a proposal by John Holt to approve a paper on the
IAAF's fight against doping, and more recent developments, such as the
introduction of the laboratory accreditation procedure.[80] Clearly, it wanted to
demonstrate to the IAAF Congress, but also to the anti-doping laboratory experts
its willingness to combat doping. At the same time, the controversy indicates the
emerging conflicts between anti-doping laboratory experts and sport
administrators (see Chapter 7).

It is important at this stage to summarise the processes within the IAAF, and
their meaning for the involvement of anti-doping laboratory experts, due to their
wide-reaching effects and at the time, unique character. Following the 1976
Montreal Olympic Games, the IAAF Medical Committee continued its policy to
include chemical experts onto the body and to grant responsibility of the
development of the doping controls to a small working group. This led to the
establishment of the permanent IAAF Doping Subcommittee, in which Manfred
Donike was included as a full member from late 1976. Under his guidance, the

---

[78] Minutes, "IAAF Council Meeting in Rome, June 7-8, 1980," archive collection "IAAF
Council Meetings," IAAF Archive, Monaco, 29.
[79] Ibid.
[80] Ibid.

body pushed for an enhanced network of anti-doping laboratories so doping tests could take place at all IAAF events. The IAAF Doping Subcommittee pursued the strict policy to have doping tests conducted only in appropriate laboratories. In order to do so, the group was prepared to contribute to the development of doping laboratories worldwide, in terms of education, accreditation and administration. The IAAF Council, who recognised the need for reliable doping controls due to increasing complaints about positive results, supported the IAAF Doping Subcommittee. With the decision to have doping tests only analysed in officially certified doping laboratories, the anti-doping laboratory experts made themselves irreplaceable in the IAAF's attempts to combat doping. Consequently, it was necessary to address the processes that led to an official IAAF laboratory accreditation procedure in so much detail.

In addition, the developments in the IAAF also reveal changes on the individual level, because Manfred Donike became the main force behind the accreditation process. Manfred Donike had drafted this document because he had doubts about the efficiency of the IOC Medical Commission. Hence, one can compare his role in the IAAF from 1977 onwards to the dominant role that Arnold Beckett occupied in the IOC Medical Commission. There is no doubt that Manfred Donike had an immediate impact. It also explains why Arnold Beckett seems to be less central when contributing to the IAAF. Simultaneously, the close work on the IAAF also enabled them to create a better network, therefore benefiting from the increasingly better possibilities within their own institutions.

ANTI-DOPING LABORATORY NETWORK DEVELOPS BY INCREASED COOPERATION

Creation of Institutional Requirements for More Doping Controls

The processes, leading to the choice of Manfred Donike and his laboratory in Cologne to become the official anti-doping laboratory for the 1972 Munich Olympic Games, have already been discussed in Chapter 3. After the Olympic Games, the BMI and the BISp maintained their decision to install a central institution for doping analysis in the FRG, although most national federations lacked interest in the issue.[81] In summer 1974, Manfred Donike officially signed a contract to become "Commissioner for Doping Analysis" of the BISp.[82] At this

---

[81] KRÜGER et al., *Doping und Anti-Doping*, 76.
[82] Letter, "August Kirsch to Presidents of National Federations, February 27, 1976," BISp-Archive, Bonn.

point, Manfred Donike was still working at the Biochemical Institute of the University of Cologne. After receiving the *venia legendi* (habilitation) in 1975,[83] he moved to the DSHS to head the Biochemical Department of the Institute of Cardiology and Sports Medicine. The initiatives to install such an institute reached back to the rectorship of Wildor Hollmann, who already in 1969, had expected, "the scale of possibilities to artificially enhance performance will increase significantly."[84] This was clearly a visionary but realistic statement at the time. However, according to his own statement, Wildor Hollmann was mainly interested in the effect of performance on catecholamines, and not in doping controls.[85] Once the anti-doping laboratory moved to the new facilities of the DSHS in 1980, organisational tasks became considerably easier for Manfred Donike because the BISp was also located at the DSHS. Earlier, he had still complained about the necessity to extend the doping analysis measures in terms of staff and equipment.[86] Therefore, Wildor Hollmann requested for the installation of an independent Institute for Biochemistry, which was eventually accepted.[87]

KRÜGER et al. also acknowledge the establishment of the central doping control laboratory, and maintain that it proved to be an important step for the FRG's anti-doping policy.[88] It enabled the sport in the FRG to test with reliable and uniform methods, whilst simultaneously conducting research on analytical procedures. The research aspect was especially important to Manfred Donike. He had realised from a very early stage that there was a constant development within the used substances, so the success of the anti-doping policy depended largely on the development of new, reliable and universal analytical procedures. This was one of his main arguments for remaining at a university location. It allowed him to conduct further research, and not solely to focus on the execution of the doping controls by himself. It is important to emphasise that Manfred Donike also

---

[83] Curriculum Vitae, "Manfred Donike," BISp-Archive, Bonn.

[84] Wildor HOLLMANN, "Sporthochschule – Heute und Morgen," in: *Dokumente zur Gründung und zum Aufbau einer wissenschaftlichen Hochschule auf dem Gebiete des Sports*, ed. Dietrich R. QUANZ (Cologne: Wienand, 1982), 121.

[85] Svenja THYSSEN, *Manfred Donike und das Institut für Biochemie der Deutschen Sporthochschule Köln - Geschichte und Leistung im Kampf gegen Doping*, diploma thesis, Deutsche Sporthochschule Köln, 6.

[86] Report, "Manfred Donike, Ausbau der Dopinganalytik an der Universität Köln in Kooperation mit der DSHS," January, 1979, " archive collection "Nachlass August Kirsch, File 101 "Doping (1)," CuLDA, Cologne, 1.

[87] HOLLMANN and TITTEL, *Geschichte*, 66.

[88] KRÜGER et al., *Doping und Anti-Doping*, 77.

occupied advisory roles in several national anti-doping commissions along with fulfilling organisational tasks in his role as the "Commissioner for Doping Analysis." Similar to the Scientific Commission of the IOC Medical Commission, he did not restrict himself to only dealing with doping analysis. Amongst his tasks, he compiled statistics about the situation of doping controls in the FRG, which he sent to August Kirsch annually from 1976 onwards.[89]

Manfred Donike regularly engaged on the international level as well, since he was trying to exchange knowledge with other anti-doping laboratory experts on a constant basis. For example, he did not refrain from sending letters to the IOC Medical Commission, enquiring about new developments on anabolic steroid testing that he had read about in a German newspaper.[90] His frustration with the IOC Medical Commission originated from these exchanges. Apart from the international contributions on the personal level, there was also increased cooperation on the institutional level between anti-doping laboratories and their staff members to ensure the reliability of the doping controls. Between 1976 and 1980, there are several examples, mainly instigated by the decision of the IAAF Medical Commission, to appoint medical delegates for preparing and supervising doping controls. In the majority of the cases, the medical delegates were Arnold Beckett, Manfred Höppner and Manfred Donike. The latter also supervised the doping controls at the 1978 European Athletics Championships in Prague.[91] For the preparations, he visited the competition sites and the selected laboratory in Prague twice, but also announced that Dr. Jan Chundela, the medical doctor in charge at the event, should visit the Cologne laboratory with staff members for one week for educational purposes.[92] Importantly, the conducted controls in Prague led to five positive cases on the anabolic steroid nandrolone.[93] There had been a sixth positive sample but it had stemmed from Manfred Donike himself, who wanted to assure the validity of the tests.[94] Despite the involvement of

---

[89] Letter, "Manfred Donike to August Kirsch, Situation der Dopingkontrollen bei den deutschen Fachverbänden, December 7, 1976, "archive collection "Nachlass August Kirsch," File 091 "Doping von 1968 - 1977," CuLDA, Cologne.

[90] Minutes, "Meeting of the Medical Commission of the International Olympic Committee, May 7-8, 1977," 2.

[91] Minutes, "IAAF Council Meeting in Dakar, April 26-28, 1979," archive collection "IAAF Council Meetings," 26.

[92] Letter, „Manfred Donike to August Kirsch, Dopingkontrolle Prag [Bericht der Medizinischen Kommission der IAAF], October 17, 1978," archive collection "Nachlass August Kirsch," File 101 "Doping (1)," CuLDA, Cologne, 1.

[93] Ibid., 4.

[94] Ibid.

Manfred Donike however, there were complaints by the delegations of athletes who tested positive. As in previous cases, these complaints focused on possible flaws in the sampling procedures, whereas officials stressed that the doping analysis produced the correct result. This attitude, to be found in almost all official complaints about positive results at the time, Manfred Donike described, "known scheme: no doubts on the analytical results, but doubts the control procedure." [95] Obviously, individuals within sport increasingly accepted the analytical procedures, but it also reflects how the anti-doping laboratory experts had no control over the correct sampling procedure. The delegations seemed to be well aware of this and sought the possibility to criticise this aspect. Consequently, the activities that took place also in Cologne had an impact on the entire world of sport. The increased efforts to improve anti-doping laboratories and to educate its staff members all over the world resulted in the growing belief in the results of the doping analysis. Moreover, the fact that the DSHS even established an own institute accounts for the increasing reputation of doping analysis amongst academics from within the field of sport.

Common Efforts to Educate and Equip Laboratories

Preparations for the 1980 Winter Olympic Games in Lake Placid

Not only the laboratory in Cologne cooperated closely with other institutions and attempted to inform about the standards of the IAAF Medical Committee. The INRS also undertook considerable efforts in the preparation of the doping controls for the 1980 Winter Olympic Games. In fact, the Organising Committee of the 1980 Winter Olympic Games in Lake Placid (LPOOC) had decided to use the equipment and the staff of the INRS for the doping analysis. Dr. Georges Hart, the chair of the Medical Services and representative of LPOOC on the IOC Medical Commission,[96] based this decision on the experience of the INRS, their validity and the close proximity between the two cities of Lake Placid and Montreal.[97] Consequently, the INRS became the first institution to conduct the doping analysis at two subsequent Olympic Games, and LPOOC profited greatly

---

[95] Ibid., 5.

[96] ORGANISING COMMITTEE OF THE XXIIITH OLYMPIC WINTER GAMES, *Official Report of the XIIIth Olympic Winter Games in Lake Placid 1980* (Lake Placid: Organising Committee of the XXIIIth Olympic Winter Games, 1980), 186.

[97] The distance between the City of Montreal and Lake Placid is less than 200 miles. Individual Minutes, "Meetings of the IOC Medical Commission in Lake Placid, June 17-19, 1978," archive collection "IOC Medical Commission," folder "Medical Commission: Meeting in Lake Placid 1978," IOC Archive, Lausanne, 3.

from the advanced technologies and experienced staff. Nevertheless, Georges Hart still suggested setting up and maintaining regional laboratories around the world because "it will become very difficult for future cities to select facilities to run the program."[98] One main reason for this was the rising costs for the doping controls, caused by the increasing number of substances on the banned list. Georges Hart explained that each doping test cost $800.[99] Whereas some members of the IOC Medical Commission subsequently proposed to reduce the number of tests, Arnold Beckett and Robert Dugal defended the high costs. The heads of anti-doping laboratories did not want a reduction of doping tests or costs because their institutions profited financially from it. This money could eventually be invested into new research as confirmed by Michel Bertrand and Robert Dugal. They stated that the technical equipment was not that costly, but research for new compounds was.[100] Eventually, the IOC Medical Commission agreed with this argument whilst confirming that the main aim was to protect the health of the athletes.[101] Thus, it regarded a potential reduction of the number of tests a "crime",[102] which would not lead to a considerable reduction of the costs anyway. Clearly, the anti-doping laboratory experts enforced their demands concerning the argument.

Despite the experience of the INRS and Robert Dugal, the laboratory was still dependent on the cooperation with other institutions in the preparation of the doping controls as the complications shortly before the competitions reveal. Raymond Brooks, and his team from the St. Thomas Hospital, still produced the 17-α-methyl and 19-nortestosterone labels and antisera, which were necessary for the conduction of the anabolic steroid test for all anti-doping laboratories worldwide (see Chapter 4). However, they had technical difficulties in the synthezisation process in January 1980 and provided the label H^3 instead.[103] As reported by Robert Dugal, the new label required entirely different technical equipment (precisely a liquid scintillation counter), and Raymond Brooks was not

---

[98] Ibid.

[99] Ibid., 15.

[100] Ibid., 5.

[101] Minutes, "Meetings of the IOC Medical Commission in Lake Placid, June 17-19, 1978," archive collection "IOC Medical Commission," folder "Medical Commission: Meeting in Lake Placid 1978," IOC Archive, Lausanne, 8.

[102] Ibid.

[103] Individual Minutes, "Meetings of the IOC Medical Commission in Lake Placid, June 17-19, 1978," 5.

available to instruct the application of the new method.[104] Robert Dugal described that after considerable efforts, he found a scintillation counter at the Trudeau Biological Research Centre at Saranac Lake, and that the laboratory staff members undertook crash tests to use the new label. He argued that, "this incidentally requires testing actual biological samples, defining detection limits, testing for biological background noise and determining cross-reactivity potential with other steroids."[105] Only a very short period was available to this in order to be prepared for the start of testing at the Olympic Games. The detailed descriptions and the wording in the document, reveals that the scientific setting of the INRS once again proved to be crucial: Robert Dugal had all of the biological and chemical experts at his institution to train the laboratory staff members dealing with the new equipment.[106] At the same time, it demonstrates the interdependency of doping analysis on the London anti-doping laboratory.

The IOC Medical Commission accepted the laboratory in October 1979, based on the official accreditation of the INRS through the IAAF and the conduction of additional ad-hoc excretion experiments.[107] Thus, in contrast to previous Olympic Games, the IOC Medical Commission did not undertake detailed quality assurance by itself. One can relate this to the experience of the laboratory staff and the involvement of Robert Dugal. Furthermore, the IOC indirectly integrated the IAAF laboratory standards, clearly a first step towards acknowledgment of the accreditation procedure.

Preparations for the 1980 Moscow Olympic Games

The integration of the anti-doping laboratory experts and the IAAF standards becomes evident in the preparation and approval process of the anti-doping laboratory for the 1980 Moscow Olympic Games as well. Importantly, in Victor Rogozkin, the OCOG-80 had a representative on the IOC Medical Commission. He made the first proposal on the doping controls in 1977, when he outlined all the technical details to the IOC Medical Commission in a written report.[108] He anticipated that laboratory staff from the IAAF-accredited institution in

---

[104] Letter, "Robert Dugal to Alexandre de Mérode, February 12, 1980," archive collection "IOC Medical Commission," folder "Medical Commission: Correspondence january-june 1980," IOC Archive, Lausanne.

[105] Ibid.

[106] Ibid.

[107] Minutes, "Meetings of the IOC Medical Commission, October 8-12, 1979," archive collection "IOC Medical Commission," folder "Meeting in Moscow on October 8-12, 1979," IOC Archive, Lausanne, 3.

[108] Minutes, "Meeting Medical Commission Scientific Committee, March 19-20, 1977," 5.

Leningrad conducted the tests. They would be working in Moscow with the same equipment. Viktor Rogozkin foresaw testing anabolic steroids only with the RI method.[109] If there was a positive test, would the analysis of the second sample be done with GC and MS.[110] In order to do so, one of the main proposed research projects included the development of a RI method, which would enable to analyse for the presence of anabolic steroids within eight hours. [111] This became necessary, because the IOC Executive Board, on the back of the controversies following the 1976 Montreal Olympic Games, had decided that all doping control processes should be finished by the end of the Olympic Games. [112] However, written exchanges between Manfred Donike and Victor Rogozkin show that the latter was not able to conduct research and install doping tests for anabolic steroids independently. In October 1977, Victor Rogozkin had approached Manfred Donike, via Wildor Hollmann, to get support.[113] He was particularly interested in getting information on the GC-MS methods and the available steroids to educate staff members. According to Victor Rogozkin, Soviet companies could not produce these.[114] Manfred Donike showed his support, and provided Victor Rogozkin with a detailed list of the available anabolic steroids in Europe and informed him about the equipment used. [115] Curiously, Manfred Donike also voiced his concern about the preparations in a letter to Willi Daume, IOC member of the FRG. He expressed that the many questions, which Victor Rogozkin had sent him, displayed a high degree of insecurity.[116] Manfred Donike mainly considered the RI method outdated. Although there is no proof for further communication between Victor Rogozkin and Manfred Donike, the approach demonstrates that direct support between heads of anti-doping laboratories was now increasing. Correspondence did not necessarily take place via the IOC Medical Commission anymore.

---

[109] Ibid.

[110] Ibid., 6.

[111] Ibid.

[112] Minutes, "Executive Board, October 13-17, 1976," 32.

[113] Letter, "Manfred Donike to Victor Rogozkin, October 24, 1977," archive collection "Nachlass August Kirsch," File 101 "Doping (1)," CuLDA, Cologne.

[114] Letter, "Victor Rogozkin to Manfred Donike, November 24, 1977," archive collection "Nachlass August Kirsch," File 101 "Doping (1)," CuLDA, Cologne.

[115] Ibid.

[116] Letter, "Manfred Donike to Willi Daume, December 22, 1977," archive collection "Nachlass August Kirsch," File 101 "Doping (1)," CuLDA, Cologne.

The laboratory successfully underwent its pre-games test analysis procedure ahead of the Games on July 9, 1980.[117] Importantly, Manfred Donike undertook the test according to the IAAF standards, meaning that he prepared and supervised the analysis of the ten control urine samples. The IOC reported about the successful control tests in a press release on July 14, 1980.[118] In the announcement, the IOC Medical Commission claimed to have undertaken the final control by itself. However, whereas it is correct that the official request to test the anti-doping laboratory came from Alexandre de Mérode, it is significant that Manfred Donike approved the laboratory according to the official IAAF accreditation procedure. In fact, the control samples even had an official IAAF stamp.[119] One has to consider this as further acknowledgement of the IAAF accreditation procedure.

On the individual level, the accreditation procedure is an indication for the increasing influence of Manfred Donike, due to his role in the development of the GC-MS method and as main person behind the IAAF accreditation procedure. His appointment is an indirect approval of his expertise in these fields. Nevertheless, in 1976 it would have been unimaginable that a person outside the IOC Medical Commission would supervise the final check of an Olympic anti-doping laboratory. This demonstrates that the significance of his scientific work and knowledge had increased considerably through his involvement in the IAAF. Especially since there was no real expert for GC-MS on the IOC Medical Commission, he increasingly began to fill this role.

Because of their gaining influence, the CoE also took notice of the anti-doping laboratory experts in the late 1970s. George Walker, general secretary of the CoE's Committee for the Development of Sport (CDDS), wrote to Arnold

---

[117] Report, "The results of the analysis of the IOC Medical Commission control samples, carried out by Doping Laboratory of the Organising Committee 'Olympiad 80' by Victor Rogozkin," archive collection "Summer and Winter Olympic Games: Medical Files," folder "Medical matters at the 1980 Summer Olympic Games in Moscow: Correspondence," IOC Archive, Lausanne.

[118] Press Release, "Dope Control Laboratory, July 14, 1980," archive collection "Summer and Winter Olympic Games: Medical Files," folder "Medical matters at the 1980 Summer Olympic Games in Moscow: Correspondence," IOC Archive, Lausanne.

[119] Report, "The results of the analysis of the IOC Medical Commission control samples, carried out by Doping Laboratory of the Organising Committee 'Olympiad 80' by Victor Rogozkin."

Beckett in June 1979.[120] He explained that although the CoE's fight against doping was based on ethical reasons, he shared Arnold Beckett's opinion that doping controls should be pragmatic and practical. One can relate his approach to the CoE's "Recommendation No. R(79)8" on doping in sport. The 1978 Ministerial Conference had prompted this recommendation, which stressed the need for more standardised anti-doping laboratories and training for laboratory staff members in Europe.[121] Importantly, in a letter to Manfred Donike, George Walker noted his desire to arrange the meeting in Cologne, to discuss arrangements for testing substances in anti-doping laboratories and for training laboratory staff from other countries.[122] Regarding the nature of his requests, it seems reasonable to address anti-doping laboratory experts.

Finally, one has to highlight the acknowledgment of sport organisations of the role of the anti-doping laboratory experts in the preparation of the doping controls for the 1980 Moscow Olympic Games. The IAAF Medical Committee officially thanked Arnold Beckett and Manfred Donike for their support.[123] A press release of the Organising Committee specifically named the support of Manfred Donike, Arnold Beckett and Robert Dugal: "Both the recommendations of the IOC Medical Commission and the experience of famous scientists in the field of doping control of athletes A. Beckett, P. Dugal, M. Donike were taken into account at the equipment of the centre."[124] Considering Victor Rogozkin's complaint during the 1976 Montreal Olympic Games, that Arnold Beckett solely made all decisions and preparations (see Chapter 4), this appears not to be the case in 1980 because of the increasing involvement of Manfred Donike. Importantly, there is further evidence for the increasing exchange of information on scientific aspects of the doping controls. As intended by the Scientific

---

[120] Letter, "George Walker to Arnold Beckett, June 29, 1979," archive collection "IOC Medical Commission," folder "Medical Commission: Correspondence January-may 1979," IOC Archive, Lausanne.

[121] HOULIHAN, *Dying*, 159.

[122] Letter, "George Walker to Manfred Donike, October 23, 1980," archive collection "IOC Medical Commission," folder "Medical Commission: Correspondence July-December 1980," IOC Archive, Lausanne.

[123] Minutes, "IAAF Medical Committee Meeting, July 17, 1980," archive collection "Nachlass August Kirsch," File 101 "Doping (1)," CuLDA, Cologne.

[124] Press Release, "Information on the work of the Antidoping Center during the Games of the Olympiad XXII, July 15, 1980," archive collection "Summer and Winter Olympic Games: Medical Files," folder "Medical Commission matters at the 1980 Olympic Games in Moscow: Reports and minutes of the IOC Medical Commission," IOC Archive, Lausanne.

Committee, an international symposium for doping controls was held in Moscow in October 1979. Although the conference proceedings are not available in full, there is evidence for presentations of Manfred Donike, Arnold Beckett and Robert Dugal.[125] Certainly, the staging of the conference confirms the ongoing processes of the profile change of Olympic anti-doping towards more involvement of anti-doping laboratory experts. One hoped to achieve even more reliable analytical results for an increased set of substances, which served their own interest.

PUSH FOR IOC ACCREDITATION SYSTEM AND FOUNDATION OF A NEW SUBCOMMISSION TO REPRESENT ANTI- DOPING LABORATORY EXPERTS

The IAAF and individuals on the IAAF Doping Subcommittee became increasingly dominant in anti-doping politics because of its accreditation procedure. However, despite their involvement in the IAAF, Manfred Donike and Arnold Beckett felt that the IOC Medical Commission was the appropriate body for laboratory accreditation. Arnold Beckett in particular pushed for changes in the IOC. Informed about the efforts in the IAAF through Arnold Beckett, Lord Killanin made an enquiry with Alexandre de Mérode about the possibility to install "certain [doping control] centres on a continental basis."[126] At the time, Alexandre de Mérode rejected this and reasoned that the IOC did not have sufficient financial resources to accredit laboratories.[127] However, Arnold Beckett was insistent about the matter. In a memorandum sent to Lord Killanin and Alexandre de Mérode, he increased the pressure on the IOC to become active. He emphasised the efforts of the IAAF and confirmed that this task should be controlled by the IOC in order to impose an accreditation procedure also to other IFs:

---

[125] One can find several references from the Congress proceedings in a publication by Victor Rogozkin on anabolic steroids: Victor ROGOZKIN. *Metabolism of Anabolic Androgenic Steroids* (Boca Raton: CRC Press, 1991), 178ff.

[126] Letter, "Lord Killanin to Alexandre de Mérode, May 1, 1978," archive collection "IOC Medical Commission," folder "Medical Commission: Correspondence 1977 - june 26, 1978," IOC Archive, Lausanne.

[127] Letter, "Alexandre de Mérode to Lord Killanin, October 15, 1979," archive collection "IOC Medical Commission," folder "Medical Commission: Correspondence June - December 1979," IOC Archive, Lausanne.

Doping control involves not only the sampling of the athlete and the control of samples but also complex and sometimes highly sophisticated methods of analysis.

It is important to use laboratories for testing which have demonstrated their competence in dope control. It is essential to have the appropriate apparatus and staff as well as the appropriate reference compounds. Furthermore the staff should have gained experience on the determination of drugs and metabolites after examples of the banned classes of drugs have been given to man.

The IAAF have recognised this problem and have now commenced an accreditation system for laboratories. This is a demanding but fair procedure. However other federations are not so advanced in their control measures and there is a danger that innocent people could be disqualified because laboratories are being used which are not really competent in doping control.

I suggest that the I.O.C. Medical Commission now proceeds to lead and help the international federations in dope control not only at the Olympic Games but between the Games. It is essential that continued research is carried out in the field of doping controls and this necessitates co-ordination at international level. Also the I.O.C. Medical Commission should be in a position to give continued guidance and leadership and come to the aid of international federations as required.[128]

Arnold Beckett attempted to persuade Lord Killanin and Alexandre de Mérode by building on their main fields of interest. One the one hand, he tried to make clear to Alexandre de Mérode that the IOC Medical Commission was not leading the fight against doping anymore. Due to the introduced accreditation procedure, the IAAF had overtaken the IOC. He knew that Alexandre de Mérode, who was still regularly trying to strengthen the position of his body, would react to this opinion. Arnold Beckett was successful, because the IOC Medical Commission included the following statement on its agenda after a meeting in October 1979:

---

[128] Letter, "Arnold Beckett to Lord Killanin and Alexandre de Mérode, June 1, 1979," archive collection "IOC Medical Commission," folder "Medical Commission: Correspondence June - December 1979," IOC Archive, Lausanne.

The Commission estimated that its role and authority would be enhanced if it had the power and means to control laboratories every 2 years throughout the world, and also help in the setting up of new ones. The IFs, otherwise, will act by themselves, which could lead to severe problems, as they do not all follow the same rules. This could also preserve laboratories from pressures from various domains, which endanger the necessary confidence which everyone should have in them.[129]

On the other hand, Arnold Beckett tried to convince Lord Killanin that without certified laboratories, wrong results would be possible. Arnold Beckett was probably targeting Lord Killanin's concern following the controversies at the 1976 Montreal Olympic Games (see Chapter 4). In light of the present crisis within the Olympic Movement, caused in particular by the financial disaster of the 1976 Montreal Olympic Games,[130] Lord Killanin wanted to avoid more controversy about flaws in the doping control procedures. Arnold Beckett believed that anti-doping laboratory standards were necessary to reduce mistakes in all aspects of the doping controls. Based on Arnold Beckett's initiative, the IOC Medical Commission voiced its concerns in the report to the IOC Session in 1979, asking for financial support "to recognise a number of recognised laboratories geographically dispersed throughout the world to which these Organising Committees [of Regional Games] may refer should the need arise."[131] One has to attribute key value to the letters by Arnold Beckett as they demonstrate the intent with which he now wanted to enforce a profile change of the IOC's fight against doping towards more inclusion of anti-doping laboratory experts. Clearly, he hoped to have more doping tests because of it. The fact that the IAAF had installed the accreditation procedure was in his favour and he used it to demonstrate the need for action from the side of the IOC.

His initiatives eventually came to fruition at the meetings during the 1980 Winter Olympic Games in Lake Placid. In collaboration with Manfred Donike and Robert Dugal, Arnold Beckett had submitted a "Proposal with regard to the acceptance of qualified laboratories in the fight against doping" to the IOC

---

[129] Minutes, "Meeting Medical Commission Scientific Committee, March 19-20, 1977," 7.
[130] PAYNE, *Olympic Turnaround*, 9.
[131] Minutes, "81st Session of the IOC in Montevideo, April 5-7, 1979," Annex 11.

Medical Commission.[132] In the proposal, he urged the IOC again to take over more responsibility. He claimed that doctors, athletes and coaches were aware of the lack of technical requirements in many laboratories: "this situation throws a permanent discredit on the controls and constitutes an intolerable discrimination in the world of sport."[133] Hence, the IOC should actively become involved in the accreditation of anti-doping laboratories. The proposal also included a concrete request to change the organisational structure of the IOC Medical Commission, recommending the installation of a "doping control sub-committee." [134] He envisaged that the new anti-doping body would consist of five members: three from the IOC Medical Commission and two heads of anti-doping laboratories. The subcommittee's main task should be to take over the technical and administrative steps of the anti-doping laboratory accreditation. In contrast to the Scientific Committee, which had a similar set-up but only actually met once, Arnold Beckett proposed a permanent installation of the "doping control sub-committee" with its own budget. [135] Furthermore, it should have discretionary competence concerning the accreditation of doping laboratories and all aspects of the doping analysis. Evidently, this proposal is of major importance for the ongoing developments since Arnold Beckett attempted to create an anti-doping body for experts in doping analysis only, to represent their interest in a more powerful way.

As one would expect, there were intensive discussions within the IOC Medical Commission on the proposal. Ludwig Prokop especially opposed some of the proposed responsibilities because he did not think research was part of such a body.[136] In light of the previous Scientific Committee of the IOC Medical Commission, which dealt with all aspects of doping and anti-doping and which Ludwig Prokop had criticised, these concerns appear understandable. Showing awareness of the medical experts, who were likely to feel excluded, Arnold Beckett argued that the new body was designed to combat doping and not entering any medical fields.[137] However, scientific research was necessary to

---

[132] Proposal, "Proposal with regard to the acceptance of qualified laboratories in the fight against doping by Arnold Beckett," archive collection "IOC Medical Commission," folder "Medical Commission: Correspondence January-February 1980," IOC Archive, Lausanne.

[133] Ibid., 3.

[134] Ibid., 4.

[135] Ibid.

[136] Minutes, "Meeting of the IOC Medical Commission, February 12, 1980," archive collection "IOC Medical Commission," folder "Meeting in Lake Placid on 1980," IOC Archive, Lausanne, 4.

[137] Ibid.

investigate into the effects of doping substances and especially ways to detect them. He regarded it essential to have a central body to coordinate such research.[138] Moreover, Arnold Beckett – as in previous attempts – campaigned for Alexandre de Mérode's support by stressing, "if the I.O.C. Medical Commission did not decide on the need for centralising doping control practices, an independent organisation would almost certainly set up."[139] He touched again on Alexandre de Mérode's constant concern about the standing of the IOC Medical Commission within the IOC and the world of sport.

Although he was at first hesitant, Arnold Beckett's arguments must have convinced Alexandre de Mérode. On the very same day, Alexandre de Mérode informed Lord Killanin about the plan of the IOC Medical Commission to become active in the official accreditation of doping laboratories through the installation of the "doping control sub-committee."[140] Interestingly, although there is no documentation on the final decision within the IOC Medical Commission available, he also forwarded Arnold Beckett's proposal to Monique Berlioux[141] for approval within the IOC Executive Board.[142] Eventually, the IOC Executive Board agreed on the "proposal concerning doping control centres," which also included the installation of the "doping control sub-committee" in April 1980.[143] At its 83rd Session, the IOC members then also accepted the proposal after Alexandre de Mérode had emphasised the significance of a central doping committee:

> He proposed the creation of a sub-commission on doping which would ensure that the important question of compliance with all the various regulations was fully ensured, and not only partially, as had recently

---

[138] Ibid.

[139] Ibid.

[140] Letter, "Alexandre de Mérode to Lord Killanin, February 12, 1980," archive collection "IOC Medical Commission," folder "Medical Commission: Correspondence January-February 1980," IOC Archive, Lausanne

[141] Monique Berlioux (born 1925), a French champion in swimming in the 1940s and competitor at the 1948 London Olympic Games, became the IOC's director of Press and Public Relations in 1967 before she became its director in 1971. Joanna DAVENPORT, "Monique Berlioux: Her association with three IOC presidents," *Citius, Altius, Fortius* (became *Journal of Olympic History* in 1997) 4, no. 3 (1996), 11.

[142] Letter, "Alexandre de Mérode to Monique Berlioux, February 19, 1980," archive collection "IOC Medical Commission," folder "Medical Commission: Correspondence January-February 1980," IOC Archive, Lausanne

[143] Minutes, "Executive Board, April 21-23, 1980," archive collection "IOC Executive Board Meetings 1921-1982," IOC Archive, Lausanne, 33.

been the case. The Prince de Mérode felt that the work of such a commission would be of value not only to these Games, but in the future for international meetings and regional Games.[144]

Curiously, the plan of the new "doping control sub-committee," accepted by the IOC Executive Board and the 83rd IOC Session, was exactly the same draft that Arnold Beckett had submitted to the IOC Medical Commission.[145] In addition, Alexandre de Mérode also suggested the creation of two more Subcommissions: one dealing with sports medicine and orthopaedics, the other with biomechanics and physiology.[146]

The processes that led to the ultimate creation of a sub-committee for doping clearly demonstrate the power shift within the Olympic anti-doping system in the years between 1976 and 1980. In this period, experts, based on their professional competencies in doping analysis, increasingly purposefully expanded their advisory role. This process began with the introduction of the accreditation system by the IAAF Medical Committee, where anti-doping laboratory experts had significantly more influence. It legitimised them to create consistent testing procedures within all sports. Arnold Beckett in particular, made IOC officials continuously aware of the need for standardised doping techniques and educated laboratory staff. Curiously, this was exactly the proposal Gottfried Schönholzer had already made eight years before (see Chapter 3). Alexandre de Mérode eventually supported Arnold Beckett, recognising the need to give anti-doping laboratory experts more influence.

NO POSITIVE DOPING RESULT AT THE TWO OLYMPIC GAMES IN 1980: SUCCESS OR FAILURE?

Doping Controls at the 1980 Winter Olympic Games in Lake Placid

The doping tests analysed at the 1980 Winter Olympics in Lake Placid became the first ones dealt with by an officially accredited anti-doping laboratory. For this process, the Organising Committee transferred the entire equipment from Montreal to the O'Donnell laboratory at the Will Rogers Hospital in Lake

---

[144] Minutes, "83rd Session of the IOC in Moscow, July 15 – August 3, 1980," archive collection "IOC Sessions 1894-2009," IOC Archive, Lausanne, 25.
[145] Minutes, "Executive Board, April 21-23, 1980," Annex 21.
[146] Ibid.

Placid.[147] In total, it installed twelve gas chromatographs and four mass spectrometers.[148] The doping control officers took 440 samples but there were no positive results.[149] Moreover, the laboratory correctly identified the five control samples that Arnold Beckett had prepared and contained banned substances. The laboratory staff tested all samples for stimulants and 350 additionally for anabolic steroids.[150] The controls also showed an increase in the involved chemists and biochemists, which included 25 people from these scientific fields, which confirms the outlined developments.[151] As in Montreal, a local pharmacologist supported the anti-doping work. However, the absence of positive doping test results indicates that the drug cheats were still beating the doping control system, including the anti-doping laboratory experts.

Nevertheless, Robert Dugal and Michel Bertrand felt very positive about the installed methods, arguing in the *New York Times* that due to their research, the doping system had become more sophisticated.[152] Michel Bertrand went even further by saying, "the technologists can develop new tests faster than the athletes and their trainers can develop new doping techniques."[153] Importantly, Arnold Beckett was more realistic about the state of anti-doping affairs. He accused sport medicine specialists and sport officials of supporting the usage of performance-enhancing substances.[154] It is important to revisit this statement following the revelation of his strategy to change the approach to the doping problem by the installation of a "doping control sub-committee." He therewith targeted towards sport officials to allow more control for anti-doping laboratory experts, and make them aware of different areas of responsibilities between anti-doping laboratory experts and sport medicine specialists. Moreover, it shows awareness that despite Arnold Beckett pursuing a strict testing policy, the athlete's entourage and the

---

[147] Minutes, "Executive Board, June 26-29, 1979," archive collection "IOC Executive Board Meetings 1921-1982," IOC Archive, Lausanne, 17.

[148] TODD and TODD, "Significant Events," 77.

[149] ORGANISING COMMITTEE OF THE XIIITH OLYMPIC WINTER GAMES, *Official Report*, 72.

[150] Albert DIRIX and Xavier STURBOIS, *The First Thirty Years of the International Olympic Committee Medical Commission* (Lausanne: International Olympic Committee, 1998), 59.

[151] Report, "Medical Report of the Services, Equipment, Personnel and Feminity Performed by the Medical Dept. for the Lake Placid Olympic Organising Committee, by George G. Hart, 1980," archive collection "Summer and Winter Olympic Games: Medical files," folder "Minutes and medical report of the Olympic Winter Games of Lake Placid 1980," IOC Archive, Lausanne, 28ff.

[152] HUNT, *Drug Games*, 64.

[153] BARNES, "Olympic Drug Testing," 23.

[154] HUNT, *Drug Games*, 65.

entire sport system played a key role in solving the doping problem of sport. A careful reading of George Hart's final report of the medical report reveals that he supported the installation of worldwide-accredited laboratories and a centrally organised doping control programme: "I would strongly recommend that the IOC considers in some fashion the selection of three or four laboratories around the world, which can do this service [doping analysis]."[155]

Doping Controls at the 1980 Moscow Olympic Games

Although Victor Rogozkin had originally planned to obtain anti-serums for the doping controls at the 1980 Moscow Olympic Games from the London laboratory, the intensive research within his own anti-doping laboratory eventually enabled him to produce anti-serums and H^3 radioactive hormones independently.[156] This is an indication towards the high technical standards, despite Manfred Donike's concerns. The doping control laboratory made 6868 analyses by means of GC, 2493 RIs, 220 analyses by means of MS and 43 alcohol tests from the 1645 number of samples taken at the Moscow Olympics.[157] Similar to the 1976 Montreal Olympic Games, the laboratory staff employed RI screening procedures to analyse the samples for anabolic steroids and GC-MS analysis to confirm potentially positive screening results.[158] However, as in Lake Placid the doping controllers did not find any positive doping tests. According to Victor Rogozkin, the doping controls were of the highest technical standards. He linked this to the successfully detected control samples. Arnold Beckett affirmed this point and highlighted that especially the detection of the control samples containing the anabolic steroid methandrostenolone "proves good work of the laboratory and confirms that there were no real dopings [sic] among the competitors."[159]

---

[155] Report, "Medical Report of the Services, Equipment, Personnel and Feminity Performed by the Medical Dept. for the Lake Placid Olympic Organising Committee by George G. Hart, 1980," 28ff.
[156] ROGOZKIN, "Moscow 1980," 155.
[157] Report, "Doping Control at the Games of the XXIInd Olympiad by Victor Rogozkin, 1980," 28.
[158] KAMMERER, "What Is," 4.
[159] Individual Minutes, "Meetings of the IOC Medical Commission in Moscow, July 15 – August 3, 1980," archive collection "Summer and Winter Olympic Games: Medical files," folder "Medical matters at the 1980 Summer Olympic Games in Moscow, Reports and minutes of the IOC Medical Commission," IOC Archive, Lausanne, 66.

In addition to his detailed descriptions of the applied analytical methods, Victor Rogozkin did not refrain from emphasising the increased cooperation between anti-doping laboratory experts before and during the controls at the Olympic Games: "In recent years a good reciprocal exchange of information has been established with scientists from foreign countries working in the field of athletes' doping control."[160] He suggested an even closer cooperation between anti-doping laboratory experts and made four recommendations, which stand exemplary for the eventual outcome of the observed developments from 1976 to 1980. These recommendations were the introduction of (1) an accreditation procedure; (2) the standardisation of analysis procedures and techniques; (3) the organisation of joint research by doping control specialists from all over the world; and (4) a mutual exchange of information through regularly held seminars or symposia.[161] Therefore, he reiterated Arnold Beckett's proposal to install a subcommission solely dealing with anti-doping issues. This is understandable because Victor Rogozkin was the head of an anti-doping laboratory and hoped to profit from such an installation.

Unsurprisingly, Arnold Beckett used the opportunity to stress the significance of accredited laboratories during the meetings of the IOC Medical Commission in Moscow. Considering the reinstatement of the five athletes by the IAAF, the IOC Executive Board had decided to ban positive tested athletes from subsequent Olympic Games.[162] However, on recommendation of Arnold Beckett, the IOC Medical Commission decided to delay the implementation of this rule. He based his suggestion on the following reasons:

1. The policy of accreditation of laboratories by the I.O.C. Medical Commission has only been instituted recently.

2. Some International Federations are disqualifying competitors on results of doubtful validity.

3. Laboratories with staff of suitable experience and with appropriate apparatus are not available in many regions of the world.

---

[160] Ibid., 29.
[161] Ibid., 30.
[162] Ibid., 11.

4. Sometimes the method of obtaining urine samples for analysis and their control from a security point of view at some competitions is open to challenge.

5. The I.O.C. must not act unless a positive result has been obtained by methods which are correct scientifically in all aspects.[163]

With these recommendations, he again promoted awareness of having certified laboratories.

Nevertheless, the conclusions on the "purity" of the 1980 Moscow Olympic Games were drawn far too early, and there appears to have been a considerable amount of usage of performance-enhancing substances, particularly through the administration of testosterone esters. Despite the positive statements on the successful doping controls, the IOC Medical Commission was aware of this and approved the usage of the samples taken at the Olympic Games for additional tests by Manfred Donike. The Commission actually made the decision before the start of the competition,[164] when Manfred Donike informed Alexandre de Mérode that the detection of exogenous testosterone had become possible, and that he wanted to test its validity and reliability.[165] The test was based on the quantitative determination of testosterone and epitestosterone through GC-MS, developed by Japanese researchers S. BABA, Y. SHINOHARA and Y. KASUYA: the level of epitestosterone, where the 17-epimere of testosterone does not increase when exogenous testosterone is applied.[166] Usually, the relation is about one but increases when pharmaceutical preparations of testosterone are applied.[167] Consequently, Manfred Donike set a 6:1 ration (testosterone to epitestosterone,

---

[163] Ibid.

[164] Individual Minutes, "Meetings of the IOC Medical Commission in Moscow, July 15 – August 3, 1980," 22.

[165] Letter, "Manfred Donike to Alexandre de Mérode, July 16, 1980," archive collection "IOC Medical Commission," folder "Medical Commission: Correspondence January-june 1980," IOC Archive, Lausanne.

[166] S. BABA, Y. SHINOHARA and Y. KASUYA, "Differentiation between endogenous and exogenous testosterone in human plasma and urine after oral administration of deuterium-labelled testosterone by mass fragmentography," *Journal of Clinical Endocrinology and Metabolism* 50, no. 5 (1980), 889-894.

[167] Manfred DONIKE, K.R. BÄRWALD, Karl KLOSTERMANN, Wilhelm SCHÄNZER and Johann ZIMMERMANN, "Nachweis von exogenem Testosteron," in: *Sport: Leistung und Gesundheit*, eds. Hermann HECK, Wildor HOLLMANN, Heinz LIESEN and Richard ROST (Cologne: Deutscher Ärzte Verlag, 1983), 293-300.

T/E ratio) as a positive test.[168] For the preparation of the samples, Manfred Donike travelled to Leningrad in October 1980, where Victor Rogozkin had stored the samples by order of the IOC Medical Commission.[169] The analysis of the samples took place in Cologne under the presence of Soviet laboratory staff members. This was an important aspect for Manfred Donike, who did not want to convey the impression of undertaking subjective controls. This was also a result of the problematic sport political climate. He just wanted to have an opportunity to test his newly developed methods.[170] The outcome of the analysis revealed that more than 20.0% of the samples were positive, amongst them 16 gold medal winners of the 1980 Moscow Olympic Games.[171] The consequences of the publication of the results, and the discussions surrounding the technical development are explored in Chapter 6. However, in short, the results prove that the doping control system was by no means as efficient as was widely believed by many anti-doping laboratory experts at the time. Despite their increasing efforts, there remained many loopholes for athletes. The usage of performance-enhancing substances was well-advanced in comparison with the analytical methods. Manfred Donike´s tests highlighted that change was needed. This favoured Arnold Beckett´s proposed structural amendments and played into the hands of the anti-doping laboratory experts to expand the institutional doping control system.

INTERIM RESULTS FOR THE PERIOD 1977-1980: EFFORTS TO INCREASE INFLUENCE OF ANTI-DOPING LABORATORY EXPERTS

The period between the 1976 Montreal Olympic Games and the 1980 Moscow Olympic Games was the main transition period in the history of the anti-doping laboratory experts within the Olympic Movement. In particular, it was characterised by a shift in influence that resulted in Alexandre de Mérode deciding to introduce a new "doping control sub-committee," dealing with matters of anti-doping only, thereby focusing especially on doping analysis. He finally acknowledged that, by the beginning of the 1980s, the implemented

---

[168] Ibid.

[169] Letter, "Manfred Donike to Karlheinz Gieseler, July 25, 1980," archive collection "IOC Medical Commission," folder "Medical Commission: Correspondence January-june 1980," IOC Archive, Lausanne.

[170] Ibid.

[171] HUNT, *Drug Games*, 66.

doping control system depended on the professional expertise in doping analysis by a few individuals.

Partly, this change was based on the success of the more pragmatic approach by the IAAF Medical Committee. Whereas in previous years, Alexandre de Mérode had refrained from bringing in other anti-doping laboratory experts, apart from Arnold Beckett, into the IOC's anti-doping bodies, the installation of the IOC Medical Commission's Scientific Commission in 1976 outlined the start of a more focused approach. However, the establishment of the Scientific Commission did not satisfy leading anti-doping laboratory experts such as Arnold Beckett and Manfred Donike. They believed that in order to enable for more scientific reliability, anti-doping laboratory experts needed to occupy a more important role in anti-doping bodies.

In contrast to the circumstances in the IOC Medical Commission, Arnold Beckett encountered a different situation within the IAAF Medical Committee, who had installed an IAAF Doping Subcommittee in 1977. Therein, the anti-doping laboratory experts were more influential, and possessed in Manfred Donike another dominant figure to support their case based on their scientific competencies. With his input, the IAAF Doping Subcommittee introduced the official accreditation system in 1979. Importantly, the installation resulted in the irreplaceability of the anti-doping laboratory experts within the IAAF's anti-doping policy. They, and they alone, dealt with the administration and execution of the accreditation procedure and were simultaneously the heads of the most technically advanced anti-doping laboratories. No other controlling bodies were involved because anti-doping laboratory experts were the only individuals that had the professional competencies to supervise the procedures. This gave them decisive power and clearly went beyond the sole advisory role that they had occupied before. In fact, the anti-doping laboratory standards became a crucial part of the entire anti-doping system.

Naturally, the introduction of the accreditation system also had consequences for the network of anti-doping laboratory experts. It implicated closer cooperation between the institutions in the accreditation process, but also consultation with the experts of the IAAF on the execution of the doping tests at different events. Even though only five laboratories obtained official accreditation in the first year, the interest in becoming a certified laboratory was much bigger. There is also evidence for an exchange of knowledge at small scientific congresses at the experts could discuss details on the technical advancements in doping analysis. However, this is not to say that the increased focus on scientific matters solved all the problems. On the contrary, the post-Games tests on the usage of testosterone at the 1980 Moscow Olympic Games by Manfred Donike revealed that the drug cheats were still beating the entire doping control system.

The final step in the transition phase was to convince Alexandre de Mérode about the necessity to have a more coordinated approach to doping analysis. These attempts, mainly initiated by Arnold Beckett and Manfred Donike, consisted of stressing the need for IOC-accredited anti-doping laboratories, and calling upon the leading role of the IOC Medical Commission in global anti-doping matters. Arnold Beckett especially was aware that the doping control system already depended heavily on the expertise in the field of doping analysis and he aimed for more influence within the Olympic Movement. Clearly, financial benefits were part of their motivation. The anti-doping laboratory experts were aware that a more influential role would enable them access more research funds for the development of analytical procedures. For example, the budget estimate for doping analysis in the FRG was doubled from 1978 to 1979.[172] In combination with the expanding and institutionally professionalised interconnectedness of the anti-doping laboratories, their attempts prompted Alexandre de Mérode to reconstruct the IOC Medical Commission whilst accepting Arnold Beckett's proposal to install a "doping control sub-committee." Consequently, whereas the introduction of the tests for anabolic steroids before the 1976 Montreal Olympic Games enabled anti-doping laboratory experts to occupy a stronger advisory role, the processes in the subsequent period allowed the anti-doping laboratory experts to become more significant on the decision-making level. They had intended this in order to exert more influence on the sports organisations

---

[172] KRÜGER et al., *Doping und Anti-Doping*, 122.

CHAPTER 6

Indispensable Key Players (1980-1984)

THE IOC SUBCOMMISSION ON DOPING AND BIOCHEMISTRY OF SPORT: TURNING POINT FOR THE IOC'S FIGHT AGAINST DOPING

Initial Efforts

At the IOC Medical Commission's meeting in July 1980, it officially installed the IOC Subcommission on Doping and Biochemistry (IOC MSD).[1] Importantly, this decision also caused the official dissolution of the IOC Medical Commission's Scientific Commission. Although Arnold Beckett had originally proposed the installation of an "anti-doping" body, the resolution to include "biochemistry" in the official designation of the IOC MSD demonstrates the significance given to the field of doping analysis. Moreover, it explicitly reveals that the development of analytical procedures was now a key strategy to a successful anti-doping policy. It represents the shift from medical experts to anti-doping laboratory experts to deal with doping problems.

The IOC MSD's composition gives further evidence for this. The official members were the new IOC MSD chairman Manfred Donike, Arnold Beckett, Robert Dugal, Victor Rogozkin and Claus Clausnitzer. They all had first-hand experience in doping controls, a scientific background in (bio) chemistry or pharmacy and headed an anti-doping laboratory. Consequently, the IOC MSD developed into the main organ for the network of anti-doping laboratory experts, who had now more direct influence, and it is necessary to distinguish between the dealings of the IOC Medical Commission and the IOC MSD from this point onwards. This has been neglected in previous research. Alexandre de Mérode and Albert Dirix also attended the meetings. However, they were only responsible for administrative tasks.

It is important to elaborate on the inclusion of the head of the Kreischa anti-doping laboratory, Claus Clausnitzer, who gained his doctorate in chemistry from

---

[1] Individual Minutes, "Meetings of the IOC Medical Commission in Moscow, July 15 – August 3, 1980," 18.

the Karl-Marx University in Leipzig in 1984.[2] Due to its sophisticated doping regime, officially known under as "State Plan 14.25,"[3] the GDR had a strong interest in the involvement of a GDR representative on the new IOC MSD. Claus Clausnitzer actually played a central role in the cover-up of the GDR doping system. His laboratory was not only conducting doping tests for international sport organisations, but also controlled the GDR athletes on doping substances before leaving the country.[4] Every athlete had to submit themselves to these controls to allow GDR officials controlling whether administered substances were not detectable anymore.[5] Hence, Claus Clausnitzer was one of the most powerful men within the entire GDR doping system, and the only person authorised to transport the results of the doping tests to Manfred Höppner.[6] GDR officials also had interest in other anti-doping laboratories. In fact, the GDR's Ministry of State Security (Ministerium für Staatssicherheit, MfS) accused Manfred Donike of undertaking "pro-doping research" in at least one case.[7] It based these accusations on the practices in the GDR itself and the assumption that other countries were also investigating into the systematic usage of doping. However, the accusations remain unconfirmed until today. Despite the sophisticated strategy of the GDR doping system, the historical records of the GDR's NOC illustrate that it was Alexandre de Mérode, who suggested the inclusion of a GDR representative on

---

[2] Brigitte BERENDONK, *Doping. Von der Forschung zum Betrug* (Reinbek: Rowohlt Taschenbuch Verlag, 1992), 55f. Despite various attempts and intensive inspection of the historical sources, it was not possible to obtain information on his biographical data.

[3] "State Plan 14.25" was the official term for the state specifications of the GDR to establish an extensive system of government-funded doping. The system led to the systematic development and usage of performance-enhancing substances. Although there were doping practices already before 1974, the "State Plan 14.25" was only put in place in October 1974 due to the SED increasingly losing control over the doping practices and the improved doping testing techniques, particularly the introduction of anabolic steroid testing. Steven UNGERLEIDER, *Faust's Gold. Inside the East German Doping Machine* (New York, NY: St. Martin's Press, 2001), 44f.

[4] Brigitte BERENDONK, *Doping Dokumente. Von der Forschung zum Betrug* (Berlin: Springer Verlag, 1991), 109.

[5] Ibid.

[6] UNGERLEIDER, *Faust's Gold*, 91.

[7] SPITZER, *Doping in der DDR.*, 71.

the IOC Medical Commission.[8] The GDR's leading sport officials took advantage of this suggestion immediately and made several suggestions. However, Alexandre de Mérode rejected the first two proposals, to include Professor Stanley-Ernest Strauzenberg[9] and Manfred Höppner, because they did not have any experience in doping analysis.[10] This is evidence for the realignment of the IOC Medical Commission's strategy. Hence, the vice-president of the GDR's NOC, Günther Heinze, recommended Claus Clausnitzer to Alexandre de Mérode.[11] The GDR regime anticipated that he could spy on the IOC's means of controls and forward the information to the MfS. This strategy was successful since the MfS translated many documents discussed within the IOC MSD immediately and brought them to the attention sport officials.[12] However, Claus Clausnitzer contributed rarely to the discussions and did not actively oppose main decisions. In this way, the GDR regime hoped to raise no suspicions about its doping practices.

Clearly, the driving forces in the IOC MSD were Manfred Donike, Arnold Beckett and Robert Dugal. Under their leadership, the IOC MSD committed itself to carrying out four specific tasks from the very beginning. These were the accreditation procedure, the acquisition of standard reference compounds for the

---

[8] Memo, talk between Alexandre de Mérode, Manfred Ewald and Günther Heinze in Lake Placid, March 3, 1978, archive collection "DR 510 Nationales Olympisches Komitee der DDR," folder "DR 510/966, Band 4, Medizinische Kommission des IOC, 1977-1987," Bundesarchiv, Berlin-Lichterfelde. Manfred Ewald occupied a central role in the doping system of the GD. He was president of the central sport organisation in the GDR, the GDR's Gymnastic and Sports Union, from 1961 until 1988. He was also president of the GDR's NOC from 1973 until 1990. He was found guilty of assisted assault in 20 cases through the administration of anabolic steroids in 2000. Helmut MÜLLER-ENBERGS, Jan WIEGOHLS, Dieter HOFFMANN, eds., *Wer war wer in der DDR. Ein biographisches Lexikon* (Berlin: Christoph Links Verlag, 2001), 354.

[9] Profssor Dr. Stanley-Ernest Strauzenberg (born 1914) was head of the Central Institute of the SMD in Kreischa. The doping laboratory in Kreischa was under control of the SMD. Letter, "Günther Heinze to Alexandre de Mérode, April 5, 1978," archive collection "DR 510 Nationales Olympisches Komitee der DDR," folder "DR 510/966, Band 4, Medizinische Kommission des IOC, 1977-1987," Bundesarchiv, Berlin-Lichterfelde.

[10] Letter, "Günther Heinze to Alexandre de Mérode, July 7, 1979," archive collection "DR 510 Nationales Olympisches Komitee der DDR," folder "DR 510/966, Band 4, Medizinische Kommission des IOC, 1977-1987," Bundesarchiv, Berlin-Lichterfelde.

[11] Letter, "Günther Heinze to Alexandre de Mérode, May 16, 1980," archive collection "DR 510 Nationales Olympisches Komitee der DDR," folder "DR 510/966, Band 4, Medizinische Kommission des IOC, 1977-1987," Bundesarchiv, Berlin-Lichterfelde.

[12] There are several such documents available from the Bundesarchiv, mainly within the collection "DR 510 Nationales Olympisches Komitee der DDR".

accreditation, research on analytical methods and educational activities for laboratory staff members.[13] In terms of adding substances to the banned list, the IOC MSD members focused not as much on whether a drug had a performance-enhancing effect, but rather on the availability of analytical methods. For example, in November 1980, the IOC MSD still decided to refrain from adding beta-blockers to the banned list in view of high costs anticipated for the analysis.[14] Similarly, Robert Dugal informed the other members about his continuous research into the problem of blood doping.[15] However, due to the lack of analytical methods, blood doping could not yet be determined or proven.

The IOC MSD defined the establishment of a wider anti-doping laboratory network as its main field of work. This seems to be obvious because it was the motivation for the installation of the new body in the first place. Arnold Beckett again highlighted the significance of the anti-doping laboratories and the correct analysis in a comment attached to the official minutes of the IOC MSD meeting.[16] The anti-doping laboratory experts on the IOC MSD were in particular dissatisfied about an accreditation process installed by the UCI. In fact, the UCI had registered 44 institutions and the IOC MSD reasoned that the high number of

---

[13] Minutes, "Meeting of the IOC Subcommittee on Doping and Biochemistry in Cologne, November 29 and 30, 1980," archive collection "IOC Medical Commission," folder "Medical commission: Sub-commission doping and doping and sporting biochemistry 1980-1982," IOC Archive, Lausanne, 6.

[14] Ibid., 4.

[15] Ibid.

[16] Minutes, "Meeting of the IOC Subcommittee on Doping and Biochemistry in Cologne, November 29 and 30, 1980," Annex 3.

laboratories did not allow for a control of the technical standards.[17] At the same time, it perceived the UCI system a threat for the exclusivity of the anti-doping laboratories headed by the members of the IOC MSD. Thus, they did not want IFs to accredit their own laboratories but instead (as intended through the installation of the IOC MSD), have a central accreditation body to control the network.[18] As

---

[17] Laboratoire Biochimie et Toxicologie (Algier, Algeria), Facultad de Ciencias Exactas y Naturales (Buenos Aires, Argentina), Chemische Abteilung Institut für Gerichtliche Medizin der Universität (Vienna, Austria), Analytical Reference Laboratories Pty Ltd (Victoria, Australia), Institute of Drug Technology (Victoria Australia), Faculte de Medicine Veterinaire (Ghent, Belgium), Centre National de Medicine Sportive (Sofia, Bulgaria), INRS (Montreal, Canada), Laboratorio de Control del Doping Sociedad Hipodromo Chile (Santiago, Chile), Laboratorio de Farmacologia (Cali, Colombia), Laboratorio de Medicine Deportiva (Medellin, Colombia), Laboratoire de Toxicologie (Bogota, Colombia), Laboratorio de Toxicologia (Santander, Colombia), Instituto de Medicina Legal (Medellin, Colombia), Centro Nacional Investigaciones Cientificas (Havanna, Cuba), Laboratorio de Bioquimica Investigacion (Madrid, Spain), Laborario de Analisis (Barcelona, Spain), Laboratorio de Colegio Oficial de Farmaceuticos de Guipozcoa (San Sebastian, Spain), Allentown Sacred Heart Hospital (Allentown, USA), Laboratoire de Toxicologie (Clichy, France), Chelsea College (London, Great Britain), Biological Materials Analysis Unit (Salford, Great Britain), Laboratoire Central de l'Institut de Sante Sportive et de la Culture Physique Nationale (Budapest, Hungary), Equine Forensic Unit (Dublin, Ireland), Institut Superieur des Medicines Sportives (Rome, Italy), Laboratorio Antidoping di Firenze delle FMSI (Florence, Italy), Division of Chemical Pathology (Wellington, New Zealand), Chemical Service Laboratories (Johnsonville, New Zealand), Laboratoire de l'Universite de Panama (Panama), Institut de Pharmacologie de l'Universite de Nijmegen (Nijmegen, Netherlands), Pracownio Antydopingowa Przy (Katowice, Poland), Faculte de Pharmacie de Coimbra (Coimbra, Portugal), Institut für Gerichtliche Medizin und Kriminalistik der Humboldt Universität Berlin (Berlin, GDR), Doping-Labor des Sportmedizinischen Dienstes (Kreischa, GDR), Institut für Biochemie der Deutschen Sporthochschule Köln (Cologne, FRG), Centrul de Medicina Sportiva Bucaresti (Bucharest, Romania), Statens Rattskemiska Laboratorium (Stockholm, Sweden), Laboratoire de l'Ecole Federale de Gymnastique (Magglingen, Switzerland), Laboratory of Doping Control (Prague, Czechoslovakia), Laboratoires Unis Antidoping de l'Institut de Recherches Scientifiques de la Culture Physique de l'URSS et de l'Institut d'Etat de Recherches Scientifiques de Medicine Legales (Moscow, USSR), Universidad de los Andes (Merida, Venezuela), Toksikolojski Laboratorij za Sodno Medicino (Ljubljana, Yugoslavia), Faculte de Pharmacie (Belgrade, Yugoslavia), Laboratorija za Doping Kontrolu Institut za Medicinu Sporta (Belgrade, Yugoslavia). Letter, Michal Jekiel to Alexandre de Mérode, February 15, 1982, archive collection "IOC Medical Commission," folder "Correspondence January-April 1982," IOC Archive, Lausanne.

[18] Minutes, "Meeting of the IOC Subcommittee on Doping and Biochemistry in Cologne, November 29 and 30, 1980," Annex 3.

such, the IOC MSD decided to recognise the IAAF accredited anti-doping laboratories automatically and immediately took over the work of the IAAF, but did not to accept the UCI's system.[19] Thus, with the effect of the IOC MSD's constitution, the anti-doping laboratories in Cologne, Kreischa, Leningrad, Montreal and London also became authorised IOC anti-doping laboratories. They were informed in writing on December 18, 1980.[20] Hence, this date was the beginning of official IOC-accredited doping laboratories. The decision to overtake the five laboratories appears reasonable in light of the fact that Manfred Donike and Arnold Beckett were in charge of both accreditation processes, and members of the IOC MSD headed all authorised laboratories. Essentially, the IOC MSD members therefore accredited their own institutions for a second time, which illustrates an emerging conflict of interest. Significantly, in contrast to the IAAF procedure, the main accreditation centre was situated at Manfred Donike's offices at the DSHS.[21]

However, the agreement between the IAAF and IOC was only informal, and uncoordinated processes become apparent during Arnold Beckett's visits to Australia, New Zealand and the USA at the end of January 1981. The IAAF Medical Committee had received applications from two laboratories in Brisbane and in Sydney, and Arnold Beckett travelled there to study the testing centres. He also attended the Pacific Conference Games in Christchurch in 1981 in order to supervise the doping controls.[22] At the event, the discus throwers Ben Plunknett (USA) and Gael Mulhall (Australia) tested positive for anabolic steroids.[23] In his final report, Arnold Beckett concluded that the equipment at the laboratories in Australia and New Zealand was satisfactory, but the staff did not have any experience in the conduction of doping analysis.[24] Therefore, it was too early for

---

[19] Minutes, "Meeting of the IOC Subcommittee on Doping and Biochemistry in Cologne, November 29 and 30, 1980," 2.

[20] Letters, "Alexandre de Mérode to Arnold Beckett, Claus Clausnitzer, Manfred Donike, Robert Dugal and Victor Rogozkin, December 18, 1980," archive collection "IOC Medical Commission," folder "Correspondence July-December 1980," IOC Archive, Lausanne.

[21] Minutes, "Meeting of the IOC Subcommittee on Doping and Biochemistry in Cologne, November 29 and 30, 1980," 6.

[22] The Pacific Conference Games took place every four years between 1969 and 1985. The participants were from Australia, Canada, Japan, New Zealand and the USA. In 1981, athletes from all nations could participate in the competitions.

[23] TODD and TODD, "Significant Events," 77.

[24] Report, "Visit by Arnold Beckett to Australia, New Zealand and USA, January 23 – February 4, 1981," archive collection "IOC Medical Commission," folder "Correspondence January-April 1981," IOC Archive, Lausanne, 4.

the laboratories to seek accreditation. Nevertheless, as he argued, his visit would ensure that much closer cooperation was established. Importantly, whereas his trip to Oceania was made on behalf of the IAAF, he spontaneously planned a visit to Los Angeles (the host city of the 1984 Olympic Games), but the IAAF asked the IOC to pay for 50.0% of Arnold Beckett's travel expenses.[25] This is interesting because Arnold Beckett was not officially sent there by the IOC Medical Commission, but rather undertook the journey on his own initiative to start the preparations for the anti-doping laboratory as early as possible. Nevertheless, Alexandre de Mérode and Monique Berlioux appear to be convinced that the IOC profited from his initiative.[26] In Los Angeles, Arnold Beckett observed the working practices of potential anti-doping laboratory facilities at the Department of Pharmacology at the University of California Los Angeles (UCLA) and the Bioscience Laboratories, a commercial organisation. He summarised his impressions in a letter to the Organising Committee of the 1984 Los Angeles Olympic Games (LAOOC). Arnold Beckett favoured the UCLA laboratory because of the university environment where it was possible, so he explained, "to link the service aspects of doping control with the research aspects needed to develop methods."[27]

Another example for this period of ambiguities between the IOC and the IAAF is the accreditation of a sixth anti-doping laboratory at the Swiss Federal Institute of Sports Magglingen (EHSM) in Magglingen (Switzerland). This process had already started in 1979, when the laboratory had correctly analysed three samples, sent by Manfred Donike on behalf of the IAAF Doping Subcommittee. However, it was only granted official accreditation in March 1981.[28] In this instance, the IAAF informed the IOC officially about the processes and eventually also recognised the laboratory. Both cases illustrate the overlapping processes and reveal that in the first months after the establishment

---

[25] Letter, "John Holt to Monique Berlioux, January 16, 1981," archive collection "IOC Medical Commission," folder "Correspondence January-April 1981," IOC Archive, Lausanne.

[26] Letter, "Monique Berlioux to Alexandre de Mérode, March 5, 1981," archive collection "IOC Medical Commission," folder "Correspondence January-April 1981," IOC Archive, Lausanne.

[27] Letter, "Arnold Beckett to Anthony Daly, February 12, 1981," archive collection "IOC Medical Commission," folder "Correspondence January-April 1981," IOC Archive, Lausanne.

[28] Letter, "John Holt to Hans Howald and James Baumler, March 31, 1981," archive collection "IOC Medical Commission," folder "Correspondence January-April 1981," IOC Archive, Lausanne.

of the IOC MSD, individual efforts still existed. Furthermore, the double function of Manfred Donike and Arnold Beckett in IOC and IAAF resulted in unclear institutional responsibilities.

Although the IOC MSD had met for the first time in November 1980, the most significant summit took place during its second meeting in May 1981 in Cologne. This also included a joint meeting with the IAAF Medical Committee.[29] There are two reasons for this. First, the IAAF Medical Committee and the IOC MSD decided on a formal agreement on the official anti-doping laboratory accreditation procedure.[30] The arrangement intended that the IOC MSD should formally accept those six laboratories accredited by the IAAF, because this had only been an informal agreement before. Furthermore, those laboratories, which were in the process of being certified by the IAAF, would then automatically be accepted by the IOC, as had been the case with the EHSM laboratory in Magglingen.[31] The IOC would only completely overtake the accreditation system once appropriate resources and facilities were available.[32] Manfred Donike and Alexandre de Mérode discussed specific steps for the request for accreditation. They agreed that only the first approach, and the final letter of accreditation, were dealt with by the IOC Medical Commission chairman. The secretariat at the Institute of Biochemistry in Cologne and the IOC MSD administered and organised all other aspects.[33] It was the intent of IOC and IAAF that other IFs would accept the leading role of the IOC MSD concerning the accreditation system. Again, reference is made to the system by the UCI, which was regarded as "not stringent enough."[34]

Second, the assembly in Cologne was significant because it did not only entail the joint meeting of the IOC MSD and the IAAF Medical Committee, but also a scientific symposium and the meeting between the head of doping

---

[29] Minutes, "Meeting of the IOC Subcommittee on Doping and Biochemistry in Cologne, May 20-22, 1981," archive collection "IOC Medical Commission," folder "Medical commission: Sub-commission doping and doping and sporting biochemistry 1980-1982," IOC Archive, Lausanne.

[30] DIRIX and STURBOIS, *The First*, 33.

[31] Minutes, "Meeting of the IOC Subcommittee on Doping and Biochemistry in Cologne, May 20-22, 1981," 18.

[32] Ibid.

[33] Letter, "Alexandre de Mérode to Manfred Donike, December 30, 1981," archive collection "IOC Medical Commission," folder "Correspondence May-December 1981," IOC Archive, Lausanne.

[34] Minutes, "Meeting of the IOC Subcommittee on Doping and Biochemistry in Cologne, May 20-22, 1981," 18.

laboratories, set up by George Walker of the CoE. The symposium was staged on the initiative of Manfred Donike, who had already anticipated a more regular scientific exchange forum at the first meeting of the IOC MSD and was asked to organise a symposium with the title "Progress in Doping Analysis."[35] On his suggestion, all five members of the IOC MSD presented academic work from their respective fields of research.[36] Moreover, on invitation by Manfred Donike, the opportunity of having leading experts in doping controls present was also used to stage a workshop for other scientists, informing them about the newest developments in doping analysis. These demonstrations were done on the second day of the meeting,[37] with representatives from more than 20 countries attending.[38] This was the first educational initiative for laboratory staff members, as envisaged by the IOC MSD. The large number of participating experts highlights the apparent need for an increased knowledge distribution on testing techniques with the desire by many laboratories to gain accreditation. The meeting of "Heads of Top-Class Doping Control Laboratories" by the CoE resulted in the support of the CoE's "Recommendation No. R(79)8" on doping in sport, which placed emphasis on the need for more official anti-doping laboratories.[39] At the same time, the participants also urged CDDS to provide a

---

[35] Minutes, "Meeting of the IOC Subcommittee on Doping and Biochemistry in Cologne, November 29 and 30, 1980," 5.

[36] The presentations had the following titles: "Doping Analytic: History, State and Future" (Robert Dugal), "Polyvalent Antisera for RIA-Detection of Anabolic Steroids" (Victor Rogozkin), "Metabolites as Indicators of Doping" (Arnold Beckett), "Detection of Anabolic Steroids by GC-MS: Routine Applications and its Limits" (Claus Clausnitzer), "A new Reference System for Retentions-Index Determinations suitable for GC-MS- and GC-N-FID-Determinations", "Alkylation of acid compounds with Fluoroalkyl- and Fluoroaryl-groups". Furthermore, Raymond Brooks gave a presentation on "the problem of exogenous testosterone." "The Detection of Testosterone Abuse" and "HPLC in Dope Detection" (all: Manfred Donike and co-workers). Note, "Symposium: "Fortschritte in der Dopinganalytik, Progress in Doping Analysis, May 21, 1981," archive collection "IOC Medical Commission," folder "Correspondence May-December 1981," IOC Archive, Lausanne.

[37] Note, "Manfred Donike, Klehr und das Symposium, 1980," archive collection "Nachlass August Kirsch," File 101 "Doping (1)," CuLDA, Cologne.

[38] Report, "IAAF Medical Committee on its activities between September 1981 and September 1982," archive collection "IAAF Medical Committee," folder "Medical Committee Reports to the Congress1976-1982," IAAF Archive, Monaco, 7.

[39] Statement, "Meeting of Heads of Top-Class Doping Control Laboratories by the Committee for the Development of Sport of the CoE, May 25, 1981," archive collection "IOC Medical Commission," folder "Correspondence May-December 1981," IOC Archive, Lausanne, Annex 1.

framework and financial resources for an increased cooperation between the authorised laboratories. One has to assume that the CoE framework was considered as an alternative avenue of support due to the lack of financial resources available within sport.

One must contribute an extremely high significance to the meetings of the IAAF Medical Committee, the IOC MSD, the heads of European doping laboratories and the educational workshop. This is mainly due to the multi-dimensional exchange of the anti-doping laboratory experts. Whereas previously, they had contributed to different bodies of the sporting organisations, efforts were combined for the very first time. Their expertise in the domain of doping analysis had allowed them to become key figures in the IOC's anti-doping activities, and instantly attempted to harmonise regulations. The symposium and the workshop constituted new kinds of activities because they dealt solely with aspects of doping analysis. All initiatives presented are connected to the foundation of the IOC MSD, which allowed the anti-doping laboratory experts to have a much more scientific approach to anti-doping. This had not been the case in the IOC Medical Commission. Consequently, just one year after the installation of the IOC MSD, a new orientation, steered by anti-doping laboratory experts, became visible and went beyond the scope of mere integration on the decision-making level. Their efforts in particular regarding the accreditation of anti-doping laboratories, a process that they controlled internally, quickly strengthened their position. However, in contrast to Arnold Beckett's approach to use the IOC MSD as a global, central body for anti-doping controls, attempts to harmonise the rules of other federations were not made in the first year. Instead, it focused on administrative challenges, resulting from the structural changes.

Joint Accreditations Efforts: Same Individuals but Different Organisations

Following the joint communiqué between the IAAF Medical Committee and the IOC MSD, IOC and IAAF representatives discussed the agreement again in Rome in December 1981.[40] Although no anti-doping laboratory experts were present at this meeting, the eventual agreement is significant because it formalised the cooperation in laboratory accreditation on the sport political level. The IAAF officials were not satisfied with the proposal in its contemporary form

---

[40] Minutes, "Meeting with Members of the IAAF Council and a Delegation from the IOC in Rome, December 14, 1981," archive collection "IAAF Council Meetings," IAAF Archive, Monaco, 3ff.

and only regarded it a first step.[41] Rather, they insisted on the importance of an appropriate implementation and only a full hand-over once they were satisfied that the IOC was able to accredit appropriately. According to the minutes of the meeting, the IAAF reiterated its stance that it did not want to be the "police federation" in global anti-doping affairs, but that a decent global doping control structure was necessary. All other IFs could then follow a strict anti-doping policy.[42] In order to do so, the main concern should be the extension of the laboratory network outside Europe, but one remarked that the financial resources for this initiative should come from the IOC.[43] Arne Ljungqvist also asserted that the IAAF Medical Committee thought international anti-doping initiatives should be extended to out-of competition testing.[44] This was the first time that such measures were discussed on the decision-making level. It was agreed that this was not possible until there were more accredited laboratories. Consequently, the anti-doping laboratory experts (in their role as certifiers of official laboratories) played a key role and should implement the framework to allow out-of competition testing. As a result, IAAF president Primo Nebiolo[45] and IOC president Juan Antonio Samaranch[46] signed another communiqué, outlining the increased anti-doping cooperation between IOC and IAAF on the political level with the following intentions:

1. Other International Federations should be urged to adopt the IAAF/IOC scheme of accreditation.

---

[41] Ibid.

[42] Ibid.

[43] Ibid.

[44] Minutes, "Meeting with Members of the IAAF Council and a Delegation from the IOC in Rome, December 14, 1981," 4.

[45] Primo Nebiolo (1923-1999) was IAAF president from 1981 until 1999. Prior to that, he was an IAAF Council member from 1972. He was the president of the organising committees of the 1974 European Athletics Championships, the 1981 Athletics World Cup and the 1987 World Athletics Championships, all held in Rome. He became a member of the IOC in 1992 but also acted as IAAF representative on various commissions before 1992. INTERNATIONAL OLYMPIC COMMITTEE, *Biographies of the Members of the International Olympic Committee* (Lausanne: International Olympic Committee, 1998), 72.

[46] Juan Antonio Samaranch (1920-2010) was IOC president from 1980 until 2001. He became an IOC member in 1961, was head of protocol (1968-1975, 1979-1980), member of the Executive Board (1970-1978, 1979-2001) and vice-president (1974-1978). Following his presidency, he became honorary president in 2001. INTERNATIONAL OLYMPIC COMMITTEE, *Biographies*, 117.

2. Action against persons inciting or supplying athletes with doping substances should be increased.

3. The programme of doping control testing should be extended to include testing in domestic competitions and testing in training.

4. IAAF and IOC must have the same sanction rule against athletes found guilty in training.[47]

Alexandre de Mérode eventually undertook the final step for the official approval of the IOC-IAAF agreement on the IOC Session in Rome in May 1982. He reported:

> The Commission has strengthened its agreement with the IAAF as to the procedure for recognising laboratories and to the sanctions which can be imposed on the athlete and those in his immediate circle in the period between the Olympic Games. The Medical Commission, which has elaborated a recognition of laboratories solely for screening with the purpose of reducing costs and assisting countries that are less well equipped in this field, has decided to continue separate agreements with each IF, particularly with-regard to anti-doping controls during training.[48]

Whilst the agreements refer to the general efforts of the IOC and the IAAF, it is important to emphasise the practical consequences of the accreditation procedures for the anti-doping laboratory experts. In reality, the intended expansion of the laboratory network was not as straightforward as originally anticipated. During a meeting of the IAAF Medical Committee, Manfred Donike remarked that there was no room for optimism because it was completely necessary to have sufficient knowledge about the analytical methods to test for stimulants and steroids before laboratories could get official accreditation.[49] According to Manfred Donike, he needed more than six months to educate laboratory staff members on the methods. Consequently, the sports organisations did not accredit more laboratories until

---

[47] Note, "Communiqué on Doping Controls, December 14, 1981," archive collection "IAAF Council Meetings," IAAF Archive, Monaco.
[48] Minutes, "85th Session of the IOC in Rome, May 27-29, 1982," archive collection "IOC Sessions 1894-2009," IOC Archive, Lausanne, Annex 13.
[49] Minutes, "Meeting of the IAAF Medical Committee in Stockholm, May 15 and 16, 1982," 1.

May 1982. He stressed that in 1981 laboratories in Zagreb (Yugoslavia) and Prague (Czechoslovakia) had tried to obtain accreditation, but failed due to breakdowns in the mass spectrometers and the computers.[50] In October 1982, the laboratory in Rome had been unable to detect the compounds present in the urine samples, even after two attempts.[51] Considering the strategies to recognise more laboratories as soon as possible, Manfred Donike accordingly suggested accrediting the laboratories in two stages. They should only conduct tests for stimulants and narcotics and then – providing they achieved the required standards – they would be granted official accreditation to test for steroids two years later.[52] This proposal is another indication for Manfred Donike's pragmatic thinking and his attempt to overcome any technical problems whilst still accommodating the political strategies. However, the IAAF Medical Committee rejected his idea and instead accepted a suggestion by Arnold Beckett. He had proposed allowing, in special cases, to undertake screening tests based on GC and RI, which was easier to implement but less specific.[53] In this way, laboratories could gain experience on doping analysis. These testing centres were not allowed to announce positive findings. Only once an authorised laboratory had confirmed the results with GC-MS, were the results announced. Moreover, the accredited laboratory had to re-check the "positive" A-sample along with the B-sample under the presence of representatives from the federation and the NOC.[54] The IOC Medical Commission accepted this strategy two weeks later on its meeting.[55] This measure supported the prevalent policy to deter athletes from doping, as stated in Arnold Beckett's proposal on the accreditation of "Recognised Laboratories for Screening."[56]

The decision also favoured the already accredited anti-doping laboratories, headed predominantly by the IOC MSD members, because it maintained their

---

[50] Ibid.

[51] Letter, "Manfred Donike to Alexandre de Mérode, November 23, 1982," archive collection "IOC Medical Commission," folder "Correspondence October-December 1982," IOC Archive, Lausanne.

[52] Minutes, "Meeting of the IAAF Medical Committee in Stockholm, May 15 and 16, 1982," 2.

[53] Ibid.

[54] Minutes, "Meeting of the Medical Commission of the International Olympic Committee, May 23 and 24, 1982," archive collection "IOC Medical Commission," folder "Meeting in Rome on May 1982 and in Sarajevo on February 1982," IOC Archive, Lausanne, Annex 10.

[55] Ibid., 9.

[56] Ibid., Annex 10.

supremacy. Accordingly, Manfred Donike wrote in a letter to August Kirsch that there was actually no need for the installation of more official anti-doping laboratories in Europe. [57] He preferred that the international and national federations should invest more financial resources into the existing ones. A higher quantity of accredited institutions would result in lower quality doping controls. Manfred Donike explained that even in the case of the introduction of out-of-competition testing, the existing anti-doping laboratories would be able to cope with the increased demand, because the tests in athletics would take place in a period where they were less busy.[58] Whilst one has to acknowledge Manfred Donike´s concern for the standard of the laboratories, his suggestions also include a degree of self-interest: he was hoping for more financial resources through the execution of more tests. At the same time, he admitted that the sport organisations needed official laboratories on other continents than Europe. Hence, his letter reveals a developing dilemma for the anti-doping laboratory experts on the medical bodies. Whereas they had to exercise accountability for the increase in the network, they also attempted to maintain the exclusivity of their own laboratories to raise their funding opportunities. They were thereby opposing the political level, for which the extension of the laboratory network was too slow. IAAF President Primo Nebiolo made this very clear in an IAAF Council meeting in 1983, where he complained about the lack of suitable laboratories.[59]

Funding was again a problem for the IOC MSD that hindered the accreditation of more laboratories. Although the IAAF and members of the IOC Medical Commission, such as Miroslav Slavik, demanded that the IOC would get supreme authority of the accreditation process,[60] the IOC MSD faced financial difficulties. Hence, in contrast to the IAAF, the IOC MSD charged a fee for the accreditation. As a result, most laboratories approached the IAAF Medical Committee instead. Yet, the example of the accreditation of the Moscow anti-doping laboratory, which Manfred Donike undertook on behalf of the IAAF in

---

[57] Letter, "Manfred Donike to Prof. Dr. August Kirsch, January 18, 1982," archive collection "Nachlass August Kirsch," File 007 "Doping (002)," CuLDA, Cologne, 3f.
[58] Ibid.
[59] Minutes, "Meeting of the Meeting of the IAAF Juridical Working Group, August 5, 1983," archive collection "Nachlass August Kirsch," File 012 "IAAF 1982-1987," CuLDA, Cologne, 12.
[60] Minutes, "Meeting of the Medical Commission of the International Olympic Committee, May 23 and 24, 1982," 9.

November 1982,[61] illustrates that the IOC also granted official accreditation once the IAAF had supervised the tests.

The IAAF dealt with the cases of thirteen laboratories, seeking accreditation during its meeting in May 1982.[62] Five of them were likely to get accreditation at the time. These were the testing centres in Brisbane (only for the Commonwealth Games), Sydney, Rome, Madrid and Stockholm. The institutions in Sofia (Bulgaria), Prague, Aarhus (Denmark), Helsinki (Finland), Paris, Budapest, Zagreb and Belgrade (Yugoslavia) also raised interest. However, Arnold Beckett and Manfred Donike raised objections concerning technical and administrative difficulties with those locations.[63] This reflects his attitude of not needing more laboratories in Europe. Importantly, the list reveals that the intention to accredit laboratories from outside Europe was difficult to realise. Hence, the IAAF Medical Commission members decided to provide the IAAF representatives of Mexico, Brazil, Puerto Rico and Japan with the necessary information material that they could push for a laboratory to become certified.[64]

The large number of requests to the IAAF Medical Committee prompted Manfred Donike to approach Alexandre de Mérode about subsidisation from the IOC.[65] This is understandable because the Institute of Biochemistry at the DSHS dealt with the accreditation process, no matter whether the IOC or the IAAF initiated the tests. Until 1985, there was no financial support for Manfred Donike although Alexandre de Mérode had established a way to generate funds. He had pushed for the installation of an International Olympic Association for Research in Sports Medicine (IOARSM). Officially, the association had the intention to support the IOC Medical Commission to achieve the following aims: to develop scientific research in the medico-sports field, to allow the publication of the results obtained and to encourage the development of practical actions based on established scientific data.[66] However, the IOARSM was also a strategic model

---

[61] Letter, "Manfred Donike to Members of the IOC Medical Commission´s sub-commission on doping and biochemistry, November 8, 1982," archive collection "IOC Medical Commission," folder "Correspondence October-December 1982," IOC Archive, Lausanne.

[62] Minutes, "Meeting of the IAAF Medical Committee in Stockholm, May 15 and 16, 1982," 4.

[63] Ibid.

[64] Ibid.

[65] Letter, "Manfred Donike to Alexandre de Mérode, June 29, 1982," collection "IOC Medical Commission," folder "Correspondence May-September 1982," IOC Archive, Lausanne.

[66] Minutes, "85th Session of the IOC in Rome, May 27-29, 1982," Annex 14.

through which the IOC Medical Commission could accept sponsorships legally. Arnold Beckett contributed to the first working group of IOARSM,[67] so the anti-doping laboratory experts had a representative on this important body as well. Once the IOC officially established the association in December 1982, Alexandre de Mérode informed Primo Nebiolo that the IOC had now sufficient funds to carry out the accreditation procedure solely by itself.[68] Yet, even financial backing through IOARSM did not convince the IAAF officials to transfer all competence entirely to the IOC. At the April 1983 IAAF Council meeting, Arne Ljungqvist reported that he did not consider the IOC MSD capable of conducting the procedure independently.[69] It was only in 1985 when the IOC MSD began to organise the shipping of all reference samples and started to finance the accreditation entirely by itself.[70] Eventually, the financial obligation on the part of the IOC led to the official withdrawal of the IAAF from the accreditation procedure, originally invented by its IAAF Medical Committee.[71] Hence, the transfer of competence from the IAAF to the IOC, which had started with the indirect adoption of the laboratory standards for the 1980 Winter Olympic Games in Lake Placid, was formally executed only five years later. Consequently, a key milestone in the history of the anti-doping laboratories was reached only months after the conclusion of the 1984 Los Angeles Olympic Games. Clearly, one can contribute this achievement to the IOC MSD's efforts and the inclusion of the leading anti-doping laboratory experts on the political level.

It is necessary to note in this regard that by the end of 1982 Victor Rogozkin had handed in his resignation from the IOC MSD due to illness.[72] Dr. Vitaly

---

[67] The other members of the working group were Alexandre de Mérode, IOC director Monique Berlioux, Anselmo Lopez (Spain, honorary director of Olympic Solidarity), Adrien Vanden Eede (Belgium, advisor to the IOC President for commercial affairs) and Professor Dr. Wolfgang Baumann (FRG, member of the IOC Medical Commission's Subcommission on Biomechanics and Physiology and professor at the DSHS. Minutes, "86th Session of the IOC in New Delhi, March 26-28, 1983," archive collection "IOC Sessions 1894-2009," IOC Archive, Lausanne, Annex 24.

[68] Letter, "Alexandre de Mérode to Primo Nebiolo, January 20, 1983."

[69] Minutes, "Kurzprotokoll – Kirsch: Council Sitzung, April 23, 1983," archive collection "Nachlass August Kirsch," File 012 "IAAF 1982-1987," CuLDA, Cologne, 8.

[70] Minutes, "Minutes of the IAAF Council Meeting, March 29, 1985," archive collection "Nachlass August Kirsch," File 012 "IAAF 1982-1987," CuLDA, Cologne, 25.

[71] Ibid.

[72] Letter, "Victor Rogozkin to Alexandre de Mérode, October 27, 1982," collection "IOC Medical Commission," folder "Correspondence October-December 1982," IOC Archive, Lausanne.

Semenov[73], the new head of the Moscow anti-doping laboratory at the Research Institute of Physical Culture, replaced him on suggestion of the former president of the NOC of the USSR, Sergei Pavlov.[74] This assured Soviet representation on the IOC MSD but at the same time, he also suited the profile of head of an accredited anti-doping laboratory.

Numeric Gain in Anti-doping Laboratories between 1982 and 1985

By mid-1983, the IOC and the IAAF had accredited the laboratories in Moscow, Madrid and Prague, the latter having overcome the difficulties with its computers.[75] Consequently, there were now eight doping control laboratories jointly authorised by the IOC and the IAAF, since the laboratory in Magglingen had lost its accreditation due to changes in personnel. It was reaccredited in 1985.[76] Arne Ljungqvist attributed the low number of accreditations to the difficulty that only a few experts were able to undertake the supervision of an accreditation procedure.[77] This provides evidence for their influence and their key administrative roles. Whereas the organisational structure had been changed, those responsible were still the same small group of anti-doping laboratory experts. Furthermore, the IAAF Medical Committee incorporated an additional administrative stage, which stalled any decision: once the IAAF had received all official papers from the respective laboratory, all IAAF Medical Committee members were provided with a full report on the laboratory and the accreditation procedure before official recognition was actually granted and the IOC could be informed.[78]

Besides such extra directorial steps, organisational difficulties made the approval of laboratories outside Europe more difficult. For example, the private

---

[73] Dr. Vitaly Semenov (born 1937) took over the role of head of the anti-doping laboratory of the *Research Institute of Physical Culture* from Victor Rogozkin in 1982. At the same time, he acted as president of the Council for New Medicaments at the Ministry of Public Health of the USSR and was a member of the Medical Commission of the IWF since 1980. Letter, "Sergei Pavlov, former President of the NOC of the USSR, to Alexandre de Mérode, December 13, 1982," collection "IOC Medical Commission," folder "Correspondence October-December 1982," IOC Archive, Lausanne.

[74] Ibid.

[75] Minutes, "86th Session of the IOC in New Delhi, March 26-28, 1983," archive collection "IOC Sessions 1894-2009," IOC Archive, Lausanne, Annex 14.

[76] "Doping Control Laboratory," *Olympic Review* 215 (1985), 568.

[77] Minutes, "IAAF Medical Committee Meeting in Helsinki, May 23, 1983," archive collection "IAAF Medical Committee," IAAF Archive, Monaco, 1.

[78] Ibid.

Mitsubishi-Yuka Laboratory of Medical Science in Tokyo had already applied for official accreditation through the IOC MSD in January 1983.[79] However, problems in sending the reference samples through Japanese customs occurred, because the sport organisations needed a license to import specific drugs.[80] In the case of the Brisbane laboratory, the accreditation procedure was conducted successfully, but there were problems with the full documentation.[81] The IOC MSD eliminated the laboratory in Sydney from the list of potential testing centres because it could not undertake the analytical work without new MS equipment.[82]

Within Europe, complications were more of technical nature. Earlier in 1983, Arnold Beckett's staff member Professor Dr. David Cowan[83] had visited the National Laboratory for the Detection of Doping (Laboratoire National de Dépistage du Dopage, LNDD) run by Dr. Jean-Pierre Lafarge in Châtenay-Malabry, southwest of Paris.[84] Yet, irregularities with the samples occurred and the laboratory could not identify the substances correctly. Jean-Pierre Lafarge blamed the instability of the urine solutions.[85] However, Arnold Beckett and Manfred Donike claimed that in cases where laboratories had failed to identify substances, this was due to old screening procedures.[86] They insisted on a strict accreditation policy, to maintain the high standards of the doping analysis, but also to ensure the exclusivity of the accredited institutions. Due to the difficulties, Arne Ljungqvist proposed a revision and simplification of the process to

---

[79] Letter, "Katsuji Shibata and Yoshio Kuroda to Alexandre de Mérode, January 26, 1983," archive collection "IOC Medical Commission," folder "Correspondence October-December 1982," IOC Archive, Lausanne.

[80] Minutes, "IAAF Medical Committee Doping Sub-Committee Meeting in London, January 14, 1984," archive collection "IAAF Medical Committee," IAAF Archive, Monaco, 6.

[81] Minutes, "IAAF Medical Committee Meeting in Helsinki, May 23, 1983," 4.

[82] Ibid., 6.

[83] Prof. Dr. David Cowan became head of the Drug Control Centre at KCL in 1990, having worked with Arnold Beckett for many years. He currently holds a chair in Pharmaceutical Toxicology and is an alumnus of KCL in pharmacy. In 1998, the IOC awarded him the Trophy for Ethics in Sport. Due to the human resources policy of the KCL, it was not possible to get information on David Cowan's biographical data. Email, Alison Woffendin to Jörg Krieger, March 11, 2015.

[84] Minutes, "IAAF Medical Committee Meeting in Helsinki, May 23, 1983," 5.

[85] Ibid.

[86] Ibid.

Alexandre de Mérode.[87] However, with strong opposition from the now more powerful anti-doping laboratory experts, he did not undertake any initiatives.

Consequently, there were only two more accreditations in 1983. First, the IAAF approved the anti-doping laboratory in Rome, which was eventually successful in the identification of the control substances. Second, the private anti-doping laboratory Yhtyneet Medix Laboratoriot in Helsinki led by Professor Dr. Kimmo Kuoppasalmi, gained accreditation. It became the first official anti-doping laboratory in Scandinavia.[88] Without a doubt, it was essential to the IAAF to have an accredited anti-doping laboratory in Finland in 1983 because of the inaugural World Athletics Championships in Helsinki in that year. In contrast to this, the IOC MSD's meetings focused on the approaching Olympic Games in 1984. It approved the doping laboratories in Sarajevo and Los Angeles in January 1984 and November 1983 respectively (see later in this chapter).[89] Consequently, despite various initial difficulties, the intended wide range of accreditations was gaining momentum and the total number rose to twelve.

Further laboratories were officially approved until shortly after the 1984 Los Angeles Olympic Games. By September 1985, the institutions in Paris, Tokyo and Brisbane had overcome their earlier challenges and the sport organisations awarded them accreditation. Along with these accreditations, Arne Ljungqvist had pushed for the installation of a Swedish testing centre in Huddinge at the Division of Clinical Chemistry at the Karolinska Institute (Karolinska Institutet) led by Professor Dr. Ingemar Björkhem.[90] The Nijmegen doping control centre of IAAF Medical Committee member Jacques van Rossum was also accredited.[91] Besides, the institution in Leningrad stopped conducting doping controls because

---

[87] Minutes, "IAAF Council with the IOC Executive Board in Helsinki, August 6, 1983," archive collection "Nachlass August Kirsch," File 123, "IAAF (2)," CuLDA, Cologne, 4.

[88] Report, "Major Decisions of the International Amateur Athletic Federation World Championships in Athletics, Helsinki 1983: Council Meeting, August 4 and 5, 1983," archive collection "Nachlass August Kirsch," File 012 "IAAF 1982-1987," CuLDA, Cologne, 2.

[89] Report, "Medical Controls. Doping Controls. XIV Olympic Winter Games Sarajevo, 1984, June, 1984," archive collection "Summer and Winter Olympic Games: Medical Files," folder "Medical matters at the Olympic Winter Games of Sarajevo 1984: reports," IOC Archive, Lausanne, 2. Also see: Fax, "Arnold Beckett to Alexandre de Mérode, November 23, 1983," archive collection "Summer and Winter Olympic Games: Medical Files," folder "Medical matters at the 1984 Summer Olympic Games in Los Angeles: Correspondence," IOC Archive, Lausanne.

[90] Minutes, "Minutes of the IAAF Council Meeting, July 12, 1985," archive collection "Nachlass August Kirsch," File 012 "IAAF 1982-1987," CuLDA, Cologne, 16.

[91] "Doping Control Laboratory," *Olympic Review* 215 (1985), 568.

the Soviets had made the laboratory in Moscow their main doping control centre.[92]

Ultimately, in the period between the first IOC-IAAF agreement on dual laboratory accreditation in 1981, and the end of 1985, the number of worldwide doping laboratories rose to sixteen, due to the efforts of the anti-doping laboratory experts, who established the necessary processes (for an overview on the year of accreditation for each laboratory.[93] Nevertheless, IAAF President Primo Nebiolo commented generously on the matter and according to the official minutes was of the opinion that even more laboratories were needed.[94] Since he had complained about the slow process of the accreditation procedure on numerous occasions, there is little doubt that the announcement of more laboratories was primarily a marketing strategy for him. Furthermore, the institutional characteristics of the anti-doping laboratories also constituted a deviation compared to the original attempts of focusing on anti-doping laboratories in a university setting. For example, the laboratories in Helsinki and Tokyo were privately funded. One can attribute this to the urgency of installing an anti-doping laboratory for the 1983 World Athletics Championships in Helsinki, and the long-term desire to have a testing centre on the Asian continent.

Whilst it appears that the political level was much interested in the increase of the *quantity* of doping laboratories, the anti-doping laboratory experts attempted to retain a high *quality* through the eventual implementation of a reaccreditation process. Previously in 1979, the original IAAF process foresaw such a strategy (see Chapter 5). At the IAAF Medical Committee meeting in 1983, it becomes clear that the anti-doping laboratories in Cologne, London and Kreischa should act as "reference laboratories" and produce the samples for all other accredited doping testing centres.[95] This demonstrates the privileged status of the three laboratories. Besides being an instrument for quality control, the reaccreditation had the side effect that the reference laboratories maintained a degree of exclusivity and attained further distinction. The reaccreditation process was executed biannually and made compulsory for all accredited anti-doping

[92] Ibid.

[93] In a 1985 edition of the *Olympic Review*, the IOC argued it had accredited only fourteen institutions but in fact listed fifteen institutions. Moreover, the IOC MSD accredited the doping laboratory in Nijmengen at the end of the year and it did not appear on the official list. "Antidoping Laboratories," *Olympic Review* 213 (1985), 411.

[94] Minutes, "Minutes of the IAAF Council Meeting, July 12, 1985," archive collection "Nachlass August Kirsch," File 012 "IAAF 1982-1987," CuLDA, Cologne, 16.

[95] Minutes, "IAAF Medical Committee Meeting in Helsinki, May 23, 1983," 5.

laboratories that had been certified for more than a year prior to the reaccreditation date.[96] Although it was mainly the IAAF Medical Committee that pushed for the execution of the re-authorisation, the first overall test of all laboratories took place at the end of January 1985 under the auspices of the IOC MSD. In 1985, all originally accredited institutions passed the reaccreditation test.[97]

It becomes evident from the developments in the anti-doping laboratory network that despite unclear responsibilities, the increasingly strong role of the anti-doping laboratory experts led to the establishment of more official laboratories along with a growing set of procedures such as the reaccreditation process. Certainly, this resulted in more administrative tasks for key individuals such as Manfred Donike and Arnold Beckett, which is reflected in the rising amount of written exchanges that exist from this period. At the same time, the extending anti-doping laboratory network is proof as their progressively self-initiated indispensability.

MANFRED DONIKE BECOMES A CENTRAL FIGURE

Possibilities and Challenges in his New Role

It is important to continue investigating the proceedings surrounding the individual and institutional networks of the anti-doping laboratory experts. Within these networks, Manfred Donike increasingly progressed as central figure due to his role in the IOC MSD, his important part in the accreditation process and his expertise in testosterone testing. He used his role within the international anti-doping community to justify his growing demands for funds from his national financial backer, the BISp. He listed besides the increasing number of doping analyses, the expansion of the banned list and the introduction of new methods, as reasons for more funding.[98] Moreover, he stressed that the "Zunahme der internationalen Zusammenarbeit, Kommissionssitzungen und Laborbesuche, Demonstrationen [Increase of international collaboration, commission meetings and laboratory visits, demonstrations]," resulted in a much higher workload.[99] He

---

[96] Ibid.

[97] Minutes, "90th Session of the IOC in East Berlin, June 4-6, 1985," archive collection "IOC Sessions 1894-2009," IOC Archive, Lausanne, Annex 11.

[98] Letter, "Manfred Donike to BISp, Vertrag des Beauftragten für Dopinganalytik und Etatgestaltung in den Jahren 1983 und folgende, January 27, 1982," archive collection "Nachlass August Kirsch," File 086, "Doping (2)," CuLDA, Cologne, 1.

[99] Ibid., 2.

elaborated on this in an attached report for the Sports Committee of the government, where he remarked that the international meetings, visits by foreign scientists and travels to approve laboratories were extremely time-consuming. He requested to consider these aspects favourably within the human resource planning.[100]

Manfred Donike was successful in using his international influence to strengthen his position on the national level. However, the expansion of the doping analysis as enforced through increased influence of the anti-doping laboratory experts encountered resistance from sport medicine specialists in the FRG. KRÜGER et al. claim that the research funds for sports medicine had decreased significantly by the beginning of the 1980s, and that the focus on doping analysis had created a competitive situation between sports medicine and doping analysis.[101] This was similar on the international level. Because Joseph Keul felt overlooked on the national scene, he made abundantly clear in a letter to Arne Ljungqvist that he regarded the doping analysis to be only one of many ways to combat doping, while lobbying for a more holistic approach. [102] According to Joseph Keul, the doping control institutions were obtaining huge amounts of research funds, which were not affordable to many nations. Instead, he favoured an educational and informative approach aimed at athletes, coaches, officials and medical doctors.[103] It is interesting that Joseph Keul sought support on the international level. Whereas Manfred Donike had established himself as an important agent on the international scene who set the guidelines for national sport, Joseph Keul´s influence was restricted to the national level. Hence, the two were attempting opposing ways of communication and exerting their influence. Manfred Donike used his international influence to get financial support from within the FRG, causing Joseph Keul to complain to international sport administrators. Without doubt, Manfred Donike occupied the more important strategic position.[104] One can say this not only for the situation in the FRG, but also definitely for global anti-doping activities. For example, Arne Ljungqvist

---

[100] Report, "Entwicklung der Doping-Analytik und -Forschung, January 27, 1982," archive collection "Nachlass August Kirsch," File 086, "Doping (2)," CuLDA, Cologne, 2.

[101] KRÜGER et al., *Doping und Anti-Doping*, 120ff.

[102] Letter, "Joseph Keul to Arne Ljungqvist, Dopinganalytik, September 6, 1983," archive collection "Nachlass August Kirsch," File 086, "Doping (2)," CuLDA, Cologne, 2.

[103] Ibid.

[104] KRÜGER et al., *Doping und Anti-Doping*, 123.

constantly supported Manfred Donike, although he perceived the influence of the anti-doping laboratories as too extensive occasionally.[105]

The support on the international and national level encouraged Manfred Donike to continue acting as a strong advocate for an increasing number of doping tests. Thereby, his focus was on the addition of exogenous testosterone onto the IOC´s list of banned substances following the success of his unofficial screening at the 1980 Moscow Olympic Games. Arnold Beckett, who proposed the ban of exogenous testosterone in February 1982, supported him in his efforts.[106] Again, the IAAF acted faster in this regard and had already included testosterone and its esters as banned substances in the 1981 IAAF Handbook but did not specify a testing method for it. [107] The IOC Medical Commission eventually added exogenous testosterone to the list in 1982. [108] On Arnold Beckett´s proposal, the IOC Medical Commission installed a testing period of four months without sanctions in order to allow further research by Raymond Brooks based on RI.[109] On a subsequent meeting in May 1982, Manfred Donike presented the technical details of his GC-MS method, which he continued to advocate as more advanced than RI, because it allowed more specific screening.[110] However, Arnold Beckett insisted on using the RI for screening because its use was more widespread, but also because his institution in London employed Raymond Brooks, the leading expert of the RI method. In reality, it posed difficulties for Arnold Beckett because he realised that he was losing the leadership in the field of doping analysis to Manfred Donike. Having been the sole anti-doping laboratory expert on the IOC Medical Commission since the establishment of the body in 1967, Arnold Beckett faced more compromises through the creation of the IOC MSD. Thus, the disagreement between the two anti-doping laboratory experts on the appropriate screening method illustrates that the rise in the significance of their role also brought with it a conflict of interests,

---

[105] Minutes, "Meeting of the IAAF Medical Committee in Stockholm, May 15 and 16, 1982," 1.

[106] Minutes, "Meeting of the IOC Medical Commission in Los Angeles, February 6 and 7, 1982," archive collection "IOC Medical Commission," folder "Meeting in Moscow on July 19 and August 23, 1980, in Baden-Baden in September 1981 and Los Angeles in February 1982," IOC Archive, Lausanne, 10.

[107] Report, "Report – IAAF: Council Meeting 1981 - 1982, March 20-22, 1981," archive collection "Nachlass August Kirsch," File 010 "IAAF 1980/81," CuLDA, Cologne, 15.

[108] Minutes, "Meeting of the IOC Medical Commission, February 6 and 7, 1982," 10.

[109] Ibid., Annex 9.

[110] Minutes, "Meeting of the Medical Commission of the International Olympic Committee, May 23 and 24, 1982," 11.

as the doping analysis field became more differentiated. Whilst Arnold Beckett and Manfred Donike were eager to expand doping tests and outdo sport medicine specialists, they were both dictating terms that did not necessarily agree. In the case of the testosterone tests, Alexandre de Mérode aligned with Manfred Donike because he, as always, wanted to follow the progress of science, and acknowledged the fact that GC-MS was quicker and more precise, allowing up to 200 analyses per day.[111] Hence, the IOC Medical Commission planned GC-MS screens for the 1984 Los Angeles Olympic Games under the condition that Arnold Beckett and his colleagues did not develop a RI method with the same broad spectrum of detectable substances and the same sensitivity as GC-MS.[112] This decision was a success for Manfred Donike and a setback for Arnold Beckett.

Whereas the introduction of the exogenous testosterone test consolidated Manfred Donike´s position on the international scene, it aroused opposition from Joseph Keul again. He opposed the testosterone test because he considered the testing method insufficient.[113] He also did not agree with the addition of caffeine to the banned list, officially agreed upon in 1983, because he doubted its health-damaging effects.[114] However, the attitude of sport medicine in the FRG towards the expansion of the doping analysis was also a reason for this. From another of Joseph Keul´s letters, it becomes evident that he thought Manfred Donike´s single-handed attempt to advance the doping analysis without feedback to sport medicine was "pathetic." [115] He maintained that Manfred Donike should appreciate that individuals from sport medicine had promoted doping analysis in general, and had supported the foundation of the anti-doping laboratory in Cologne (see Chapter 3). [116] This expressly underlines the demonstrated development that the sport medicine specialists lost their commanding position in anti-doping matters to anti-doping laboratory experts by the beginning of the 1980s.

Curiously, Joseph Keul stated that the communication processes of the GDR should be used as an example, because at the 1983 World Athletics Championships, their team doctors had been strictly instructed by Manfred

---

[111] Ibid., 3.
[112] Ibid., 11.
[113] KRÜGER et al., *Doping und Anti-Doping*, 120ff.
[114] Ibid.
[115] Letter, "Joseph Keul to Manfred Donike, September 8, 1983," archive collection "Nachlass August Kirsch," File 086, "Doping (2)," CuLDA, Cologne.
[116] Ibid.

Höppner.[117] However, the stream of information amongst GDR officials was highly developed because in the GDR doping system, testosterone esters were used as undetectable alternatives for steroids for "steroid bridging" (also known as "bridging therapy") in the weeks ahead of sporting competitions.[118] Once it became clear that the sport organisations would introduce a test for exogenous testosterone, Manfred Höppner reported to the sports authorities.[119] By the time of the addition of testosterone to the list, Claus Clausnitzer had already developed solutions to circumvent the doping tests. The last injection of exogenous testosterone, which was now only a testosterone proportionate, should be given four to five days before the competition.[120] Despite these anticipatory measures, these circumstances explain why Manfred Höppner voted for a delay in the IAAF Medical Committee in 1982:[121] it gave the scientists of the GDR more time to test their new strategy.

The increasing sophistication in doping analysis in terms of the extending network and the growing list of banned substances led to multi-layered challenges but also huge possibilities for Manfred Donike. He became the main administrator of the anti-doping laboratory network because of his position as head of the IOC MSD, the introduction of the accreditation system coordinated from the DSHS and the invention of the testosterone test. Within the FRG, sport medicine specialists battling for national funding caused the problem. On the international level, Arnold Beckett attempted to retain his leading position by promoting the RI method. Their efforts to include testosterone and caffeine on the list of banned substances can also be contributed to the financial profit and public funds that the doping laboratories received. Manfred Donike and Arnold Beckett had already displayed this attitude in their attempt to establish an official laboratory accreditation system. Whereas KRÜGER demonstrate this for the national level,[122] the same applies for the international level.

---

[117] Ibid.

[118] Werner FRANKE and Brigitte BERENDONK, "Hormonal doping and androgenization of athletes: a secret program of the German Democratic Republic government," *Clinical Chemistry* 43, no. 7 (1997), 1270.

[119] Giselher SPITZER, *Doping in der DDR*, Annex 7.

[120] FRANKE and BERENDONK, "Hormonal doping," 1271.

[121] Minutes, "Meeting of the IAAF Medical Committee in Stockholm, May 15 and 16, 1982," 6.

[122] KRÜGER et al., *Doping und Anti-Doping*, 120ff.

The Installation of the Cologne Workshop

Besides the extension of the anti-doping laboratory network, educational activities were initiated, even though these efforts did not only come from within the community of the anti-doping laboratory experts. Amongst them was one suggestion (not without a high degree of self-interest) for increased internationalisation of the doping analysis at the Olympic Games from sport officials of the GDR and the USSR. The officials proposed that the doping analysis should be conducted not only by staff from the host country, but also by representatives of different participating countries. To stress their intent, they submitted a proposal of suggested doctors and professors from Socialist countries. [123] They claimed that this would make the doping controls more objective, though it is likely that the intention was to manipulate the doping tests. Werner FRANKE and Brigitte BERENDONK reveal that GDR officials such as Manfred Höppner used the manipulation of samples as a last resort to cover positive doping tests.[124] They simply exchanged the urine samples. The members of the IOC Medical Commission discussed the suggestion but eventually rejected it.[125] Instead, they favoured an approach where the members of the IOC MSD were supervising the laboratory work.[126] This gave the members of the IOC MSD even more influence in the IOC's attempts to combat doping. They suggested that only an international body, such as the IOC MSD, could grant an objective supervision.[127] Although the decision did not correspond entirely with the GDR's initial proposal, Claus Clausnitzer regarded the supervision by the five members of the MSD as a partial success.[128] Consequently, Manfred Ewald immediately

---

[123] Minutes, "Meeting of the IOC Medical Commission, February 6 and 7, 1982," Annex 2.

[124] FRANKE and BERENDONK, "Hormonal doping," 1271.

[125] Minutes, "Meeting of the IOC Medical Commission, February 6 and 7, 1982," 4.

[126] Ibid.

[127] Minutes, "Meeting of the IOC Medical Commission's Subcommisson on 'Doping and the Biochemistry of Sport', September 29, 1983," archive collection "IOC Medical Commission," folder "IOC Medical Commission: meeting of both sub-commissions Doping and biochemistry of sport and Sports medecine and orthopaedics in Cologne on 29th September 1983: minutes," IOC Archive, Lausanne, 4.

[128] Report, "Zuarbeit für Generalsekretäre des NOK der DDR durch Leiter DKL des SMD der DDR zu 'Internationalisierung Dopinkgontrollen', September 7, 1983," archive collection "DR 510 Nationales Olympisches Komitee der DDR," folder "DR 510/525, Band 5, Medizinische Kommission des IOC, 1977-1987," Bundesarchiv, Berlin-Lichterfelde.

showed his appreciation to Alexandre de Mérode.[129] The NOCs of the USSR and the GDR did not let the matter rest though, and proposed an alternative approach in November 1983. In this proposal, Manfred Ewald suggested that the doping analysis should take place in two laboratories, one situated in a socialist and one in a non-socialist country.[130] The IOC MSD also rejected this approach. The episode illustrates that the establishment of the anti-doping laboratory network was by no means detached from the politicisation of the Olympic Movement.

Furthermore, the expansion of the laboratory network and the doping controls initiated numerous requests by international laboratory workers for Manfred Donike. Consequently, he came up with a new educational format to instruct about new testing methods: the "Cologne Workshop."[131] As explained earlier in this chapter, a first workshop had already taken place in the context of the joint meeting of the IOC MSD and the IAAF Medical Committee in Cologne in May 1981. However, the Cologne Workshop was under the sole responsibility of Manfred Donike. Therefore, it is important to distinguish between the two workshops, although the location indicates the increasing institutional centralisation of the doping analysis. In the official invitation, Manfred Donike claimed that the introduction of the testosterone tests with GC-MS had made the workshop inevitable, because colleagues from all over the world wanted to visit his laboratory to learn about the new procedure:

> As I can not fulfil the individual request of each colleague out of lag [sic] of time – I apologize for this situation – I have decided to organize a workshop each year at the end of January, beginning of February. This workshop should give opportunity to all interested colleagues to work with our routine methods in detecting dope agents, the opportunity for discussions and criticisme [sic], maybe also the opportunity to

---

[129] Letter, "Manfred Ewald to Alexandre de Mérode, September 22, 1983," archive collection "DR 510 Nationales Olympisches Komitee der DDR," folder "DR 510/966, Band 4, Medizinische Kommission des IOC, 1977-1987," Bundesarchiv, Berlin-Lichterfelde.

[130] Letter, "Manfred Ewald to Alexandre de Mérode, November 9, 1983," archive collection "Summer and Winter Olympic Games: Medical Files," folder "Medical matters at the 1984 Summer Olympic Games in Los Angeles: Correspondence," IOC Archive, Lausanne.

[131] Letter, "Manfred Donike to Heiner Henze, Workshop in dope analysis, October 13, 1982," archive collection "Nachlass August Kirsch," File 086, "Doping (2)," CuLDA, Cologne.

demonstrate their own progress in dope analysis. They are also invited to make contributions.[132]

This gives further evidence for his central position within the anti-doping laboratory network, but also proves his growing workload because of ever-increasing administrative tasks. The installation of the Cologne Workshop was an attempt to maintain the central point of the anti-doping laboratory network, apart from obvious practical reasons of knowledge exchange. It enabled Manfred Donike to control the communication processes on the latest technical developments and to set the agenda. For example, he sent out invitations to selected individuals only, and he determined the topics for each talk. A consultation during IOC MSD meetings did not take place. Rather, Manfred Donike contacted its members directly. For example, he commissioned Claus Clausnitzer to speak about the identification of steroid hormones through MS.[133]

The Cologne Workshop immediately became a central element in the exchange of knowledge amongst the widening network of anti-doping laboratory experts, and is proof of its progressive professionalization. Particularly because the event allowed the inclusion of a broader community than the IOC MSD did. Manfred Donike highlighted this in the invitation.[134] In total, eighteen participants from twelve countries participated in the first Cologne Workshop, which took place between January 31 and February 4, 1983.

Whereas Manfred Donike intended the Cologne Workshop as a regular exchange forum for anti-doping laboratory experts only, the IOC MSD created a second format to notify other representatives of the sporting community about the newest developments in anti-doping matters. It is important to differentiate between the two. The "anti-doping course," which took place for the first time in Cologne at the end of September 1983, was targeted towards practising doctors from each Continental Association of NOCs to advise about the general problems of doping and to educate them on doping controls.[135] In contrast to the Cologne Workshop, the entire IOC MSD organised this course. Manfred Donike provided the facilities at the DSHS. In several communications, the IOC MSD made clear

---

[132] Ibid.

[133] Letter, "Manfred Donike to Claus Clausnitzer, Workshop in dope analysis, October 25, 1982," archive collection "DR 510 Nationales Olympisches Komitee der DDR," folder "DR 510/966, Band 4, Medizinische Kommission des IOC, 1977-1987," Bundesarchiv, Berlin-Lichterfelde.

[134] Letter, "Manfred Donike to Heiner Henze, Workshop in dope analysis," October 13, 1982."

[135] Minutes, "86th Session of the IOC in New Delhi, March 26-28, 1983," 77.

that it was an informative forum to expand knowledge on doping and anti-doping. It stressed that it was staged separately from educational seminars for heads of laboratories.[136] The official programme reveals that the members of the IOC MSD gave lectures on general topics such as "Definition of Doping," "The Pharmacology of Dope Agents," "Organisation of Dope Control" and "Routine Dope Analysis in the Laboratory."[137] For example, in contrast to his very scientific speech at the Cologne Workshop, Claus Clausnitzer advised on the functioning and working of an anti-doping laboratory.[138] Eventually, the initiative, along with the apparent need to inform about anti-doping in general, led to the installation of another IOC Medical Commission Subcommittee on "Coordination with the NOCs" in 1985.[139]

Besides the spread of information, the anti-doping course also allowed integration of another increasingly important body within the Olympic Movement: the IOC Athletes' Commission. The IOC had created this body following the decisions of the IOC Congress in Baden-Baden in 1981.[140] The

---

[136] Minutes, "Meeting of the IOC Medical Commission, February 5-19, 1984," archive collection "IOC Medical Commission," folder "IOC Medical Commission: meeting in Sarajevo on 5th-19th February 1984 : roll call, minutes, drawing of a meeting and working documents," IOC Archive, Lausanne, 16.

[137] Programme, "Course on Anti-Doping – Cologne, September 25 to October 1, 1983," archive collection "IOC Athletes' Commission," folder "Athletes' Commission: reports, statement, seminar, press release, press cuttings and leaflets of the commission," IOC Archive, Lausanne.

[138] Speech, "Claus Clausnitzer, 'Funktion und Arbeitsweise eines Dopingkontroll-Labors,' September 27, 1983," archive collection "DR 510 Nationales Olympisches Komitee der DDR," folder "DR 510/966, Band 4, Medizinische Kommission des IOC, 1977-1987," Bundesarchiv, Berlin-Lichterfelde.

[139] Minutes, "Meeting of the IOC Medical Commission, April 10 and 11, 1985," archive collection "IOC Medical Commission," folder "IOC Medical Commission: meeting of both sub-commissions Doping and biochemistry of sport, Sports medecine and orthopaedics and Coordination with the NOCs in Moscow on 10th-11th April 1985: roll call, minutes and working documents," IOC Archive, Lausanne, 2.

[140] Minutes, "Meeting of the IOC Athletes' Commission, May 24, 1982," archive collection "IOC Athletes' Commission," folder "Athletes' Commission, meeting in Roma on 24th May 1982: roll call, minutes, correspondence and recommendations," IOC Archive, Lausanne, Annex 1.

athletes stressed from the very beginning the problem of doping.[141] The IOC Athletes' Commission's suggestions included the increase of sanctions, the introduction of out-of competition tests and most importantly, assistance given for the establishment of doping laboratories around the world.[142] Consequently, the IOC MSD and the IOC Athletes' Commission began to form a close relationship. As result of the links created, Manfred Donike invited a representative of the IOC Athletes' Commission to the anti-doping course for medical doctors. Dr. Thomas Bach[143] eventually attended it. The summary of his visit reveals that the lack of appropriate anti-doping laboratories around the world was emphasised at the meeting.[144] Thomas Bach considered this largely a financial and technical problem, and highlighted that as long as the already admitted institutions were prepared to give their support, the difficulties could be minimised.[145] Thus, his report lends further evidence to the fact that the anti-doping laboratory experts with their attempt to expand their network were gaining influence. The IOC Athletes' Commission supported this because it had a strong interest in the implementation of strict and reliable doping controls.

Impact of Manfred Donike on Specific Sporting Events

Only shortly after the installation of the IOC MSD, Manfred Donike was increasingly regarded a key player within the global fight against doping. One can

---

[141] The athletes who participated in the Congres elected the following members onto the IOC Athletes' Commission: Edwin Moses (USA), Thomas Bach (FRG), Sebastian Coe (Great Britain), Ivar Formo (Norway), Svetla Otzetova (Bulgaria), Kipchoge Keino (Kenya) and Vladislav Tretyak (USSR). IOC member Peter Tallberg from Finland became its first chairman. Minutes, "Meeting of the IOC Athletes' Commission, May 24, 1982," Annex 1.

[142] INTERNATIONAL OLYMPIC COMMITTEE, *Proceedings of the XI Olympic Congress in Baden-Baden, 1980. Volume 1* (Lausanne: International Olympic Committee, 1981), 109.

[143] Dr. Thomas Bach (born 1953) is the current IOC president, elected at the 125th IOC Session in Buenos Aires in 2013. Prior to his sport political career, he was a successful athlete, who won the Olympic gold medal with the FRG fencing (foil) team at the 1976 Montreal Olympic Games. He was elected as IOC member in 1991, member of the IOC Executive Board in from 1996 to 2000, then vice-president from 2000 until 2004 and re-elected in 2006. He was the founding president of the DOSB. INTERNATIONAL OLYMPIC COMMITTEE, *Biographies*, 14.

[144] Report, "Seminar of the Medical Commission of the IOC by Dr. Thomas Bach, n.d.," archive collection "IOC Athletes' Commission," folder "Athletes' Commission: reports, statement, seminar, press release, press cuttings and leaflets of the commission," IOC Archive, Lausanne.

[145] Ibid.

confirm this with a closer look at his impact on global sporting events. In their monograph, former chief medical officer for USOC, Dr. Robert VOY, and Kirk D. DEETER have raised suspicions about unreported doping tests at the 1983 World Athletics Championships in Helsinki.[146] They state that it was highly unlikely that IAAF president Primo Nebiolo pushed for rigorous doping controls at the first global athletics championships and Richard Pound supported their doubts through further critical comments.[147] In fact, Manfred Donike admitted in 1990 that there had been unreported positive tests.[148] The enhanced body of source material allows more evidence to be brought into focus.

It is necessary to emphasise that in contrast to the statements by VOY and DEETER, Manfred Donike was not present in Helsinki to supervise the doping controls.[149] He had prepared the laboratory and educated the staff members on the analytical techniques.[150] However, the IAAF Medical Committee appointed Arnold Beckett and Grigory Vorobiev to supervise the doping analysis. They joined Arne Ljungqvist, who was the official medical delegate.[151] In the context of the first application of the new GC-MS method with which Arnold Beckett was not as familiar as Manfred Donike was, one has to stress this as an important detail.

Discussions within the IOC MSD in September 1983 reveal that there had indeed been two positive tests during the competitions.[152] However, the head of the laboratory and Arnold Beckett had not been willing to declare the samples positive because the T/E ratio was only a little higher than six.[153] Hence, they transported the samples to the anti-doping laboratory in London, where apparently the ratio was now under six.[154] Thus, the IAAF did not take any action and listed the sample as negative in the official files. Importantly, the IAAF

[146] VOY and DEETER, *Drugs,* 86ff.

[147] Charles DUBIN, *Commission of Inquiry into the Use of Drugs and Banned Practices Intended to Increase Athletic Performances* (Ottawa: Canadian Government Publishing Centre, 1990), 446.

[148] VOY and DEETER, *Drugs,* 86ff.

[149] Ibid.

[150] Minutes, "Meeting of the IOC Medical Commission's Subcommisson on 'Doping and the Biochemistry of Sport'," September 29, 1983, 6.

[151] Minutes, "Meeting of the IAAF Medical Committee in Stockholm, May 15 and 16, 1982," 9.

[152] Minutes, "Meeting of the IOC Medical Commission's Subcommisson on 'Doping and the Biochemistry of Sport', September 29, 1983," 6.

[153] Ibid.

[154] Ibid.

Medical Commission did not mention the cases in their official protocols. But there is also an explanation for this. August Kirsch´s reported that by the end of 1983, the IAAF Council still refrained from officially determining a boundary value on the T/E ratio, despite different regulations.[155] In fact, there were still discussions in the IAAF Medical Committee in January 1984 on the appropriate T/E ratio, without deciding a conclusion.[156] Consequently, it was possible to adapt such a laissez-faire approach, and provided possibilities to conceal potentially positive doping tests, as speculated by VOY and DEETER.[157]

The incidents of Helsinki had a direct effect on the doping controls at the 1983 Pan American Games in Caracas (Venezuela). VOY and DEETER reason that the escape of several athletes before the start of the competition and the positive test results of nineteen athletes (eleven of them in weightlifting), was prompted by the introduction of the testosterone test in Helsinki.[158] They suspect that although there was officially no positive doping test, the athletes realised that the testing system was working and report that, anticipating a major disaster, the NOCs of Canada, Cuba and the USA convinced ten weightlifters to hand in urine samples for doping analysis on a voluntary basis. Ten of them turned out to be positive.[159] It is also important to point out that in Caracas, Manfred Donike and the laboratory in Cologne were in charge of the doping analysis.[160] It is at this point, where it becomes significant to stress that he was *not* in charge of the doping analysis in Helsinki. Naturally, he was interested in proving the reliability of GC-MS for testosterone testing, particularly after having surpassed numerous obstacles until its eventual introduction. According to the official protocols, he emphasised that although the laboratory preparations in Caracas did not go according to plan at first, his team established a satisfying situation with all the necessary equipment.[161] Moreover, it is vital to take into account that the 1983 Pan American Games were under the patronage of the IOC, which also had an interest in demonstrating its willingness in pursuing doping offenders, especially

---

[155] Report, "IAAF-Präsidumssitzung in Manila vom 16.-18. Dezember 1983, December 24, 1983," archive collection "Nachlass August Kirsch," File 012 "IAAF 1982-1987," CuLDA, Cologne, 4.

[156] Minutes, "IAAF Medical Committee Doping Sub-Committee Meeting in London, January 14, 1984," 6ff.

[157] VOY and DEETER, *Drugs*, 86ff.

[158] Ibid., 103.

[159] Ibid.

[160] Minutes, "Meeting of the IOC Medical Commission´s Subcommisson on 'Doping and the Biochemistry of Sport', September 29, 1983," 6.

[161] Ibid.

if events were regional. These two important pre-conditions did not exist at the 1983 World Athletics Championships. The disclosure of nineteen positive doping controls at the Pan American Games highlights this.[162]

Curiously, IAAF officials criticised the entire process at the Pan American Games. The IAAF Council raised doubts about the quality of the laboratory in Caracas in December 1983. It appears that IAAF Council members, such as Amadeo Francis (Puerto Rico) and Ollan Cassell (USA), tried to find loopholes for the positive tests and connected them to the laboratory. It was in principle agreed upon that, "the tests done were invalid according to IAAF rules."[163] Nevertheless, Primo Nebiolo did not want to provoke a scandal and agreed on acknowledging the samples as positive.[164] The discussions illustrate that the IAAF Council members were not happy about the positive doping cases at the 1983 Pan American Games, which matches the suspicions about the World Athletics Championships in the same year. One considered the entire process as a rushing ahead of Manfred Donike and the IOC MSD:

> In Helsinki the President had been very outspoken about the monopoly exercised by the Doping Control Sub-Committee [of the IOC], and the procedure in Caracas was another example of this.[165]

This is a significant finding because it stresses that the immediate high impact of the IOC MSD and the anti-doping laboratory experts was not always seen as favourable.

Finally, the documents show that the revelation of the positive cases from Caracas gave Manfred Donike a high degree of recognition amongst the anti-doping laboratory experts' community, and in public. For example, according to the official minutes of the IOC Medical Commission, "Professor Beckett congratulated Professor Donike on his excellent work and added that the whole Commission was indebted to him."[166] In the public´s and in the athletes´ eyes, he earned himself a reputation as "the doping hunter," which was first mentioned

---

[162] Ibid, Annex 6.

[163] Report, IAAF-Präsidumssitzung in Manila vom 16.-18. Dezember 1983, December 24, 1983," 31.

[164] Ibid., 32

[165] Ibid.

[166] Minutes, "Meeting of the IOC Medical Commission´s Subcommisson on 'Doping and the Biochemistry of Sport', September 29, 1983," 6.

following the detection of the doping usage at the Pan American Games. [167] Hence, the event was a milestone for Manfred Donike's final recognition as a key figure in doping analysis and was evidence for the successful efforts of the entire IOC MSD. The established processes had an effect on global sporting events.

ALL INITIATIVES ESTABLISHED: DOPING CONTROLS AT THE TWO OLYMPIC GAMES IN 1984

Doping Controls at the 1984 Winter Olympic Games in Sarajevo

As with previous Winter Olympic Games, historical accounts of doping controls appear to circumvent the problem of lack of resources on the 1984 Winter Olympic Games in Sarajevo by not actually addressing the issue at all. However, one can discover some evidence in the available data, which highlight the presented developments.

First, the development to attribute more significance to the anti-doping laboratory expertise reappears by the appointment of the "medical" representative 1984 Winter Olympic Games in Sarajevo. The Organising Committee nominated Professor Dr. Branko Nikolin, who was head of the Biochemical Institute at the Faculty of Pharmacology of the University of Sarajevo. [168] Significantly, in contrast to previous appointments of that kind, Branko Nikolin was not in charge of the medical section of the Organising Committee, but occupied the position of head of the anti-doping laboratory. The institutional affiliation of Branko Nikolin also initiated the installation of the laboratory at the University of Sarajevo. In fact, the Yugoslavians did not present any other options to the IOC MSD, who visited the facilities in early 1983 and expressed their satisfaction. [169]

Second, the establishment of the IOC MSD allowed Manfred Donike to deal more directly with Branko Nikolin in the preparation phase. For example, in December 1983, two staff members of the Institute for Biochemistry in Cologne travelled to Sarajevo to support the installation of the mass spectrometer

---

[167] Richard MOORE, *The Dirtiest Race in History. Ben Johnson, Carl Lewis and the 1988 Olympic 100m Final* (London: Bloomsbury, 2012), 72.

[168] Letter, "Ahmed Karabegovic to Monique Berlioux, May 16, 1980," archive collection "Summer and Winter Olympic Games: Medical Files," folder "Medical matters at the Olympic Winter Games of Sarajevo 1984: correspondence," IOC Archive, Lausanne.

[169] Minutes, "Meeting of the IOC Medical Commission in Los Angeles, February 6 and 7, 1982," 9.

equipment.[170] The reason for the late acquisition of the technical apparatus was the predominant opinion to test the T/E ratio through GC-MS as proposed by Manfred Donike. However, because there was no decision on the official method to conduct the T/E test for the Sarajevo Games, the laboratory staff screened all samples with the RI method, and then additionally tested them using GC-MS. This necessitated that the Organising Committee purchased a high-resolution GC-MS system, whereas it only hired a second one to reduce the costs.[171] The final quality check of the anti-doping laboratory took place on January 22, 1984, two weeks before the beginning of the competitions. On behalf of Arnold Beckett, David Cowan visited the laboratory and supervised the analysis of the samples that Manfred Donike had given him.[172] It is significant that none of the IOC MSD members were present during this process. One explanation for this could be the minor importance given to doping controls at the Winter Olympic Games but also the increasing inclusion of additional staff members. Originally, Branko Nikolin had planned the installation of only one GC-MS system, and anticipated an accreditation date in summer 1983.[173] However, the late date of the quality check explains David Cowan's recommendation for accreditation, although one of the two mass spectrometers broke down during the process.[174] Moreover, David Cowan identified technical difficulties with the gas chromatograph and the training of the laboratory staff members, using the GC-MS machine. He stressed that they should "receive additional training in all aspects of MS."[175] This statement proves the anti-doping laboratory experts' interest and efficiency whilst also wanting to ensure that the staff members were educated appropriately. However, contrary to David Cowan's recommendations, and the processes of an increased strengthening of the accreditation regulations, the IOC Medical Commission refrained from making additional requirements in this case. This was a pragmatic solution made under pressure due to the upcoming Winter Olympic Games and it refrained from its usual policy of insisting on high technical standards.

---

[170] Fax, "Alexandre de Mérode to Branko Nikolin, December 9, 1983," archive collection "Summer and Winter Olympic Games: Medical Files," folder "Medical matters at the Olympic Winter Games of Sarajevo 1984: correspondence," IOC Archive, Lausanne.

[171] Branko NIKOLIN, Meliha LEKIC and Miroslav SOBER, "Introduction of the new analytical approaches to the doping control on the XIV Winter Olympic Games," *Bosnian Journal of Basic Medical Sciences* 3, no. 3 (2003), 46.

[172] Minutes, "Meeting of the IOC Medical Commission, February 5-19, 1984," Annex 5.

[173] Ibid., Annex 3.

[174] Minutes, "Meeting of the IOC Medical Commission, February 5-19, 1984," Annex 5.

[175] Ibid.

Third, at the 1984 Winter Olympic Games in Sarajevo, the five IOC MSD members undertook the supervision of the anti-doping laboratory for the first time.[176] In the daily minutes of the doping controls, they did not report any inconsistencies. 408 urine samples were taken, and the laboratory team made 6200 analyses from them.[177] Amongst the four positive samples were three control samples provided by the members of the IOC MSD and one positive doping test on an anabolic steroid by the Mongolian athlete Batsukh Purevjal.[178] Since the analysis of the B-Sample was also positive, the IOC Medical Commission disqualified the athlete.[179]

The three arguments illustrate that the Sarajevo Winter Olympic Games did reflect the general developments about doping analysis and the increasing influence of the anti-doping laboratory experts. Indeed, it was at in Sarajevo that they applied the first doping controls for testosterone misuse. However, the efforts did not yet have an effect as there was not positive test on it in Sarajevo. Clearly, the preparation and the accreditation of the laboratory indicate that the IOC did still not consider Winter Olympic Games as a field for wide-ranging usage of doping substances.

Doping Controls at the 1984 Los Angeles Olympic Games

Anti-doping Laboratory Experts in the Preparation Phase

LAOOC selected orthopaedic surgeon and head of the Olympic Health Services for the Los Angeles Games Dr. Anthony Daly[180], as representative to the IOC Medical Commission. He had been involved with the USOC for a long period, having been the team doctor for several Olympic teams in the years prior to his LAOOC appointment. In fact, the nomination was by the controversial president

---

[176] Minutes, "Meeting of the Medical Commission of the International Olympic Committee, February 12-14, 1983," 14.

[177] Report, "Medical Controls – Doping Controls. XIV Olympic Winter Games Sarajevo, 1984," archive collection "Summer and Winter Olympic Games: Medical Files," folder "Medical matters at the Olympic Winter Games of Sarajevo 1984: correspondence," IOC Archive, Lausanne, 37.

[178] Ibid., 39.

[179] Minutes, "Meeting of the IOC Medical Commission, February 5-19, 1984," 53.

[180] The orthopaedic surgeon Dr. Anthony Daly (1933-2008) was a military doctor before he started to work in sports medicine. He was the US basketball's team doctor in 1976 and 2004 and the medical director of the 1994 FIFA World Cup in the USA. Bill DWYRE, "Doctor attended to sports stars," *Los Angeles Times*, July 7, 2008; http://articles.latimes.com/2008/sep/07/local/me-daly7 [accessed February 11, 2015].

and general manager of LAOOC Peter Ueberroth personally, providing an indication for the close relationship between the two.[181] As opposed to Branko Nikolin, Anthony Daly played an active role in the meetings of the IOC Medical Commission, mainly because it attached particular importance to the doping controls in Los Angeles. This also explains the significance that another representative regularly participated in the IOC Medical Commission meetings. This was Professor Dr. Don H. Catlin, who was more directly involved with the doping controls, and emerged as a key player within the community of anti-doping laboratory experts. Although Don Catlin had a medical background, he had occupied a position as assistant professor at the Department of Pharmacology at UCLA from 1972 onwards, and had published numerous papers on drug addiction and methods for the detection of drugs.[182]

Arnold Beckett had already established the first contact to UCLA in 1981 (see earlier in this chapter). In Los Angeles, he had met with the chairman of the Department of Pharmacology at UCLA, Donald J. Jenden, who transferred all responsibilities to Don Catlin once LAOOC had officially chosen UCLA as the institution to conduct the doping analysis for the Olympic Games. This was on February 3, 1982.[183] Significantly, Don Catlin contributed to all meetings of the IOC MSD following his appointment. In view of the specific objectives of the IOC MSD, this seems understandable. Whereas Anthony Daly occupied a more organisational role and was competent to give a ruling, Don Catlin was responsible for the actual execution of the doping analysis. Alexandre de Mérode quickly acknowledged Don Catlin's contribution and wrote about him in a very positive manner to Monique Berlioux, already recommending him as a potential

---

[181] Letter, "Peter Ueberroth to Monique Berlioux, May 12, 1980," archive collection "Summer and Winter Olympic Games: Medical Files," folder "Medical matters at the 1984 Summer Olympic Games in Los Angeles: correspondence," IOC Archive, Lausanne. Peter Ueberroth revolutionised the Olympic Movement through the almost entirely privately funded Olympic Games, based on the sale of television rights and an innovative marketing concept. He limited the number of corporate sponsors to 30 in order to guarantee exclusivity for bidders and aim for higher bids. According to BARNEY, WRENN and MARTIN, the 1984 Olympic Games and the marketing concepts initiated through Peter Ueberroth "ushered in the formalization of relations between the world of business and the Modern Olympic Movement." BARNEY, WRENN and MARTIN, *Selling,* 160.

[182] "Proposal for the Olympic Analytical Laboratories in the Louis Factor Health Sciences Building at UCLA," Private Archive Don H. Catlin, Los Angeles, 41ff.

[183] Minutes, "Meeting of the IOC Medical Commission in Los Angeles, February 6 and 7, 1982," 6.

future member of the IOC MSD in 1982.[184] Moreover, Don Catlin undertook visits to the doping laboratories of Manfred Donike, Arnold Beckett and Robert Dugal in early April 1982 in order to get more insights on the execution of doping controls in sport, which he did not have much prior experience of.[185] One can consider this further proof for the increasing exchange of knowledge.

Certainly, the efforts of the IOC MSD members to advise Don Catlin and his staff members appropriately were also due to their desire to establish a sustainable testing centre in the USA. This did not exist at that time. Arnold Beckett based his recommendation of UCLA on this argument, along with the interest of UCLA to undertake permanent research in the field of doping analysis.[186] Don Catlin's team proved their future-oriented interest through the submission of an extensive research proposal to LAOOC in 1982. It consisted of the development of a centre for education of laboratory staff, and the continuation of chemical analyses for doping in sport.[187] This long-term approach suited the interests of the anti-doping laboratory experts and their intentions to expand doping controls globally.

The understanding between Don Catlin and the members of the IOC MSD comes to the fore with the decision to test for testosterone and caffeine at the 1984 Los Angeles Olympic Games. In fact, Anthony Daly and Peter Ueberroth strongly objected testosterone testing because they feared that a potentially high number of positive test results could negatively influence the entire reputation of the Olympic Games.[188] The date of the signing of the contract with the UCLA laboratory played an important role in this episode. The official agreement was made only a few days before an IOC Medical Commission meeting, where discussions concerning the testosterone and caffeine issues were on the agenda.[189] It is likely that Anthony Daly (who must have been aware of the possibility to introduce the testosterone and caffeine tests), wanted to sign the contract before a

---

[184] Letter, "Alexandre de Mérode to Monique Berlioux, April 23, 1982," collection "IOC Medical Commission," folder "Correspondence May-September 1982," IOC Archive, Lausanne.

[185] Minutes, "Meeting of the Medical Commission of the International Olympic Committee, May 23 and 24, 1982," 2.

[186] Letter, "Arnold Beckett to Anthony Daly, February 12, 1981."

[187] Report, "Proposal for the Olympic Analytical Laboratories in the Louis Factor Health Sciences Building at UCLA," 2.

[188] HUNT, *Drug Games*, 72ff.

[189] Minutes, "Meeting of the IOC Medical Commission in Los Angeles, February 6 and 7, 1982," 6.

decision was made, so that he could later argue that it was not part of the agreement with UCLA. For example, he argued in the following statement:

> Our contract with UCLA was signed on the basis of the information available prior to the February meeting in Los Angeles. This contract contained limitations on financing and on numbers of samples. We most object, therefore, to the addition of the quantitative testing of testosterone and caffeine this time because:
>
> a) It has not been scientifically validated that such tests are in fact a proof of the administration to an athlete of a banned substance
>
> b) We have received a cost estimate from UCLA that adding these additional tests would involve the expenditure of over $500,00.00 beyond our basic contract. This is a cost we are not willing to undertake.[190]

Consequently, Alexandre de Mérode accused LAOOC of purposely picking the wrong moment to sign the contract, since the IOC Medical Commission had not yet made important decisions.[191] He even went to the lengths of bringing the issue in front of the IOC Executive Board, where Peter Ueberroth and Anthony Daly reiterated their stance that the proposed methods were not scientifically validated. In an official statement, Anthony Daly used the different opinions of Arnold Beckett and Manfred Donike (see earlier in this chapter) of whether to use RI or GC-MS as an argument to demonstrate that even within the IOC MSD, the incorporation of the methods could not be resolved. [192] In contrast to this statement, Manfred Donike regarded LAOOC's approach as insulting, and suggested that its attitude was offensive "to all the people who have been engaged in dope analysis in the past and have made contribution in this field." [193] He referred to his own contribution to the IOC's fight against doping through the

---

[190] Minutes, "Meeting of the Medical Commission of the International Olympic Committee, May 23 and 24, 1982," Annex 4.

[191] Ibid., 4.

[192] Minutes, "Meeting of the Medical Commission of the International Olympic Committee, May 23 and 24, 1982," Annex 4.

[193] Note, "Comments of Professor M. Donike regarding the LAOOC report to the IOC Medical Commission, February, 1984," archive collection "Summer and Winter Olympic Games: Medical Files," folder "Medical matters at the 1984 Summer Olympic Games in Los Angeles: correspondence," IOC Archive, Lausanne.

technical development of the GC-MS method, and listed the analytical developments at previous Olympic Games since the installation of the first Olympic anti-doping laboratory in Munich in 1972.[194]

Notwithstanding the criticism, Anthony Daly attempted to undermine Manfred Donike´s scientific approach by getting a second scientific opinion of American pathologist and toxicologist Dr. Michael Lubran, who questioned the scientific validity of the testosterone test.[195] However, according to Manfred Donike, Michael Lubran made several mistakes in his report and he assumed that LAOOC had withheld important documents.[196] For example, LAOOC had not informed Michael Lubran about the exact routine analytical procedure for anabolic steroids, and he was not aware of the technical details of the testosterone test. Consequently, Manfred Donike rejected Michael Lubran´s criticism and suspected that LAOOC officials had changed parts of the report: "the questions and remarks are mixed in a way that I cannot believe that this is the diction of a scientist."[197] Manfred Donike saw in the resistance from LAOOC another challenge to his enduring attempt to introduce the test, having overcome considerable confrontation before. Hence, his evaluation of Michael Lubran´s statement must have been written with a high degree of self-interest. One can also see this by the emotional wording in the letter.

Other than the substantial mistakes in Michael Lubran´s report, Manfred Donike also criticised LAOOC´s way of proceeding.[198] There seemed to be a conflict between the UCLA laboratory of Don Catlin and LAOOC/Anthony Daly, because LAOOC had asked an external reviewer to compile a report. Manfred Donike maintained that LAOOC should rely on the laboratory for a scientific report:

---

[194] Ibid.

[195] Letter, "Anthony Daly to Alexandre de Mérode, June 8, 1983," archive collection "Summer and Winter Olympic Games: Medical Files," folder "Medical matters at the 1984 Summer Olympic Games in Los Angeles: correspondence," IOC Archive, Lausanne.

[196] Letter, "Manfred Donike to Alexandre de Mérode, July 14, 1983," archive collection "Summer and Winter Olympic Games: Medical Files," folder "Medical matters at the 1984 Summer Olympic Games in Los Angeles: correspondence," IOC Archive, Lausanne.

[197] Ibid.

[198] Ibid.

> In my eyes Dr. Catlin and his staff supported by the Medical and Pharmacological Department of UCLA, have not lost their scientific reputation and their scientific qualification in the last year and a half.[199]

Moreover, Don Catlin made very clear that he had no doubt about the scientific correctness of Manfred Donike's methods.[200] He favoured GC-MS as general screening method, thus enabling easy execution of the testosterone test. As a result, Don Catlin faced opposition from LAOOC a few months later, as the Committee did not provide the necessary funds to acquire technical equipment.[201] Clearly, this demonstrates the apparent conflict of interest. Whereas LAOOC had only contemplated the success of the Olympic Games, Don Catlin wanted to establish the anti-doping laboratory as a long-term testing centre. Similar to the other anti-doping laboratory experts, Don Catlin realised great financial benefits connected to doping analysis because he later admitted:

> I thought it was too complex for me. I'm in internal medicine. I'm not a chemist. And it wasn't clear to me at the beginning what funding there'd be for it. But it became clear after a while that they were talking about a lot of money. And I was just a junior professor.[202]

More official involvement eventually solved the issue. In September 1983, Alexandre de Mérode reported to the IOC MSD that Juan Antonio Samaranch had reached an agreement with Peter Ueberroth, and LAOOC was now prepared to test for caffeine and testosterone.[203] This occurred after Manfred Donike gave another scientific presentation to LAOOC officials on the analytical procedure.[204] Consequently, LAOOC finally provided Don Catlin with the much-needed financial resources, and acquired eight GC-MS instruments.[205] For public

---

[199] Ibid.

[200] Minutes, "Meeting of the Medical Commission of the International Olympic Committee, May 23 and 24, 1982," 11.

[201] Minutes, "Meeting of the Medical Commission of the International Olympic Committee, February 12-14, 1983," 17.

[202] Don Catlin in: MOORE, *The Dirtiest Race*, 103.

[203] Minutes, "Meeting of the IOC Medical Commission's Subcommisson on 'Doping and the Biochemistry of Sport', September 29, 1983," 7.

[204] HUNT, *Drug Games*, 163n17.

[205] Report, "Medical Services Games of the XXIII Olympiad" by the Los Angeles Organising Committee – Olympic Health Services, 1984," archive collection "Summer and Winter Olympic Games: Medical Files," folder "Medical matters at the 1984 Summer Olympic Games in Los Angeles: Reports," IOC Archive, Lausanne, 3.

relations work, Anthony Daly ultimately adopted a different stance in July 1984 and refrained from what REINOLD rightly labelled as an "obstructionist policy regarding testing from the side of the Organising Committee." [206] In a news conference, Anthony Daly asserted that the doping control equipment was highly sensitive and would not allow any athletes to beat the doping control system. [207] He must have been aware of pre-Olympic controls, which were analysed at the UCLA laboratory and revealed 86 positive results but were not announced by USOC because it wanted to avoid bad publicity. [208]

The dispute on testosterone testing also influenced the late date of the laboratory accreditation. It was only in October 1983 when Don Catlin requested the control samples. [209] He did so by contacting Arnold Beckett, who visited the laboratory in November 1983 to bring the control samples and to supervise the tests. Curiously, Arnold Beckett recommended accreditation instantly, arguing that the laboratory had demonstrated its scientific competence in the analysis of the control samples. [210] However, the follow-up check of the code numbers at the Cologne laboratory revealed incorrect results. [211] Consequently, Manfred Donike visited the UCLA laboratory again in mid-December 1983 to supervise a second test where it appeared that there had only been a mix-up with the code numbers, but that the results of the analysis had in fact been correct. [212] This provides evidence for the accuracy and seriousness of the IOC MSD's approach to technical details, and particularly Manfred Donike's role.

The outlined debates and conflicts demonstrate the common approach of the anti-doping laboratory experts to make instant use of the scientific advancements. Manfred Donike, Arnold Beckett and Don Catlin appeared as proponents of the testosterone test. They played an important role in the enforcement of the new procedure, thus highlighting their significance. Simultaneously, the dispute between LAOOC and Manfred Donike proves that the political level increasingly considered the anti-doping laboratory experts a threat. The conflict can be compared to the disagreement between Manfred Donike and Joseph Keul on the national level. In both cases, Manfred Donike faced considerable resistance to the

---

[206] REINOLD, "Arguing," 40.

[207] TODD and TODD, "Significant Events," 82.

[208] Ibid., 79.

[209] Diary, "Laboratory Research Note Book – Department of Pharmacology, D. Catlin," Private Archive Don H. Catlin, Los Angeles, 41.

[210] Fax, "Arnold Beckett to Alexandre de Mérode, November 23, 1983."

[211] Diary, "Laboratory Research Note Book – Department of Pharmacology, D. Catlin," 78.

[212] Interview with Don H. Catlin, November 12, 2012.

introduction of the testosterone test its validity. Peter Ueberroth feared the increasing control of doping tests within the Olympic Movement and he made his opinion clear in a letter to Juan Antonio Samaranch, when he wrote "drugs and doctors are not only controlling the Games of the XIIIrd Olympiad, they are beginning to gain control of the whole Olympic Movement."[213] Whereas Joseph Keul´s concerns were more of a financial nature, Peter Ueberroth wanted to avoid bad press during the Olympic Games. However, the anti-doping laboratory experts were eventually successful in expanding their influence by the installation of the testosterone tests on both levels. Moreover, through Don Catlin and the UCLA laboratory, the experts were gaining another knowledgeable addition to their growing network in the USA. Thus, after the 1983 World Athletic Championships and the 1983 Pan American Games, the IOC MSD had an even bigger impact on the preparations of the doping controls at the 1984 Los Angeles Olympic Games.

Execution of Doping Controls and Doping Analysis

Researchers have explored the doping incidents and the attempted involvements through officials at the 1984 Los Angeles Olympic Games.[214] Therefore, the focus in this section is on the anti-doping laboratory experts´ role during the Games and their involvement in various controversies. Ultimately, the doping control teams took 1,510 different urine samples, which underwent 9,440 screening analyses.[215] In all cases, the staff used combined GC-MS to confirm results of the screening procedures. The IOC officially declared twelve positive doping tests and disqualified eleven athletes and one team official. The positive samples came from the following athletes: weightlifter Serafim Grammatikopoulos (Greece, nandrolone), discus thrower Vésteinn Hafsteinsson (Iceland, nandrolone), wrestler Thomas Johansson (Sweden, methenolone), weightlifter Stefan Laggner (Austria, nandrolone), weightlifter Göran Petterson (Sweden, nandrolone), volleyballer Eiji Shimomura (Japan, testosterone),

---

[213] Letter, "Peter Ueberroth to Juan Antonio Samaranch, November 14, 1983," archive collection "Summer and Winter Olympic Games: Medical Files," folder "Medical matters at the 1984 Summer Olympic Games in Los Angeles: correspondence," IOC Archive, Lausanne.

[214] See for example John GLEAVES recent article on blood doping at the 1984 Los Angeles Olympic Games: John GLEAVES, "Manufactured Dope," 89-107.

[215] Don H. CATLIN, Craig KAMMERER, Caroline K. HATTON, Michael H. SEKERA and James L. MERDINK, "Analytical Chemistry at the Games of the XXIIIrd Olympiad in Los Angeles, 1984," *Clinical Chemistry* 33, no. 2 (1987), 319. Also see: HEMMERSBACH, "History," 843.

weightlifter Ahmed Tarbi (Algeria, nandrolone), weightlifter Mahmud Tarba (Lebanon, nandrolone), hammer thrower Gianpaolo Urlando (Italy, testosterone), long distance runner Martti Vainio (Finland, methenolone) and javelin thrower Anna Verouli (Greece, nandrolone).[216] Japanese volleyballer Mikiyasu Tanaka tested positive for ephedrine, but the IOC Medical Commission ruled that the Japanese team doctor was responsible for the incident and did not disqualify the athlete.[217] If one considers the individual cases in detail, the success of the anti-doping laboratory experts since the foundation of the IOC MSD, becomes again apparent. First, the IOC MSD did not refrain from attempts to expand knowledge on the execution of doping controls. In Los Angeles, it requested LAOOC's Olympic Health Services together with the public relations department to develop a multi-faceted film to educate the doping control staff and the NOC team doctors, but also the athletes on all aspects of the doping controls.[218] The IOC had made such a film already before the 1984 Winter Olympic Games in Sarajevo. However, with posed scenes to inform the team doctors about the doping controls.[219] In contrast to this earlier film, the actual doping procedures were filmed in Los Angeles, including the laboratory work. The IOC MSD used the video for educational purposes during workshops outside of the Olympic Games.[220] Moreover, there was a great deal of information exchange between Manfred Donike, Arnold Beckett and Don Catlin on the work within the laboratory. Not only did the members of the IOC MSD supervise the laboratory work, but the Don Catlin constantly involved them in the analytical processes, too. A scrapbook of Don Catlin evidences this, outlining the very close cooperation, aiming to increase the reliability of the doping analysis.[221]

---

[216] Individual Minutes, "Meetings of the IOC Medical Commission, July 24 to August 12, 1984," archive collection "IOC Medical Commission," folder "IOC Medical Commission: meeting in Los Angeles on 24th July - 12th August 1984 : roll call, minutes and working documents," IOC Archive, Lausanne.

[217] Ibid., 27.

[218] Report, "Medical Services Games of the XXIII Olympiad by the Los Angeles Organising Committee – Olympic Health Services, 1984," archive collection "Summer and Winter Olympic Games: Medical Files," folder "Medical matters at the 1984 Summer Olympic Games in Los Angeles: Reports," IOC Archive, Lausanne, 26.

[219] Minutes, "Meeting of the IOC Medical Commission, February 5-19, 1984," 7ff.

[220] Report, "Medical Services Games of the XXIII Olympiad by the Los Angeles Organising Committee – Olympic Health Services, 1984," 25.

[221] Diary, "Laboratory Research Note Book – Department of Pharmacology, D. Catlin," 78.

Second, the discussions in the IOC Medical Commission meetings reveal an ongoing debate whether to disqualify athletes with a T/E ratio of more than six, with Manfred Donike pushing for a strict application of the rules. For example, the analysis of the A- and B-sample of the urine sample by Eiji Shimomura had shown a T/E ratio of around ten.[222] It was the first case of a positive test on exogenous testosterone at any Olympic Games. However, several IOC Medical Commission members, such as Ludwig Prokop, still voiced concerns, arguing that the IOC should only disqualify athletes if it were 100% sure that it was purposeful doping.[223] Anthony Daly also claimed, "the case was not a good first testosterone case for the Olympic Games."[224] In contrast to Anthony Daly's statement, Manfred Donike, obviously still convinced of the validity of his test, adopted a different and more rigorous stance, trying to demonstrate that the results of the analysis were a clear violation of the IOC's anti-doping regulations. He rejected the execution of additional tests, arguing that the same calibrations had been used in previous sporting events and in the leading anti-doping laboratories in London and Cologne.[225] Arnold Beckett supported Manfred Donike and assured the members that there was no question as to the scientific validity of the results obtained by the laboratory. As in previous cases, the majority of the IOC Medical Commission members went along with the expertise of the IOC MSD members, and disqualified Eiji Shimomura. They did not take sanction against the Japanese volleyball team.[226] In the second case of a high T/E ratio by Giampaolo Urlando, the members of the IOC Medical Commission agreed on the disqualification.[227] However, Anthony Daly also contested this decision and asked the IOC Medical Commission to record his opposition.[228] In fact, he became increasingly anxious about the increasing number of positive tests and began to question the entire doping control set-up halfway through the Olympic Games.[229] He even went as far as to ask questions why there had been no positive tests during the Moscow Games.[230] One has to consider this as another attempt to demonstrate LAOOC's perceived injustice through the

---

[222] Individual Minutes, "Meetings of the IOC Medical Commission, July 24 to August 12, 1984," 50.

[223] Ibid., 51.

[224] Ibid.

[225] Ibid.

[226] Ibid.

[227] Ibid., 60.

[228] Ibid.

[229] Ibid., 51.

[230] Ibid.

introduction of more sophisticated testing methods. Anthony Daly was not the only individual who appeared to prevent the publication of positive doping tests. IAAF president Primo Nebiolo also intended to prolong the publication of his fellow Italian citizen Giampaolo Urlando's positive testing result. According to POUND, IOC President Juan Antonio Samaranch supported him in his efforts.[231] Primo Nebiolo's attitude adds to the speculation that he did not want his sport to get negative press. As Andreas SINGLER and Gerhard TREUTLEIN suggest, he did not take his responsibility seriously to convict positive tested athletes at other events such as the Universiade either.[232] Manfred Donike complained extensively about such behaviour. Several written exchanges between August Kirsch and Manfred Donike regarding the "incomprehensible" attitude of Primo Nebiolo highlight that they had already discussed the issue during their stay in Los Angeles.[233] August Kirsch allied with Manfred Donike, promising him to address the matter during the IAAF Council meeting in November 1984. This demonstrates that Manfred Donike became increasingly involved in political debates because of his professional abilities in doping analysis, and his willingness to convict as many athletes as possible. It is indicative for his success that he enforced his demand that led to the disqualification of Eiji Shimomura and Giampaolo Urlando.

Third, the discussions on the positive doping cases reveal that the strong influence of the anti-doping laboratory experts enabled the IOC Medical Commission to analyse the laboratory reports in a more detailed manner. They retraced the time and the method of the drug administration. REINOLD has already identified the three following cases from the Los Angeles Olympic Games,[234] but it is important to emphasise that the interpretation of the results came predominantly from Manfred Donike. The Algerian Ahmed Tarbi, who had tested positive for the anabolic steroid nandrolone, reasoned that he had taken the substance orally several months prior to the Olympic Games. However, Manfred Donike proved that the substance had been injected, and that this had been done much later than on the suggested date.[235] Similarly, he indicated that Göran

---

[231] POUND, *Inside*, 67ff.

[232] SINGLER and TREUTLEIN, *Doping*, 141.

[233] Letter, August Kirsch to Manfred Donike, August 27, 1984, archive collection "Nachlass August Kirsch," File 086, "Doping (2)," CuLDA, Cologne. Also see: Letter, "Manfred Donike to August Kirsch, December 7, 1984," archive collection "Nachlass August Kirsch," File 086, "Doping (2)," CuLDA, Cologne.

[234] REINOLD, "Arguing," 23ff.

[235] Individual Minutes, "Meetings of the IOC Medical Commission, July 24 to August 12, 1984," 37ff.

Petterson had not taken steroids six months prior to the Olympic Games, as claimed, but rather six weeks prior.[236] Finally, Arnold Beckett and Manfred Donike uncovered the lies of Vésteinn Hafsteinsson from Iceland. They asserted that the allegedly taken drug could not possibly include steroids, that it must have been injected (not orally administered), and that the date of administration was around three to five weeks before the positive test result.[237] Thus, REINOLD is correct in his evaluation that the discovery of detailed pharmacological facts led to "several disclosures of false information given by athletes and functionaries."[238] One has to add the important detail that the discoveries were largely based on Manfred Donike's extensive level of knowledge on the interpretation of the GC-MS results. His inclusion in the IOC MSD clearly left less scope for excuses by the convicted athletes at the 1984 Los Angeles Olympic Games, which were Manfred Donike's first Olympic Games as a member.

Fourth, Manfred Donike constantly attempted to expand the doping controls and was looking for evidence of unknown drugs at the Olympic Games. This becomes obvious with the case of beta-blockers. Professor Dr. Wilhelm Schänzer[239] calculated in his Ph.D. dissertation that by 1984 it was possible to screen and identify 90.0% of available beta-blockers through GC-MS.[240] Wilhelm Schänzer, who focused his research on steroid metabolism, worked in the Cologne anti-doping laboratory, and became an important staff member for Manfred Donike. In contrast to testosterone and caffeine, LAOOC had successfully resisted the introduction of tests for beta-blockers. Although the test did not actually entail additional work for the anti-doping laboratory, LAOOC argued in its official report that additional costs would be involved and decided not to screen for beta-blockers.[241] Consequently, the IOC Medical Commission introduced its own class of substances, used for medical reasons if athletes notified about the usage prior to the start of the Olympic Games. Beta-blockers,

---

[236] Ibid., 62.

[237] Ibid., 64ff.

[238] REINOLD, "Arguing," 23.

[239] Professor Dr. Wilhelm Schänzer (born 1951) became head of the Institute of Biochemistry at the DSHS in 1997 following the death of Manfred Donike, after he habilitated in 1995. Previously in 1984, he had concluded his doctoral studies at the DSHS in biochemistry and physiology. His dissertation supervisor was Manfred Donike.

[240] Wilhelm SCHÄNZER, *Untersuchungen zum Nachweis und Metabolismus von Hormonen und Dopingmitteln, insbesondere mit Hilfe der Hochdruckflüssigkeitschromatographie,* Dissertation at the German Sport University Cologne (Cologne, 1984), 194.

[241] Report, "Medical Services Games of the XXIII Olympiad by the Los Angeles Organising Committee – Olympic Health Services, 1984," 4.

local anaesthetics, corticosteroids and beta-agonist belonged to this group. The introduction of this new class of banned substances was the impetus for the introduction of the Therapeutic Use Exemptions (TUEs) that allow athletes to participate in sport despite taking drugs for genuine medical conditions.[242] However, Manfred Donike was not satisfied with this solution and advised Don Catlin to undertake his own research with the samples of Olympic athletes and he used some samples himself to check for beta-blockers.[243] This led to the discovery of a high number of athletes in the modern pentathlon, who took the substances without giving prior notification. Therefore, Manfred Donike announced that the drug would go on the banned list following the Olympic Games.[244] On the IOC Session in Berlin in 1985, the IOC then officially added beta-blockers to the list,[245] following additional revelations about its usage by entire teams during the Los Angeles Olympic Games.[246] In addition to the case of beta-blockers, Manfred Donike undertook investigations into the content of "Chinese tablets," too. The Austrian weightlifter Stefan Laggner had claimed to use these "tablets," leading to a positive test on nandrolone.[247] However, Manfred Donike asserted that he did not know about nandrolone in tablet form and tested the pills. He revealed that the present steroid was methyltestosterone, which cannot produce nandrolone and he concluded that Stefan Laggner must have taken additional substances.[248] Besides these analytical investigations into medication, it also results that the anti-doping laboratory experts did not refrain from taking substances themselves in order to test the technical equipment. For example, Robert Dugal had taken a capsule of a medicament and his colleagues had analysed his urine.[249] Don Catlin confirmed this episode, arguing that Manfred Donike had regularly provided his colleagues with potential doping

---

[242] David R. MOTTRAM, "The evolution of doping and anti-doping in sport," in *Drugs in Sport*, eds. David R. MOTTRAM and Neil CHESTER (London: Routledge, 2015), 26.

[243] Individual Minutes, "Meetings of the IOC Medical Commission, July 24 to August 12, 1984," 64.

[244] TODD and TODD, "Significant Events," 82.

[245] Minutes, "90th Session of the IOC in Berlin (GDR), June 4-6, 1985," archive collection "IOC Sessions 1894-2009," IOC Archive, Lausanne, Annex 11.

[246] Minutes, "Meeting of the IOC Medical Commission, April 10 and 11, 1985," 4.

[247] Individual Minutes, "Meetings of the IOC Medical Commission, July 24 to August 12, 1984," 63.

[248] Ibid.

[249] Individual Minutes, "Meetings of the IOC Medical Commission, July 24 to August 12, 1984," 27.

substances.[250] These findings establish that the increased efforts of the IOC MSD did not eradicate doping at all. However, it provides evidence of the IOC MSD's awareness of the usage of more substances, and its members used the opportunity to obtain a high number of samples to conduct their research.

Fifth, it is important to address the role of the anti-doping laboratory experts in the case of the disappearance of the identification numbers of several supposedly positive urine samples. LAOOC and Alexandre de Mérode, in whose hotel room the documents were stored, have blamed each other for the loss of the papers. Whereas it is not possible to uncover the mystery of the disappearance, the role of the anti-doping laboratory experts has to be addressed and facts have be added to previously stated assumptions. Amongst the main writers to report about the mysterious incident is Andrew JENNINGS, who reiterates a television interview in 1994, where Arnold Beckett had talked about the destroyed codes for the positive tests and mentioned a meeting in Cologne at the end of 1984.[251] At this meeting, so Arnold Beckett argued, he had drafted a letter together with Manfred Donike, Robert Dugal and Alexandre de Mérode, assuring Alexandre de Mérode's innocence. This letter is available and illustrates that the members of the IOC MSD supported Alexandre de Mérode's claim that LAOOC destroyed the documents.[252] Moreover, they argue:

> The behaviour of Dr. Anthony Daly, Chief Medical Officer at the Olympic Games, and most of his staff during the Games amounted to deliberate obstruction of the working of the IOC Medical Commission.[253]

Considering the conflicts during and prior to the Olympic Games, this stance appears comprehensible. The IOC MSD, who was supervising the laboratory work, had decided that Manfred Donike would remain in Los Angeles for three more days after the end of the Olympic Games, to review potentially positive samples.[254] Thus, the behaviour of the anti-doping laboratory experts does not provide an indication for an active participation in the conspiracy. They appear too focused on the conviction of athletes, based on their professional

---

[250] Interview with Don H. Catlin, November 10, 2012.

[251] Andrew JENNINGS, *The New Lord of the Rings* (London: Simon & Schuster, 1996), 237ff.

[252] "Report by Arnold Beckett, Manfred Donike, Robert Dugal and Alexandre de Mérode, n.d.," Private Archive Don H. Catlin, Los Angeles.

[253] Ibid.

[254] Ibid.

competencies. Therefore, the documents with the identification codes were the weakest aspect of the doping control system, because the revelation of potential drug takers depended on them. Don Catlin and his assistant Dr. Craig Kammerer have expressed their discontent with the incident on various occasions. They reported that Anthony Daly even tried to close the laboratory three days before the end of the competition, to prevent the revelation of more positive doping cases.[255] Controversially, the letter also provides evidence for the statements made by Arnold Beckett in the television interview, outlining that the anti-doping laboratory experts were not willing to speak about the incident in public. He had stated that the disclosure of the information on the destroyed documents would not have resulted in the identification of the doped athletes.[256] Instead, it would have damaged the image of the Olympic Games and LAOOC. According to the letter, they decided, "not to make the statement public but to devise plans to make impossible a repetition of this disgraceful and irresponsible action in Los Angeles."[257] According to Don Catlin, who was present during the drawing up of the statement but did not sign it because he was not a member of the IOC MSD, the members had to back Alexandre de Mérode "because he was the boss (...). The Prince could make things happen so it was very, very important for us to keep things moving."[258] Whereas Alexandre de Mérode needed Arnold Beckett, Manfred Donike and Robert Dugal to uphold the IOC's fight against doping for which he was responsible, the anti-doping laboratory experts needed a representative on the political level, who could enforce more testing and could protect their role. As reported by Don Catlin, the experts knew that in order to make a difference, "you need to have some diplomacy."[259]

In summary, the execution of the doping controls at the 1984 Los Angeles Olympic Games reveals the more powerful and influential role of the anti-doping laboratory experts, particularly on the administrative level. This was a result of the introduction of the testosterone tests, the advancement in doping analysis to have more detailed results and the increased education of laboratory staff. Their growing authority also resulted in Manfred Donike and Arnold Beckett becoming

---

[255] Craig Kammerer in John M. HOBERMAN, "How Drug Testing Fails: The Politics of Doping Control," in: *Doping in Elite Sport: The Politics of Drugs in the Olympic Movement*, eds. Wayne WILSON and Edward DERSE (Champaign, IL: Human Kinetics, 2001), 251. Also see: Don Catlin in MOORE, *The Dirtiest Race*, 103.

[256] JENNINGS, *The New Lord*, 237.

[257] "Report, by Arnold Beckett, Manfred Donike, Robert Dugal and Alexandre de Mérode, n.d."

[258] Interview with Don H. Catlin, November 11, 2012.

[259] Ibid.

progressively more involved in disputes with sport administrators. Similar to the discrepancies with Anthony Daly, IAAF President Primo Nebiolo began to be an antagonist of the anti-doping laboratory experts after the Olympic Games. Primo Nebiolo was displeased by the prevalent positions of Manfred Donike and Arnold Beckett. LJUNGQVIST's publication on the history of the anti-doping confirms this finding. He describes, "I never really believed that doping was particularly important to Nebiolo's agenda (...) He was more concerned about what the world thought about the IAAF."[260] A striking example for Primo Nebiolo's attempt to end the exertion of influence of Manfred Donike and Arnold Beckett, is his effort to exclude them from the IAAF Medical Committee. In November 1984, Primo Nebiolo wanted to introduce a new re-nomination procedure for the IAAF Medical Committee.[261] However, whereas the officially recorded statements only recite such general facts, August Kirsch stated that Primo Nebiolo explicitly did not want Manfred Donike and Arnold Beckett in the IAAF Medical Commission any longer.[262] After considerable opposition through August Kirsch (who was closely linked to Manfred Donike through his position as head of the BISp) in particular, the entire group was re-nominated. Even though one has to treat August Kirsch's subjective report with caution, the account reproduces the opposing attitude of Primo Nebiolo towards Manfred Donike and Arnold Beckett. This episode of the conflict between anti-doping laboratory experts and Primo Nebiolo, entirely new to research, adds evidence to the fact that the rise of the anti-doping laboratory experts, and the execution of the quickly advancing technical possibilities, annoyed many sport administrators. Primo Nebiolo wanted to demonstrate the IAAF's efforts to combat doping at the beginning of his presidency. However, it was only after the realization that more positive doping tests were revealed, that he began to perceive the anti-doping laboratory experts as a major threat. The attempt to acquire lucrative sponsorship and television deals played an important role in this process. Thus, it is not coincidental that the first major conflicts arose during the 1984 Los Angeles Olympic Games, which were the watershed for the evolution of the commercialization of the Olympic Movement, and a catalyst of the IOC's transition to a corporate entity.[263]

---

[260] LJUNGQVIST, *Doping's Nemesis*, 130.

[261] Minutes, "IAAF Council Meeting in Canberra, November 23-25, 1984," archive collection "Nachlass August Kirsch," File 123, "IAAF (2)," CuLDA, Cologne, 13.

[262] Report, "Sitzung des IAAF-Präsidiums in Canberra/Australien, November 23-25, 1984," archive collection "Nachlass August Kirsch," File 123, "IAAF (2)," CuLDA, Cologne, 6.

[263] BARNEY, WRENN and MARTIN, *Selling*, 202.

Moreover, it also shows that with Primo Nebiolo in charge, the anti-doping laboratory faced difficulties in the IAAF, which they did not encounter in the 1970s.

INTERIM RESULTS FOR PERIOD 1980-1984: ESTABLISHMENT PHASE CONCLUDED

The events and developments surrounding the members of the IOC MSD until the 1984 Los Angeles Olympic Games and its immediate aftermath distinctly illustrate the progress made by the anti-doping laboratory experts since 1980. In this period, the significance of doping analysis in general, and the particular importance of the anti-doping laboratory experts on the sport political level, raised progressively. Their expertise in doping analysis, which they had proven in various roles until 1980, finally allowed them to occupy a more central role in the IOC's anti-doping strategies. Alexandre de Mérode had recognised that the influence of anti-doping laboratory experts on the decision-making level was necessary in order to maintain the doping control system, which they had helped to install. Once the experts had reached such acknowledgment and gained more influence, they instantly made an impact through the establishment of several procedures, which were all closely linked to their domain of expertise. Therefore, it is important to distinguish between the efforts of the IOC Medical Commission and the IOC MSD. Its members had different professional competencies and one can categorise their effects in four areas.

First, it led to faster implementation of testing procedures and an addition of new techniques into the IOC regulations. In the period under investigation in this chapter, one can see this especially in the introduction of the testosterone tests. Prior to this, testosterone had given athletes a safe opportunity of enhancing their performance. With the introduction of the test, developed by Manfred Donike, the solely testing based anti-doping strategy was a significant step forward and thus, the dependence on anti-doping laboratory experts became even stronger. The IOC MSD provided an environment where the scientific aspects could be discussed, leading to an instant introduction of the test with wide-ranging effects. For example, an unproportional T/E ratio accounted for 10.0% of the positive doping controls in 1985, as revealed by the Cologne laboratory in 1985 (6 out of 60).[264] The positive doping results at the 1984 Los Angeles Olympic Games provide additional evidence for this.

---

[264] Report, "IOC-Accredited Laboratory Statistic, 1986," archive collection "Nachlass August Kirsch," File 088 "Doping (5)," CuLDA, Cologne.

Second, the IOC MSD – in cooperation with the IAAF Medical Committee – extended the anti-doping laboratory network significantly. Sixteen anti-doping laboratories had obtained official IOC accreditation, all of whom had started the accreditation process before 1985. This allowed more tests during sporting competitions worldwide. At the same time, the IOC MSD maintained control over the accreditation procedure so that its members continued regulating the standards of the approved institutions. They undertook the accreditation themselves, thereby ensuring a privileged status of their own anti-doping laboratories, as they became the supervisory institutions for all doping analysis processes. Such a principal role consolidated their leading position within the anti-doping laboratory network, which can be ascribed to their professional expertise in doping analysis.

Third, despite the expansion of the anti-doping laboratory network through more official institutions, the inner circle of the anti-doping laboratory experts remained static. Arnold Beckett, Claus Clausnitzer, Manfred Donike and Robert Dugal were involved in all the processes regarding doping analysis. The personnel turnover from Victor Rogozkin to Vitaly Semenov was of no consequence, because neither of the Soviets appeared to be heavily involved in the IOC MSD's work. Whilst the IAAF Medical Committee, and its Doping Subcommittee, remained an important forum of exchange for the anti-doping laboratory experts, the IOC MSD provided them with a more important setting for this exchange. The members had an influential supporter within the IOC in Alexandre de Mérode, who depended on the involvement of the experts even more strongly now, and key decisions were made by the IOC MSD members. During this time, their professional competencies were valued higher regarding the doping problem than those of sport medicine specialists.

Fourth, the growing network of anti-doping laboratories naturally led to more laboratory staff becoming involved with doping analysis. As a result, Manfred Donike initiated the Cologne Workshop in order to exchange latest research developments but also to educate laboratory staff members worldwide. The IOC MSD also allowed video tutorials on the laboratory work of the 1984 Los Angeles Olympic Games. Manfred Donike took his responsibility as leader of the anti-doping laboratory network seriously, and was aware of the need for education of the less technically advanced testing centres. He intended to increase the reliability of the analytical results. His policy was to employ a high quality of laboratory work so that the athletes were convicted based on completely reliable scientific-evidence.

Finally, a power shift within the network of anti-doping laboratory experts also occurred. The appointment of Manfred Donike as head of the IOC MSD caused this transfer of power. Whereas Arnold Beckett had been at the forefront of most developments in doping analysis since the establishment of the IOC Medical Commission in 1967, appointing Manfred Donike as head of the IOC MSD signified a change in leadership. His knowledge and experience with GC-MS made him and the laboratory in Cologne the undisputable leaders in doping analysis, especially with the introduction of the testosterone test, applied by Manfred Donike for the first time at the 1984 Los Angeles Olympic Games. His involvement also allowed a more detailed analysis of the testing results, to the detriment of the convicted athletes.

With the above presented interim results in mind, one can consider the 1984 Los Angeles Olympic Games as an important landmark in the history of the anti-doping laboratory experts within the Olympic Movement. Although the success of the doping controls at the Olympic Games themselves has to be called into question, the experts were now having a decisive say regarding enhancing testing procedures, controlling an extended anti-doping laboratory network and installing educational initiatives for laboratory staff worldwide. The global doping control system did not function any longer without anti-doping laboratory experts in key positions.

However, the increased responsibility also entailed a dramatic change in their scope of duties. The small group of key players, especially Manfred Donike and Arnold Beckett, now mainly dealt with political and administrative tasks. Manfred Donike highlighted this already in 1981.[265] Whereas the anti-doping laboratory experts aspired to such influential roles, it added new challenges. The attempt of Primo Nebiolo to exclude Arnold Beckett and Manfred Donike from the IAAF Medical Committee and the struggles with LAOOC are examples for such challenges. The influence of the anti-doping laboratory experts posed significant problems for the political level, because the image of a clean sport diminished at the beginning of the 1980s.

---

[265] Report, "Entwicklung der Doping-Analytik und –Forschung," January 27, 1982.

CHAPTER 7

Consequences and Challenges (1985-1992)

CONTINUATION OF IMPACT ON BASIS OF CREATED STRUCTURES

A major reason for little focus on anti-doping laboratory experts' activities within the Olympic Movement after the 1984 Los Angeles Olympic Games are embargoes required by law. However, for the purpose of this study, the IOC has lifted its statutorily regulated embargo and made all protocols of the IOC Medical Commission and its subcommissions from 1985 until 1992 available. The results presented in this chapter are based on these documents, and attempt to enhance the valuable insights of earlier academic work.

There were no major personnel alterations in the IOC Medical Commission in the period from 1985 until 1987. This extends particularly for the IOC MSD, whose membership did not change at all during this phase. Consequently, all decisions and technical questions remained in the hands of the same few individuals under the leadership of Manfred Donike. The only major significant modifications were the addition of representatives of the summer and winter sports IFs.[1] These positions were taken up from 1984 onwards, by Professor Dr. Hans Howald[2] and Dr. Wolf-Dieter Montag[3], who also attended the meetings of the subcommissions if relevant topics were discussed, but did not make any significant contributions to anti-doping debates.

Following the phase of establishment, through which the network of anti-doping laboratory experts became an indispensable element in the IOC's anti-doping policy, the IOC MSD undertook additional initiatives. Its members attempted to build upon their increasing significance in political discussions, as introduced in Chapter 6. Thereby, their expertise in doping analysis remained at

---

[1] INTERNATIONAL OLYMPIC COMMITTEE, *Répertoire. Directory. '84* (Lausanne: International Olympic Committee, 1984), 23.

[2] Professor Dr. Hans Howald (born 1937) was professor at the medical institute at the EHSM in Magglingen and head of its anti-doping laboratory from 1972 until 1988.

[3] Dr. Wolf-Dieter Montag (born 1924) was an orthopaedist, who specialised in sport medicine. He was chief medical officer of several German Olympic teams and president of the German Ice Skating Union. INTERNATIONAL OLYMPIC COMMITTEE, *Commission Médicale*, 15.

the forefront of their decisions and strategies. Consequently, they continued to have a major effect on the sporting system with wide-ranging effects, particularly for sport administrators and athletes.

Challenges through the Development of Testing Techniques for New Substances

As in previous periods, the members of the IOC MSD dealt intensively with the development of new testing methods for a growing number of performance-enhancing substances. First, Arnold Beckett and the research team of the Drug Control and Teaching Centre at the KCL pushed for the addition of human chorionic gonatropin (hCG) and human growth hormone (hGH) to the banned list and urged Alexandre de Mérode to include the two substances.[4] According to the laboratory team, it was illogical to ban testosterone whilst the IOC allowed a drug that stimulated testosterone production. Moreover, Arnold Beckett regarded the possible addition an opportunity to continue with the usage of RI, because he wrote, "I fully realise the problem with the analysis and that we will have no alternative but to use the RI method."[5] Hence, one also has to consider the proposal in light of the previously addressed terminating relevance of RI. However, due to the perceived outdated RI technology, mainly advocated through Manfred Donike in the IOC MSD at the time, Arnold Beckett appeared to be alone in his opinion even in 1985 when his fellow IOC MSD members had an opposing view.[6] In 1987, when David Cowan and Raymond Brooks reported that during their investigations they had found 19.0% of hCG substances in the urine of male competitors,[7] there was still considerable concern about the identification procedure.[8] Consequently, the IOC MSD only added the substances to the banned

---

[4] Letter, "Arnold Beckett to Alexandre de Mérode, December 9, 1983," archive collection "IOC Medical Commission," folder "IOC Medical Commission: sub-commission Doping and biochemistry of sport: correspondence," IOC Archive, Lausanne.

[5] Letter, "Arnold Beckett to Alexandre de Mérode, December 9, 1983."

[6] Minutes, "Meeting of the IOC Medical Commission, April 10 and 11, 1985," 10.

[7] Letter, "David Cowan and Raymond Brooks to Mike McGee, June 16, 1987," archive collection "IOC Medical Commission," folder "IOC Medical Commission: sub-commission Doping and biochemistry of sport: correspondence," IOC Archive, Lausanne.

[8] Minutes, "Meeting of the IOC Medical Commission's Subcommission Doping and Biochemistry of Sport, September 28 and 29, 1987," archive collection "IOC Medical Commission," folder "IOC Medical Commission: sub-commission Doping and biochemistry of sport : meetings in Calgary on 23rd February 1987 and in Moscow on 28th-29th September 1987: roll call, minutes and working documents," IOC Archive, Lausanne, 7.

list in 1989, when it created the new doping class of "Peptide Hormones and Analogues."[9] Significantly, there was still no convincing testing procedure available at that time, but there were indications for athletes turning to alternative performance-enhancing substances, and the IOC MSD had to react to this development. Nevertheless, this cautious attitude confirms the continuation of the dedicated approach to develop reliable testing techniques before adding substances to the list of banned substances, which in the case of hCG and hGH unquestionably favoured the drug cheats. The majority of the IOC MSD members agreed that this was better than making use of an unreliable method though.

Second, as opposed to hGC and hGH, Manfred Donike supported the prohibition of diuretics, which could be identified with the GC-MS method. Vitaly Semenov's report showed 70.0% of the competitors at the 1984 World Weightlifting Championships were tested positive on diuretics,[10] confirming Manfred Donike's urgency. Eventually, the IOC banned diuretics in 1987.[11] Manfred Donike also recommended corticosteroids stay on the list of banned substances. A key reason for this had been that he was conducting research on their detection in Cologne, supported by the IOC Medical Commission.[12] Moreover, Manfred Donike urged for ephedrine to remain on the banned list. On the IAAF Medical Committee, Arnold Beckett and David Cowan had claimed that ephedrine was present in many "over-the-counter" medical products for the treatment of colds, and that the possibility of unconscious usage of the substance was likely.[13] Manfred Donike rejected this stance, arguing that any findings of ephedrine should be considered as a positive test. Consequently, the IAAF Medical Committee decided upon a compromise solution for the 1986 athletic season, which determined that laboratories should not report a concentration of ephedrine of less than 1µg/ml.[14] However, Manfred Donike was not content with

---

[9] Minutes, "Meeting of the IOC Medical Commission, April 15 and 16, 1989," archive collection "IOC Medical Commission," IOC Archive, Lausanne, 7.

[10] Minutes, "Meeting of the IOC Medical Commission, April 10 and 11, 1985," 8.

[11] Minutes, "Meeting of the IOC Medical Commission, February 24-26, 1987," archive collection "IOC Medical Commission," folder "IOC Medical Commission: meeting in Calgary on 24th-26th February 1987: roll call and minutes," IOC Archive, Lausanne, 12.

[12] Minutes, "Meeting of the IOC Medical Commission in Seoul, April 20-22, 1986," archive collection "IOC Medical Commission," folder "IOC Medical Commission : meeting in Seoul on 20th-22nd April 1986 : roll call, minutes and working documents," IOC Archive, Lausanne, 9.

[13] Letter, "Manfred Donike to August Kirsch, April 4, 1986," archive collection "Nachlass August Kirsch," File 87, "Doping (3)," CuLDA, Cologne.

[14] Ibid.

this solution and eventually proposed to penalise all concentrations of ephedrine, but suggested introducing staggered sanctions: for ephedrine and its derivates a minimum of three months (first offence), two years (second offence) and a life ban (third offence), for all other substances three years (first offence) and a life ban (second offence). Being protective about his policy based on scientific evidence, and due to his previous experiences with the political level, he wanted to avoid an ambiguous clause, which, so he claimed, "would turn the technical decision into a political decision."[15] This remarkable quote stresses his continuous strategy that the basis for a successful anti-doping policy had to have solid scientific methods, which only the anti-doping laboratory experts with their professional competencies in doping analysis could guarantee. One indication for this strategy is that the IAAF Medical Committee accepted his proposal. Therefore, the anti-doping laboratory experts kept control over the processes.[16] Manfred Donike´s attitude confirms the previous finding that after the establishment of a rigid testing regime under his leadership, he did not want to give sport administrators any chance of influencing anti-doping decisions. He evidently interpreted his role beyond the mere development of testing techniques but of a more wide-reaching nature through the recommendations of the bans. However, all of his statements are based on his professional expertise in doping analysis.

Third, none of the leading anti-doping laboratory experts excelled in the prohibition of blood doping. They did not have any detailed experience in the application of blood testing,[17] even if there had been revelations about extensive usage of blood transfusion by the US Cycling team, under the guidance of its coach Eddie Borysewicz, after the 1984 Los Angeles Olympic Games. As

---

[15] Letter, "Manfred Donike to the members of the IAAF Medical Committee, August 26, 1986," archive collection "Nachlass August Kirsch," File 87, "Doping (3)," CuLDA, Cologne.

[16] Letter, "Manfred Donike to August Kirsch, January 26, 1987," archive collection "Nachlass August Kirsch," File 98, "Doping (4)," CuLDA, Cologne. This is despite the fact that the IAAF Council changed Manfred Donike´s proposal so that a two-year ban for a first offense on any substance (except ephedrine) came into force. Minutes, "IAAF Council Meeting, March 27, 1987," archive collection "Nachlass August Kirsch," File 123, "IAAF (2)," CuLDA, Cologne, 17.

[17] It was only in 2004, that a scientific testing method to reveal blood transfusion doping was introduced in world sport, based on the following study: Michael JOYNER, "VO2MAX, blood doping, and erythropoietin," *British Journal of Sports Medicine* 37, no. 3 (2003), 190-191.

GLEAVES convincingly demonstrates,[18] the case eventually caused the IOC Medical Commission to ban blood doping in April 1985,[19] therewith abandoning its previous policy to ban only detectable substances. It also replaced the term "drugs" with the term "substance" in order to include genetic modifications such as blood doping into its doping definition. Manfred Donike regularly stated his disbelief about the extent of blood doping. He stressed that due to strict international regulations on the transportation of blood, it would not occur on a large scale.[20] He shared this view with other members of the IOC Medical Commission and the body decided against the introduction of alternative ways to detect blood doping. Consequently, "the detection of prohibited substances in the athlete's body by scientific tests remained the only accepted doping proof."[21] This was certainly in the interest of the anti-doping laboratory experts and Don Catlin confirmed this assumption, claiming, "it annoyed Manfred Donike in particular that he was not an expert in blood doping and was consequently not interested in research on possible detection methods."[22] This led to conflicts in later years (see later in this chapter). Interestingly, because the leading anti-doping laboratory experts were not as interested and knowledgeable in blood testing, other scientists began to investigate into the issue on the IOC MSD's behalf. Arne Ljungqvist approached Alexandre de Mérode in February 1985 about the possibility to obtain a research grant for a project on blood doping at the Karolinska Institute.[23] The IOC Medical Commission approved this request but after the presentation of the first results at the end of 1985, IOC MSD members raised considerable concerns about the nature of the research, because it focused on the harmful effects of blood doping. Arnold Beckett believed that the research should instead concentrate on the development of detection methods.[24] Hence, the members of the IOC MSD dealt with the challenge of increasing usage of blood doping in a

---

[18] GLEAVES, "Manufactured Dope," 13ff.

[19] Minutes, "Meeting of the IOC Medical Commission, April 10 and 11, 1985," 6.

[20] Ibid.

[21] REINOLD, "Arguing," 54.

[22] Interview with Don H. Catlin, November 11, 2012.

[23] Minutes, "Meeting of the IOC Medical Commission, April 10 and 11, 1985," Annex 6.

[24] Minutes, "Meeting of the IOC Subcommittee on Doping and Biochemistry in Strasbourg, November 17 and 18, 1985," archive collection "IOC Medical Commission," folder "IOC Medical Commission: sub-commission Doping and biochemistry of sport: meetings on 17th February 1984, in Cologne on 18th-19th February 1985 and in Strasbourg on 17th-18th November 1985: roll call, minutes and working documents," IOC Archive, Lausanne, 5.

restrictive manner only, yet their room for manoeuvre appears to have been limited even when consulting other researchers.

Fourth, the anti-doping laboratory experts concurred on the issue of international, standardised out-of competition tests and their willingness to undertake the analytical controls in their laboratories. They had expressed such a need earlier (see Chapters 4 and 6). Following the 1984 Los Angeles Olympic Games, they continuously voiced these intentions again in an attempt to convince sport officials that they could only eradicate the anabolic steroids misuse in this way. They were encouraged in their attempts by the efforts of national initiatives that intended out-of competition tests, such as an agreement between the Nordic sports confederations.[25] This arrangement appears to be the first international treaty to determine training controls. In 1987, Manfred Donike confirmed that of about 33,000 doping analyses undertaken in accredited laboratories, 23.6% were from samples taken outside of competitions, and conducted by national federations.[26] However, his efforts went unheeded on the national level at that time, due mainly to continuing opposition from Joseph Keul, who listed organisational, financial and judicial reasons to justify his objection towards comprehensive out-of competition controls.[27] KRÜGER et al. come to the conclusion that he mainly wanted to avoid an expansion of the doping analysis.[28] Manfred Donike did not mind this opposition and promoted an increase of out-of competition tests on the international scene. During a meeting of the IAAF Doping Subcommittee, he pushed for a change of the IAAF statutes to include a recommendation on out-of competition controls. He proposed the following points:

> a) general endorsement of the introduction of out-of competition doping controls. Change of the IAAF statues in this regard so that athletes can be tested by the IAAF or national athletic federations 'in or outside competition'

> b) Urge the member federations to conduct out-of competition doping controls

---

[25] FINISH CENTRAL SPORTS FEDERATION, *Nordic Anti-Doping Convention* (Helsinki: Finish Central Sports Federation, 1983).

[26] Letter, "Manfred Donike to August Kirsch, Trainingskontrollen, March 16, 1987," archive collection "Nachlass August Kirsch," File 98, "Doping (4)," CuLDA, Cologne.

[27] Letter, "Joseph Keul to August Kirsch, November 25, 1985," archive collection "Nachlass August Kirsch," File 087, "Doping (3)," CuLDA, Cologne.

[28] KRÜGER et al., *Doping und Anti-Doping*, 136.

c) Give the IAAF Medical Committee the task to undertake random controls on occasion of national championships

d) Raise the number of controlled competitions and raise the number of urine samples at some competitions without announcement

e) Inaugurate a "volunteer doping control programme," for elite athletes, for which Arne Ljungqvist should hold talks with the IAAF Athletes' Commission.[29]

The IAAF Congress gave its approval to all of the above points during its meeting in Rome in 1987 and adopted a ten-point plan. One point referred specifically to the encouragement of out-of competition controls.[30] Although the IOC Medical Commission did not make such recommendations (because it did not have any national federations to deal with), Manfred Donike and Robert Dugal expressed strong interest in the development of a similar proposal.[31] Clearly, international out-of competition controls would have allowed an extension of their influence.

The processes reveal that the anti-doping laboratory experts undertook efforts to advance the already existing analytical methods to allow testing for more substances. They considered this task their main priority, particularly because they continued to pursue the policy to add only detectable substances to the banned list. From 1985 onwards, blood doping was a notable exception, caused by the revelation of extensive misuse at the 1984 Los Angeles Olympic Games. One has to contribute the reason for the addition without a reliable detection technique to the fact that none of the leading anti-doping laboratory experts had

---

[29] Letter. "Manfred Donike to August Kirsch, January 26, 1987." The IAAF Athletes' Commission was founded officially at the IAAF Council meeting in Madrid in February 1986. It's original members were: Joan Benoit-Samuelson (USA), Darren Clark (Australia), Sebastian Coe (Great Britain), Joachim Cruz (Brazil), Omar Khalifa (Sudan), Marita Koch (GDR), Edwin Moses (USA), Merlene Ottey-Page (Jamaica), Yuriy Sedykh (USSR), Toshihiko Seko (Japan), Sara Simeoni (Italy), Thierry Vigneron (France) and Thomas Wessinghage (FRG). Minutes. "IAAF Council Meeting, February 19-21, 1986," archive collection "Nachlass August Kirsch," File 123, "IAAF (2)," CuLDA, Cologne. Also see: "International Federations." *Olympic Review* 225 (1986), 414.

[30] Minutes. "IAAF Council Meeting, December 20, 1987," archive collection "Nachlass August Kirsch," File 123, "IAAF (2)," CuLDA, Cologne, Appendix E.

[31] Minutes. "Meetings of the IOC Medical Commission, February 9-28, 1988," archive collection "IOC Medical Commission," folder "IOC Medical Commission: meeting in Calgary on 9th-28th February 1988: roll call, minutes and working documents," IOC Archive, Lausanne.

specific expertise in this field. They faced this problem because on the one hand, they did not want to incorporate other individuals into the leading circle, but on the other, those external experts consulted were unable to provide satisfying results. Certainly, the heads of the laboratories regarded the introduction of out-of competition tests another opportunity to increase the number of doping tests, and hence generate more income for their institutions. The argument for more research in testing techniques also gave more substance to disapproval from the field of sports medicine. Confronted with complaints about the large amounts of research funds going into doping analysis, Manfred Donike did not refrain from sharply criticising sport medicine specialists. He claimed, "had all doctors, who are involved in sport, attended their two semesters of ethics lectures, there would not be any research funds for doping analysis."[32] Thus, he clarified that sport medicine specialists played a decisive role within the doping system. Other members of the IOC Medical Commission supported him in his stance. For example, Hans Howald stated that not the athletes, but certain sport medicine specialists were the real enemies of the doping inspectors.[33]

Strengthening of Guidelines to Maintain High Quality Standards

Efforts to Standardise Procedures

Efforts to install more administrative procedures, and the developments of updated testing guidelines for the evolving laboratory network dominated the period after the 1984 Los Angeles Olympic Games. Following his experience with the involvement of the political level from Los Angeles, Manfred Donike tried to speed up processes. By December 1984, he had already persuaded August Kirsch to support him and put forward a request by the IAAF to the IOC that the IOC Medical Commission could make official announcements on positive controls without approval through the IOC Executive Board as well.[34] Essentially, this was another attempt for more trust in the scientific results and the work of the anti-doping laboratory experts.

A first result of modernised guidelines came out of the IAAF Doping Subcommittee, who had produced a publication summarising all aspects of doping controls. The IAAF released the publication *Doping Control Regulations*

---

[32] Manfred Donike in Steffen HAFFNER, "Wenn der Spitzensport zum Spritzensport wird," *Frankfurter Allgemeine Zeitung,* July 5, 1985, archive collection "Nachlass August Kirsch," File 087, "Doping (3)," CuLDA, Cologne.

[33] Ibid.

[34] Letter, "Manfred Donike to August Kirsch, December 7, 1984."

and Guidelines for Procedure in January 1985, to inform all stakeholders within the world of athletics about the IAAF's regulations.[35] Significantly, the brochure did not include detailed information on the doping analysis and the equipment of the laboratory anymore. Instead, it contained the remark, "only laboratories accredited or approved by the IAAF on the advice by the Medical Committee may be used to carry out the analysis in connection with doping control."[36] This is an important difference, resulting from the introduction of the accreditation system. Moreover, the IAAF adopted a regulation concerning the ratification of world records. The new rule provided confirmation of a world record only after an accredited laboratory had analysed an athlete's sample. [37] However, the practical implementation of the new rule proved to be challenging. In September 1986, the javelin thrower Klaus Tafelmeier (FRG) achieved a new world record during an international sporting competition in Como (Italy). In contrast to the regulations introduced, the organisers did not test him, and he only provided a urine sample after the DLV intervened. Manfred Donike analysed the sample in the Cologne laboratory and presented a negative result. He maintained that the sampling procedure had not been conducted according to IAAF standards and the world record should not stand.[38] Manfred Donike thought it was necessary to have scientifically valid doping controls, even if it was to the advantage of a potential doping offender. Such an attitude was the result of the raison d'être of the anti-doping laboratory experts and hence understandable. This is an indication of the need for more international regulation in doping control processes.

The introduction of an official "reference substance bank" is another example for increased standardisation. With this, the IOC MSD wanted to overcome complicated customs regulations that hindered the shipment of samples for the accreditation and reaccreditation procedures. Unsurprisingly, the London laboratory of Arnold Beckett drove this initiative because it was the main laboratory for the distribution of the reference samples. Arnold Beckett and Alexandre de Mérode visited the United Nations' International Narcotics Control Board (INCB) in Vienna to seek assistance for the official constitution of such a

---

[35] Report, "IAAF: Doping control regulations and guidelines for procedures, January 1985," archive collection "Nachlass August Kirsch," File 087, "Doping (3)," CuLDA, Cologne.

[36] Ibid., 7.

[37] Press Release, "Procedures for Doping Control, 1985," archive collection "Nachlass August Kirsch," File 087, "Doping (3)," CuLDA, Cologne.

[38] Letter, "Heiner Henze to August Kirsch, March 10, 1987," archive collection "Nachlass August Kirsch," File 087, "Doping (3)," CuLDA, Cologne.

reference sample bank at the KCL and the legal distribution of samples between countries in 1987.[39] However, the INCB advised them to provide the NOCs of the countries concerned (with priority for those countries with accredited laboratories) with a list of the reference drugs required annually. In a second step, the NOCs had to inform their governments, which would then submit the list to the INCB for approval.[40] Regarding the storage of the reference substances in London, the INCB advised Arnold Beckett to get national permission from the British Home Office. Once this step was successfully undertaken, he compiled a list of all available reference substances.[41] Although it was not possible to collect samples of all substances on the banned list,[42] the IOC MSD informed accredited anti-doping laboratories in a letter in 1988 about the new possibility to obtain reference substances easily.[43] Therein it becomes evident that non-controlled agents were delivered in quantities of 100mg, and that controlled agents needed prior approval from the respective government control authority.[44] Hence, the reference bank became a simplification of processes within the network. Simultaneously, it enabled the protagonists to keep control over it through its internal set-up.

Another new installation was the so-called "positive list," that Robert Dugal had compiled. This list included a large number of medical products, containing banned substances.[45] Although there were some concerns that certain drugs were banned in different countries, the IOC eventually added the list to the medical control brochures of the Olympic Games.[46] Robert Dugal also worked intensively on the establishment of a computer data bank for drug synonyms and commercial names, along with scientific literature related to doping and doping control from 1985 onwards.[47] Alexandre de Mérode very much welcomed this initiative but the

[39] Minutes, "92nd Session of the IOC in Istanbul, May 9-12, 1987," Annex 9.
[40] Ibid.
[41] Minutes, "Meeting of the IOC Medical Commission's Subcommission Doping and Biochemistry of Sport, September 28 and 29, 1987," Annex 18.
[42] Minutes, "Meetings of the IOC Medical Commission, February 9-28, 1988," 17.
[43] Individual Minutes, "Meetings of the IOC Medical Commission, September 14 to October 1, 1988," archive collection "IOC Medical Commission," folder "IOC Medical Commission: meeting in Seoul on 14th September - 1st October 1988: minutes and working documents," IOC Archive, Lausanne, Annex 4.
[44] Ibid.
[45] Minutes, "Meeting of the IOC Medical Commission, February 24-26, 1987," 14.
[46] Ibid., 15.
[47] Minutes, "Meeting of the IOC Medical Commission, April 20-22, 1986," Annex 32.

IOC Medical Commission did not put it into practice at that time, since it was unsuccessful to establish a link with an intended IOC platform.[48]

The Code of Ethics

The two most significant new introductions amongst the network of anti-doping laboratory experts were the "Code of Ethics" and the "Good Laboratory Practice Guide" (GLP). The IOC MSD discussed them under the headline of "information flow between the laboratories," and were a result of the perception that an increased exchange of information between the testing centres became imminent. The two documents differed extensively from each other. The "Code of Ethics" aimed to prevent laboratories from pre-testing in individual countries based on ethical grounds, whereas the GLP generally addressed all technical and organisational issues of the work in the anti-doping laboratory. Because the "Code of Ethics" was developed and adopted prior to the GLP, it is discussed in this chapter, while the GLP is addressed later in this chapter.

The IOC MSD held the first discussions on the "Code of Ethics" in November 1986.[49] It appears that the members of the IOC MSD were aware of the pre-tests ahead of the 1984 Olympic Games. They condemned such practices and wanted to obtain a degree of control to avoid unofficial pre-testing in the future. This is despite the fact that some anti-doping laboratory experts had been involved in pre-testing ahead of the Los Angeles Games too, albeit not as systematic as in the USA. KRÜGER et al. demonstrate how Armin Klümper treated the cyclist Gerhard Strittmatter (FRG) with the substance primobolon and tested positive around one month prior to the 1984 Los Angeles Olympic Games.[50] However, due to the depot effect, the FRG's Cycling Federation (Bund Deutscher Radfahrer, BDR) was looking for solutions to investigate whether the cyclist would still test positive in Los Angeles. Hence, the BDR turned to Manfred Donike, who agreed to test the cyclist and found changeable amounts of metabolites in his urine, although he had predicted otherwise.[51] This resulted in

---

[48] Minutes, "Meetings of the IOC Medical Commission, February 9-28, 1988," 18.

[49] Minutes, "Meeting of the IOC Medical Commission's Subcommission Doping and Biochemistry of Sport, November 12 and 13, 1986," archive collection "IOC Medical Commission," folder "IOC Medical Commission : sub-commission Doping and biochemistry of sport: meeting in Rome on 12th-13th November 1986: roll call, minutes and working documents," IOC Archive, Lausanne, 2.

[50] KRÜGER et al., *Doping und Anti-Doping*, 113.

[51] Report, "Zusammenfassende Analyse Huber: Fall Strittmatter by Georg Huber, September 10, 1984," archive collection "Nachlass August Kirsch," File 086, "Doping (2)," CuLDA, Cologne.

the exclusion of Gerhard Strittmaier from the Olympic Games. Curiously, Arnold Beckett and the laboratory in London were also involved in the episode. Dissatisfied about the results from the laboratory in Cologne, the athlete turned to the German magazine *Stern*, who arranged for a test of his samples and those of two reporters in London. [52] The results were negative, but the laboratory in London only tested for the pure substance, whereas the Cologne laboratory also analysed for metabolites, which resulted in the positive findings. This incident illustrates that the leading anti-doping laboratory experts were not free from guilt either, and in light of such controversies, the introduction of the "Code of Ethics" demonstrates awareness of their ethical responsibilities.

In February 1987, Robert Dugal and Manfred Donike presented a first draft of the "Code of Ethics" to the IOC Medical Commission. [53] The proposal was still very vague and only addressed main issues, such as the receipt of samples from "known" sources and the follow-up sanctions in case of a positive finding. A second draft, discussed in September 1987, did not address other aspects either. [54] However, the IOC Medical Commission eventually adopted a more detailed version in February 1988. [55] It included two separate sections for competition and out-of competition testing, and stated that doping analysis was only allowed if ordered by national or international federations, NOCs, national sport organisations, universities or similar organisations. [56] Moreover, it was emphasised that the laboratories did not accept samples from athletes, intermediaries or of a commercial nature, and it condemned the support of unofficial laboratories for athletes in their endeavours to circumvent the doping regulations. Importantly, all accredited laboratories had to sign the "Code of Ethics," and its signature was included into the IOC's requirements for laboratories seeking accreditations. [57] This is an example of dealing with the challenges that resulted from the rising number of anti-doping laboratories and to remind the heads of the laboratories about their ethical responsibilities.

Despite these favourable efforts, it was impossible to control the compliance with the code. The most obvious example for the undetected exploitation of an accredited anti-doping laboratory for the execution of a doping programme was

---

[52] Ibid.

[53] Minutes, "Meeting of the IOC Medical Commission, February 24-26, 1987," Annex 5.

[54] Minutes, "Meeting of the IOC Medical Commission's Subcommission on Doping and Biochemistry, September 28-29, 1987," Annex 3.

[55] Minutes, "Meeting of the IOC Medical Commission, February 24-26, 1987," Annex 5.

[56] Ibid.

[57] Ibid.

the laboratory of IOC MSD member Claus Clausnitzer in Kreischa. Consequently, REINOLD is correct, when he writes:

> The laboratory in Kreischa on the one hand seemed to meet the highest technological standards. On the other hand, the technological capability was not used for anti-doping but totally the contrary: It operated as an important part of the GDR's state-run doping program which pre-tested its own athletes in order to determine when to stop taking drugs and avoid detection in competitions abroad. Kreischa shows that the established code of ethics constitutes an ethical code, which was actually uncontrollable by current (re)accreditation procedures.[58]

Thus, whilst the "Code of Ethics" was a commendable and important initiative that shows awareness for their ethical responsibility, it evidently displays that once the anti-doping laboratory experts had obtained a control function through the IOC MSD, they faced challenges that went beyond their traditional areas of expertise.

Implications from the Sandra Gasser Case

In addition, the political level still found ways to undermine the anti-doping laboratory experts' initiatives. Besides the continuation of criticism from the sport medical field on the overly blinkered approach by Manfred Donike,[59] such attempts on the international level came from within the IAAF. This becomes evident at an incident prior to the 1987 World Athletics Championships in Rome. At the first edition of the IAAF's flagship event, the federation had only undertaken limited efforts to ensure the application of tight doping control procedures (see Chapter 6). Curiously, this happened again in 1987, when the

---

[58] REINOLD, "Arguing," 48.

[59] KRÜGER et al., *Doping und Anti-Doping*, 113. Written exchanges of complaints concerning international efforts to install out-of competition controls in Germany, in which Manfred Donike was involved, are: Letter, "Lebenslange Bestrafung; Unangemeldete Kontrolle; Dopingaufklärungsschrift der Aktiven," Joseph Keul to August Kirsch, November 25, 1985. Opposition against the addition of diuretica onto the banned list is revealed in: Letter, "Joseph Keul to Manfred Donike, July 2, 1987," archive collection "Nachlass August Kirsch," File 098, "Doping (4)," CuLDA, Cologne. However, it was not only Joseph Keul, who voiced criticism. Wildor Hollmann argued that too much money was invested into doping analysis, which could be used for other purposes. Wildor Hollmann in Gregor DERICHS, "Die Doping-Spirale," *SID*, January 30, 1986, archive collection "Nachlass August Kirsch," File 087, "Doping (3)," CuLDA, Cologne.

IAAF Council thwarted Manfred Donike and Arnold Beckett. Originally, the IAAF Medical Committee had selected the two to act as medical representatives at the event.[60] However, the IAAF Council overruled this decision and appointed IAAF Medical Committee member Dr. Virginia Mikhaylova from Bulgaria to supervise the doping controls instead.[61] This led to criticism from Manfred Donike, who commented:

> Ein schwaches Labor, eine (nur) in Dopingfragen schwache Delegierte der Medizinischen Kommission, ein taktierender Präsident der Medizinischen Kommission der IAAF und ein starker IAAF-Präsident auf heimatlichem Boden, was wollen Sie von einer solchen Konstellation erwarten?

> [A weak laboratory, an (only) in doping questions weak medical representative, a tactical president of the IAAF Medical Committee and an IAAF president on home soil, what do you expect from such a constellation?][62]

He made abundantly clear that politically influenced conditions were not preferable to allow reliable scientific results.

Apart from Manfred Donike's suspicions about inconsistencies, other researchers have outlined that the change in doping personnel was a clear indication to keep the event clear from positive doping cases.[63] However, there was one positive doping test for methyltestosterone by Swiss runner Sandra Gasser. HOBERMAN, who discusses Sandra Gasser's positive doping test, demonstrating the political behaviour of the IAAF, already stressed the decisive role of the laboratory staff in Rome.[64] Importantly, after the detection of the banned substance in Sandra Gasser's A-sample, the B-sample was analysed at the laboratory in Rome under the presence of Wilhelm Schänzer from Cologne. However, whilst the analysis of the B-sample revealed the presence of methyltestosterone metabolites as well, the steroid profile of the sample was found to be different from the one of the A-sample, and in itself unusual for a

---

[60] Minutes, "Meeting of the IAAF Medical Committee, August 20, 1986," Appendix E.
[61] Letter, "Manfred Donike to August Kirsch, January 26, 1987".
[62] Ibid.
[63] VOY, *Drug*, 108.
[64] HOBERMAN, *Mortal*, 229ff.

steroid profile.[65] Moreover, Wilhelm Schänzer noted in his report that the lack of urine – a doping officer had spilled parts of it during the sampling procedure – made it impossible to conduct further research. Hence, the samples should not have been accepted by the laboratory and the sampling officers in the first place.[66] An explanation for the different analytical results was found some days later when it transpired that the head of the laboratory in Rome had used different undistilled ether for the analysis of the B-samples. This had prevented an important chemical reaction from taking place.[67] Since the IAAF had made the personnel changes in the area of the doping analysis, Manfred Donike used the opportunity to blame the IAAF for the entire episode. He reasoned that it all started with the removal of Arnold Beckett and himself as supervisors for the doping controls: "[the Rome laboratory was] one of the weaker IOC and IAAF accredited laboratories, and due to the internal structure, they need help in critical situations (...) the outcoming result is a disaster, both for the laboratory and the IAAF."[68] HOBERMAN correctly asserts that the Rome laboratory temporarily lost its accreditation in the following year.[69] However, this was officially due to "unacceptable documentation" from the reaccreditation procedure (see later in this chapter), and therefore to be regarded separately from the incident involving Sandra Gasser.

The controversy of the doping controls at the 1987 World Athletics Championships went beyond the ongoing dispute between IAAF officials, who appeared to control the amount of positive tests, and Manfred Donike, who wanted controls to be as scientifically reliable as possible. He thought that the flaws in the doping analysis were a danger for the system of doping testing, for whose establishment and implementation he was in charge. Hence, he also opposed the final decision of the IAAF (which was the first case debated at the

---

[65] Report, "World Championships, 1987, Rome – Doping Control," September 23, 1987, archive collection "Nachlass August Kirsch," File 084, "[Doping] Birgit Dressel und Sandra Gasser," CuLDA, Cologne.

[66] Extract from report, "Schänzer: Statement to the 2nd test 23rd of September 1987, by Wilhelm Schänzer, September 25, 1987," archive collection "Nachlass August Kirsch," File 084, "[Doping] Birgit Dressel und Sandra Gasser," CuLDA, Cologne.

[67] Letter, "Zweite Analyse von Gasser Rom," Manfred Donike to Arne Ljungqvist, September 26, 1987.

[68] Ibid.

[69] HOBERMAN, *Mortal*, 233.

IAAF's internal arbitration panel),[70] to uphold the disqualification of Sandra Gasser.[71] He maintained that that from a scientific point of view, he could not accept the irreproducible results with strong differences in the A- and the B-sample.[72] His participation in the panel is evidence for the importance of the anti-doping laboratory experts for the existing doping control system because they were the only ones professionally qualified to comment on the doping analysis.

Notably, the Sandra Gasser case was not the only example in this list of controversies. Before the 1985 European Athletics Indoor Championships in Athens, a laboratory in Athens had undertaken the doping analysis and declared eighteen positive tests (fourteen from athletics and four from other sports) on behalf of the Hellenic Athletics Federation.[73] However, the laboratory was not officially recognised and a second test by the laboratory in Cologne showed that only one sample actually contained a substance banned by the IAAF.[74] As in the case of Sandra Gasser, Manfred Donike had raised concerns about this procedure. He argued that such unconfirmed announcements would undermine the confidentiality of the anti-doping laboratory work, and counteract quality assurance processes.[75] Significantly, Primo Nebiolo publicly praised the Hellenic Athletics Federation for its procedure and the positive results, because after the announcement it would be impossible to cover up any further positive results.

---

[70] Sandra Gasser (born 1962) was successful in her appeal to seek special injunctive relief in a Swiss court to lift the ban on her in December 1987. Unmoved by this decision, the IAAF threatened in January 1988 that all athletes, who competed against her, would also be banned. As a result, Sandra Gasser sued the IAAF at the British High Court in London but she did not succeed in her effort to get a lifting of the ban. According to Aaron N. WISE and Bruce S. MEYER, the case was wrongly decided because "strict liability drug rules of sports governing bodiesare contrary to natural justice and possibly an unlawful restraint of trade". Aaron N. WISE and Bruce S. MEYER, *International Sports Law and Business* (The Hague: Kluwer Law International, 1997), 1468f.

[71] Fax, "Informationsschreiben Fall Gasser, John Holt to all members of the IAAF Council, June 15, 1988," archive collection "Nachlass August Kirsch," File 084, "[Doping] Birgit Dressel und Sandra Gasser," CuLDA, Cologne.

[72] Letter, "Manfred Donike to August Kirsch, January 9, 1988," archive collection "Nachlass August Kirsch," File 084, "[Doping] Birgit Dressel und Sandra Gasser," CuLDA, Cologne.

[73] Minutes, "IAAF Council Meeting, May 20, 1985," archive collection "Nachlass August Kirsch," File 123, "IAAF (2)," CuLDA, Cologne, 3

[74] Ibid.

[75] Letter, "Manfred Donike to August Kirsch, May 28, 1985," archive collection "Nachlass August Kirsch," File 087, "Doping (3)," CuLDA, Cologne.

Consequently, Manfred Donike blamed the IAAF president for not understanding the significance of scientific proof.[76]

Both cases emphasise that the attempts to strengthen the guidelines for anti-doping laboratories, in order to maintain high-quality standards, were not random. On the contrary, the regulations dealt with the challenges of an expanded network of institutions involved in doping analysis. Clearly, the inappropriate handling of Sandra Gasser's sample in the Rome laboratory is evidence for this. Manfred Donike's opinion to reject the results proves that he thought results based on bad scientific work discredited the anti-doping system. Clearly, leading IAAF figures saw in the increasingly powerful role of Arnold Beckett and Manfred Donike a danger for portraying a clean image of athletics. Their professional competencies had been essential for the establishment of the global doping control system, while the procedures they had employed since 1981 were acknowledged by sport administrators. However, as soon as they began to exert wide-reaching influence on the decision-making level, they faced increased opposition from high-ranking individuals. They saw in the anti-doping laboratory experts not only support, but also a danger for the ongoing commercialisation of sport and the attempt to attract sponsors. This is not surprising if one looks at the growing numbers of doping cases in the sport, which can also be contributed to the increased number of doping controls, and more reliable analytical procedures. For example, from 1984 until 1988, the percentage of positive doping tests in the laboratory in Cologne raised from 1.49% to 5.59%.[77]

Further Extension of Personal and Institutional Networks with Increased Differentiation and Emphasis on Quality

In Chapter 6, the extreme numeric gain in official IOC and IAAF doping laboratories between 1981 and 1985, reaching up to sixteen institutions by the end of 1985, was illustrated. However, the political level still urged for the accreditation of more institutions in the period leading up to the 1988 Olympic Games. In 1987, the IOC Executive Board and the IAAF Council released a statement, where they referred specifically to the creation of new doping

---

[76] Letter, "August Kirsch to Arne Ljungqvist, May 22, 1985," archive collection "Nachlass August Kirsch," File 087, "Doping (3)," CuLDA, Cologne.

[77] Report, "Jahresstatistik 1992 des Beauftragten für Dopinganalytik, 1993" BISp-Archive, Bonn.

laboratories.[78] The sport organisations regarded the number of doping laboratories as proof for the anti-doping activities on the political level at the time.

Accordingly, the IOC MSD continued its efforts in the extension of the anti-doping laboratory network although not as capaciously. After it awarded Magglingen its reaccreditation in 1985, the laboratory at the Department of Pharmacology and Toxicology at the Medical Investigation Institute of the Hospital del Mar (Institut Municipal d'Investigacio Médica, IMIM) under the leadership of Professor Dr. Jordi Segura applied for accreditation. The Bidding Committee for the 1992 Barcelona Olympic Games initiated the process to get an official anti-doping laboratory in Barcelona, despite the presence of one in Madrid. In fact, the other contenders for the 1992 Olympic Games – Paris and Brisbane – already had accredited anti-doping laboratories.[79] This reveals that anti-doping laboratories became relevant for the bidding process. Consequently, the Barcelona Bidding Committee addressed IMIM, where scientists conducted research on drug testing, with the intention to set up a laboratory. As a result, the hospital employed Jordi Segura, who had experience in drug metabolism and laboratory work but not in sports drug testing, from January 1985, with the specific aim trying to obtain the accreditation for anti-doping in the shortest time possible.[80] By the end of 1985, the laboratory successfully passed the admission test, and Spain became the first country to have two officially accredited doping laboratories.

When the IOC awarded Barcelona the 1992 Olympic Games in 1986,[81] Jordi Segura became a powerful figure amongst the head of anti-doping laboratories and, together with Don Catlin, extended the group of most influential anti-doping laboratory experts. The two became regular participants of the IOC MSD meetings, although they were not official members. Whilst Jordi Segura dealt particularly with the preparation for the 1992 Barcelona Olympic Games, the IOC MSD assigned Don Catlin to undertake important research projects on the effects

---

[78] Minutes, "Meeting of the IAAF Council with the IOC Executive Board, August 29, 1987," archive collection "Nachlass August Kirsch," File 123, "IAAF (2)," CuLDA, Cologne, 3.

[79] The other cities that were bidding for the 1992 Olympic Games were Belgrade (Yugoslavia), Birmingham (Great Britain) and Amsterdam (Netherlands). KLUGE, *Olympische Sommerspiele. Die Chronik III*, 344.

[80] Jordi SEGURA, "Antidoping Control, Cross Road Between Chemistry and Other Life Sciences," *Actualidad Analitica* 34 (2011), 16: http://www.seqa.es/ActualidadAnalitica/Ano2011Numero34.pdf [accessed February 11, 2015].

[81] KLUGE, *Olympische Sommerspiele. Die Chronik III*, 344.

and detection of controversial substances, because he had a highly developed research environment with sufficient financial resources at UCLA. His research on contraceptive pills containing norethisterone, which allowed female competitors to mask the usage of nandrolone, is an example for this.[82] The IOC Medical Commission first added the substance to the banned list in early 1987,[83] but removed it a couple of months later after considerable complaints from the North American continent where the percentage of contraceptive pills containing norethisertone was very high.[84] The basis for this change in opinion provided Don Catlin´s research, where he proposed the introduction of statistical confirmation studies on all analytically positive samples.[85] Jordi Segura and Don Catlin fitted into the traditional field of research of the leading anti-doping laboratory experts. Clearly, this was a reason for the IOC MSD members to include them more actively, rather than experts on blood doping, who would have brought a more uncontrollable dimension to their field.

In view of increasingly tightened accreditation standards and the awareness that the political level wanted to see an increase in official doping testing centres, Alexandre de Mérode seized the suggestion of the "screening laboratories" again in 1985, which Arnold Beckett had already proposed in 1982.[86] In contrast to the accredited laboratories, the IOC MSD did not demand doping analysis with GC-MS from the "screening laboratories", but only with RI. In case of a positive finding, the staff sent the sample to an accredited laboratory. According to Alexandre de Mérode, institutions from more countries could become involved in anti-doping, and prepare to become finally an accredited laboratory.[87] However, it is important to emphasise that after receiving the applications to become screening laboratories, the IOC MSD members argued that all institutions would be capable of becoming fully accredited laboratories with assistance from the already existing institutions anyway. Amongst them were the laboratories at the Department of Pathology at the Indiana University Medical Centre in

---

[82] Minutes, "Meeting of the IOC Medical Commission, February 24-26, 1987." 10f.

[83] Ibid.

[84] Minutes, "Meeting of the IOC Medical Commission´s Subcommission on Doping and Biochemistry, September 28-29, 1987," archive collection "IOC Medical Commission," folder "IOC Medical Commission : sub-commission Doping and biochemistry of sport: meetings in Calgary on 23rd February 1987 and in Moscow on 28th-29th September 1987: roll call, minutes and working documents," IOC Archive, Lausanne, 5.

[85] Ibid.

[86] Letter, "Walter Tröger to August Kirsch, April 17, 1985," archive collection "Nachlass August Kirsch," File 087, "Doping (3)," CuLDA, Cologne.

[87] Ibid.

Indianapolis (USA), the Institute for the Control of Drugs in Zagreb (Yugoslavia) and the Laboratory for Doping Analysis and Biochemistry of the Ministry of Education and Culture in Lisbon (Portugal). The IOC MSD granted all of them accreditation status in 1987.[88] As a result, it suspended the idea of the "screening laboratories" again.

The most important tool to maintain a good quality of doping tests amongst the already recognised doping laboratories remained the reaccreditation procedure. Whereas in 1985, all laboratories had successfully met the requirements, this was no longer the case during the second procedure in January 1987. Two of the eighteen laboratories, Brisbane and Sarajevo, were provisionally suspended, pending a further reaccreditation test. They got the opportunity to repeat the entire procedure within a period of three months.[89] Branko Nikolin claimed that the Sarajevo anti-doping laboratory had financial problems, and was in the process of moving its equipment to the University of Sarajevo.[90] The IOC MSD notified the sports federations not to conduct any doping analysis by the two institutions in that time. However, some federations continued to send urine samples to the anti-doping laboratory in Brisbane in particular.[91] As the laboratories were also not able to provide the correct analysis of the second set of samples, they lost their accreditation eventually.[92] With Brisbane the only laboratory in the Oceania region, this became a major concern. The new IOC Medical Commission member Professor Dr. Kenneth Fitch[93] (Australia), who became responsible for working with the NOCs, attempted to

---

[88] Minutes, "Meeting of the IOC Medical Commission's Subcommission on Doping and Biochemistry, September 28-29, 1987," 2.

[89] Minutes, "Meeting of the IOC Medical Commission, February 24-26, 1987," 3.

[90] Minutes, "Meeting of the IOC Medical Commission's Subcommission Doping and Biochemistry of Sport, September 28 and 29, 1987," Annex 2.

[91] THE PARLIAMENT OF THE COMMONWEALTH OF AUSTRALIA, *Drugs in Sport. An Interim Report of the Senate Standing Committee on Environment, Recreation and the Arts* (Canberra: Australian Government Publishing Service, 1989), 110f.

[92] Minutes, "Meeting of the IOC Medical Commission's Subcommission on Doping and Biochemistry, September 28 and 29, 1987," 3.

[93] Professor Dr. Kenneth Fitch (born 1933) is a medical doctor, who worked at the Royal Perth Hospital following his doctorate in Adelaide. He established a sports and soft tissue injury clinic in 1969. From 1972 oonwards, he became heavily involved with the Australian Olympic team and eventually a member of the IOC Medical Commission in 1986. "Royal Perth Hospital Emeritus Consultant Biographies," *Royal Perth Hospital*; http://www.rph.wa.gov.au/~/media/Files/Hospitals/RPH/PDFs/Emeritus%20Consultant%20Biographies%20vol%203.ashx [accessed February 17, 2015], 16.

convince his colleagues that such a situation was very unlucky, but the IOC MSD retained its policy to have no results, rather than unreliable data.[94]

The installation of quality improvement measures did not stop there. Following the review of the reaccreditation, the IOC MSD also sent out samples to assist with the establishment of quantitative analysis standards for caffeine and testosterone, and to support all laboratories in the correct identification of these substances.[95] Although the laboratories also had to report their results to the IOC MSD, they were only evaluated for training purposes, and not used for an official check. In 1988, Manfred Donike reported that the results of the proficiency test for testosterone marked an improvement, although he still considered more efforts necessary to increase "inter-laboratory reproducibility and accuracy."[96]

The period between 1985 and 1988 was also defined by attempts to increase the knowledge exchange between the laboratories. In 1987, the Norwegian sports official Dr. Hans Skaset[97] urged for more organised meetings of the heads of laboratories.[98] This appears logical in light of the growing number of anti-doping laboratories involved. Apart from the Cologne Workshop, regularly held at the DSHS, focusing increasingly on questions of pharmacokinetics and metabolism, Manfred Donike began to compile annual statistics on the conducted doping tests within the international community of anti-doping laboratories. In 1986, he demanded that the international anti-doping laboratories provide him with all information, "to improve the information between the accredited laboratories and to update the knowledge of the drug misuse which will be useful for the work of all laboratories."[99] He considered it his duty to establish a constant dialogue with the other actors. Manfred Donike also undertook the responsibility to inform all heads of laboratories directly about inconsistencies of doping controls. In 1987,

---

[94] Minutes, "Meeting of the IOC Medical Commission, February 24-26, 1987," 4.

[95] Minutes, "92nd Session of the IOC in Istanbul, May 9-12, 1987", archive collection "IOC Sessions 1894-2009," IOC Archive, Lausanne, Annex 9.

[96] Minutes, "Meetings of the IOC Medical Commission, February 9-28, 1988," 2.

[97] Professor Dr. Hans Skaset (born 1935) was a professor at the Norwegian School of Sport Sciences from 1975 to 1991. He was the chair of the Norwegian Athletics Federation from 1976 to 1983 and president of the Norwegian Confederation of Sports from 1984 to 1990. In 1991, he became member of the IOC Medical Commission to represent national governing bodies on the IOC Medical Commission's Subcommission for Out-Of Competition Testing. INTERNATIONAL OLYMPIC COMMITTEE, *Commission Médicale*, 41f.

[98] Minutes, "Meeting of the European Sports Conference Working Group on Effective Anti-Doping Measures, November 16 and 17, 1987," archive collection "Nachlass August Kirsch," File 098, "Doping (4)," CuLDA, Cologne, 3.

[99] Letter, "Manfred Donike to Don Catlin, February 2, 1986," Private Archive Don H. Catlin, Los Angeles.

suspicions about manipulated urine samples arose.[100] Whereas the laboratory in London only suspected that five to six athletes had used diuretics, Manfred Donike explained that the urine contained probenecide to cover up the usage of the banned substance.[101] He immediately informed all accredited anti-doping laboratories about the incident and requested them to check samples for probenecid.[102] This enabled the IOC MSD to act swiftly and to add probenecid immediately to the list of banned substances at the end of 1987.[103]

Besides the Cologne Workshop, the anti-doping laboratory experts planned additional educational initiatives. During an IAAF Doping Subcommittee meeting, Manfred Donike proposed the organisation of an IAAF seminar on doping control for 1986.[104] In view of the technical problems that were arising in several laboratories, but also during the sampling procedures, he maintained that the IAAF needed to show more interest in the teaching of technical/IAAF personnel about the doping control procedures. The IAAF eventually merged the seminar with the third IAAF Medical Congress into the "International Athletic Foundation World Symposium on Doping in Sport," held in Florence in May 1987.[105] Whilst doping was still the only topic discussed at the congress, Manfred Donike complained vehemently about the fact that the event had developed into a scientific conference, which, so he argued, "was not the original principle for organising such a conference."[106] According to him, such a setting did not allow for the appropriate training of laboratories anymore. Having been successful in revealing the difference between the unlike domains of anti-doping laboratory experts and medical experts, he thought there was potential risk to mix the two fields again. He suspected that Arne Ljungqvist had changed the original plan, because he wanted to attract a bigger audience.[107]

[100] Letter, "Manfred Donike to August Kirsch, June 25, 1987," archive collection "Nachlass August Kirsch," File 098, "Doping (4)," CuLDA, Cologne.
[101] Letter, "Manfred Donike to all accredited laboratories, June 22, 1987," Private Archive Don H. Catlin, Los Angeles.
[102] Ibid.
[103] Minutes, "Meeting of the IOC Medical Commission's Subcommission on Doping and Biochemistry, September 28 and 29, 1987," 8.
[104] Letter, "Manfred Donike to August Kirsch, April 4, 1986," archive collection "Nachlass August Kirsch," File 087, "Doping (3)," CuLDA, Cologne, 3.
[105] Minutes, "Meeting of the IAAF Medical Committee, August 20, 1986," archive collection "Nachlass August Kirsch," File 012, "IAAF 1982-1987," CuLDA, Cologne, 4.
[106] Letter, "Manfred Donike to August Kirsch, July 21, 1987," archive collection "Nachlass August Kirsch," File 098, "Doping (4)," CuLDA, Cologne, 2.
[107] Letter, "Manfred Donike to August Kirsch, January 26, 1987".

Finally, the growing institutional network and intensifying political dimension within the work of the anti-doping laboratory experts also resulted in disturbances amongst its key figures. The criticism focused specifically on Manfred Donike, whose attempts to control the network rigorously caused tensions. Whereas previously the disputes between Manfred Donike and Arnold Beckett had been of a technical nature (see Chapter 6), they discussed more procedural and personal matters in a written exchange in March 1987. Arnold Beckett prompted this through a letter to the chief medical officer of the 1988 Winter Olympic Games in Calgary, Professor Dr. Bruce Challis[108], a medical doctor.[109] Therein, Arnold Beckett commented on the state of the laboratory in Calgary, addressing issues such as the available apparatus, personnel and the status of the accreditation, which he had also done with doping laboratories at previous Olympic Games. However, the correspondence brought Manfred Donike into the arena, who felt overlooked and who heavily criticised Arnold Beckett for his manner of proceedings. He stressed that he and Robert Dugal should have been informed.[110] Manfred Donike also took the opportunity to remind Arnold Beckett that he had instigated the RI method for the 1980 Moscow Olympic Games and had wanted to use it in Los Angeles. Manfred Donike stressed, "even today one year before the 1988 the next Olympic Year, I see no RI method."[111] Hence, Manfred Donike blamed Arnold Beckett for thwarting the work of the IOC Medical Commission, reasoning that he was, "not willing to cooperate with the other members of the subcommission because you [Arnold Beckett] are counteracting our moves to implement a high standard of the IOC accredited laboratories."[112] Besides rejecting all claims made by Manfred Donike (especially that he was counteracting the work of the IOC Medical Commission), Arnold

---

[108] Professor Dr. Bruce Challis (born 1930) graduated as medical doctor from the University of Toronto in 1956. Following employment at several Canadian universities, he became professor and head of the Department of Family Medicine at the University in Calgary in 1981. Email, Bruce Challis to Jörg Krieger, March 7, 2015.

[109] Letter, "Arnold Beckett to Bruce Challis, March 4, 1987," archive collection "Summer and Winter Olympic Games: Medical Files," folder "Medical matters (laboratory) at the 1988 Calgary Winter Olympic Games: correspondence and report," IOC Archive, Lausanne.

[110] Letter, "Manfred Donike to Arnold Beckett, March 17, 1987," archive collection "Summer and Winter Olympic Games: Medical Files," folder "Medical matters (laboratory) at the 1988 Calgary Winter Olympic Games: correspondence and report," IOC Archive, Lausanne.

[111] Ibid.

[112] Ibid.

Beckett accused him of not accepting the opinion of others and of having a too narrow a perspective on anti-doping matters to maintain his leading position within the anti-doping network:

> What I attempt to do is to get balance and scientific credibility in the application of methods and the treatment of problems. You are well aware that there are many problems facing us which will not be solved if you adhere to your blinkered approach to the applications of science to biological problems.
>
> As you will be aware from the contents of my letter, I am very annoyed indeed. You seem to operate as though no other than your point of view is correct. For the last twenty years I have been dealing with scientists whose experience is much broader than those involved in dope control. (…) I think my work has given me the advantage of keeping matters in perspective using flexibility and ability to accept new approaches and new ideas. (…)
>
> My final point is that dope control is one aspect of our approach to prevent the misuse of drugs in sport. Please realise that the function of the testing is deterrence. Please do not let one aspect of the work obscure what is the approach to the total problem. Do not become a scientist for which it could be said 'he could not see the wood for the trees'.[113]

The written exchange exemplifies the development of the perception of Manfred Donike as powerful leader of the network since his appointment as head of the IOC MSD in 1981. Certainly, Arnold Beckett, who had been the main consultant of sports organisations until the beginning of the 1980s, must have felt particularly offended by this process. Don Catlin confirmed such conflicts for the set-up of the Cologne Workshop:

> A complicated issue arose for a few years. Some people felt that Cologne had too much power in the whole business and they stopped supporting the Cologne meeting. (…) They felt that Manfred was too controlling. He controlled the entire agenda, which was true, and only

---

[113] Letter, "Arnold Beckett to Manfred Donike, March 23, 1987," archive collection "Summer and Winter Olympic Games: Medical Files," folder "Medical matters (laboratory) at the 1988 Calgary Winter Olympic Games: correspondence and report," IOC Archive, Lausanne.

his own people could speak and others couldn't speak. (...) He even required abstracts, read them and presented the work as his. (...) Probably 1986, 1987, there was a discussion doing away with the Cologne Workshop because it was Cologne. We wanted a place for everybody to meet but we wanted a different city or to rotate, which the Prince wanted. But there were certain advantages to Cologne and in the final analysis, it remained the Cologne Workshop.[114]

To conclude, under Manfred Donike's strong influence, the IOC MSD continued to increase its efforts in quality assurance and improvement. After the intensive period of the establishment of an anti-doping laboratory network, more institutions were added to the network. Together with the improved testing techniques for an increasing number of performance-enhancing substances, this resulted in the application of more doping tests worldwide. Due to the introduced measures for quality control, the anti-doping laboratory experts believed that their testing results were also more reliable. However, with the rising number of institutions and laboratory staff involved, the challenges for the key figures also rose considerably, resulting in internal conflicts.

Integration of Anti-Doping Laboratory Experts in Supranational Meetings

After the 1988 Seoul Olympic Games, governments began to adopt a more active role in the fight against doping, and increased their initiatives mainly through bilateral, multilateral and supranational contexts.[115] There was an increase in the number of international forums to discuss doping policy at the end of the 1980s and the beginning of the 1990s.[116] However, it is important to note that individual attempts to harmonise anti-doping efforts had already commenced prior to the Seoul Olympic Games. Anti-doping laboratory experts assisted these efforts.

Most notably, this accounts for initiatives to organise a world conference on doping control, first attempted during the 1988 Winter Olympic Games in Calgary in February 1988. Representatives of several countries and organisations held a meeting, with the goal of organising a world conference on doping

---

[114] Interview with Don H. Catlin, November 12, 2012.

[115] KRÜGER et al., Doping und Anti-Doping, 149.

[116] HOULIHAN, Dying, 177.

control.[117] The initiative followed the appeal of the "36th Meeting of Leaders of Sports Organisations in Socialist Countries" and activities by the European Sports Conference.[118] The participants of the meeting agreed that the objective of the conference would be to adopt an international anti-doping charter. Significantly, besides Alexandre de Mérode, Manfred Donike represented the IOC in his function as head of the IOC MSD.[119] Thus, anti-doping laboratory experts had a strong voice in the early stages of this important international political forum, particularly because Arnold Beckett, Don Catlin and Robert Dugal participated as national representatives as well. They were regarded as essential, because the doping control system could not function without their contribution, based on their competencies in doping analysis, any longer.

It would go beyond the scope of this paper to address in detail the outcomes of the First Permanent Anti-Doping Conference, eventually staged in Ottawa from June 26 to June 29, 1988.[120] However, the basic result, of enforcing the introduction of out-of competition controls, favoured the anti-doping laboratory experts. Furthermore, the importance of the IOC accredited doping laboratories was mentioned in the final declaration and the "International Olympic Charter Against Doping in Sport," published by the IOC in November 1988. [121] Importantly, the document encouraged governments to invest into anti-doping laboratories, while the recognition of the laboratories stayed with the IOC MSD. The document confirmed the IOC MSD´s influential role as controlling body over the accreditation procedure, and emphasised the role of the anti-doping laboratory experts in the global doping control system. Point 24 lists the approved laboratories, stating, "sports organisations should make full and efficient use of

---

[117] Letter, "Lyle Makosky to Alexandre de Mérode, March 16, 1988," archive collection "IOC Medical Commission," folder "Correspondence on 1st World Anti-Doping Conference in Sport," IOC Archive, Lausanne.

[118] Press Release, "VIII European Sports Conference – Athens '87," archive collection "Nachlass August Kirsch," File 098, "Doping (4)," CuLDA, Cologne.

[119] Letter, "Lyle Makosky to Alexandre de Mérode, March 16, 1988."

[120] Final Report, "First permanent world conference on antidoping in sports," archive collection "IOC Medical Commission," folder "Correspondence on 1st World Anti-Doping Conference in Sport," IOC Archive, Lausanne.

[121] The Charter was ratified by UNESCO´s Conference of Sports Ministers in Moscow in November 1988. "International Olympic Charter Against Doping in Sport," *Olympic Review* 253 (1988), 628-631. For the remarks on the anti-doping laboratories, see page 630.

the IOC accredited laboratories."[122] Moreover, due to the importance given to the doping laboratories in the entire doping control process, Manfred Donike and Don Catlin attended an informal meeting of the Working Group on the International Anti-Doping Charter (IWG), which evolved from the Ottawa Conference. They became members of the IWG in November 1988.[123] Hence, the two got the possibility to represent the interests of the anti-doping laboratory network.

Within this context, one has to stress that Manfred Donike had already become involved in continental working groups and forums on anti-doping from the mid-1980s onwards. This enabled him to emphasise the significance of doping analysis, to strengthen the position of the IOC MSD and to assure his own position as the leading expert in doping analysis within the international political arena. In 1983, Manfred Donike was still somewhat sceptical towards his duties in a multinational working group that aimed for the standardisation of doping regulations within Europe, along with general anti-doping standards.[124] At the time, so he wrote in a letter to the FRG′s Ministry of the Interior, the Cologne laboratory through his involvement in the IOC and the IAAF had coordinated all efforts concerning the harmonisation of analytical procedures and the accreditation of laboratories.[125] This is an indication for his self-perception as central figure for international anti-doping activities. Nevertheless, he regarded an immediate resolution necessary so that other doping control centres could adjust to the requirements of the IAAF and the IOC. However, the initiative only led to a very general "European Anti-Doping Charter for Sport" in 1984.[126]

Due to the developments, which progressively led him to face more administrative and sport political challenges, he had realised by the mid-1980s that his contribution was necessary to ensure that the IOC MSD would keep control over the laboratory accreditation process and the regulation over analytical methods. For example, during a meeting of the "Working Group on Effective Anti-Doping Measures" at the European Sports Conference (he became

---

[122] Final Declaration, "First permanent world conference on antidoping in sports, June 1988," archive collection "Nachlass August Kirsch," File 088, "Doping (5)," CuLDA, Cologne, 6.

[123] Letter, "Proposed agenda; paper on International Anti-Doping Charter advancement strategy; index page of Charter Annexes, Lyle Makosky to Manfred Donike, n.d.," archive collection "Nachlass August Kirsch," File 088, "Doping (5)," CuLDA, Cologne.

[124] Letter, "Manfred Donike to German Ministry of the Interior, October 10, 1983," archive collection "Nachlass August Kirsch," File 086, "Doping (2)," CuLDA, Cologne.

[125] Ibid.

[126] HOULIHAN, *Dying*, 158.

a member in 1985), pushed for an increase of the analytical capacities of the doping laboratories.[127] He explained that fewer laboratories with a higher capacity were more useful than an inflation of official institutions that could not produce high-quality analytical results. Moreover, he also continuously defended the high IOC standards for laboratories and the work of the IOC MSD in the accreditation process, outlining that other initiatives should not influence their work.[128] This gives the impression that he became increasingly aware of the climatic interest of governments and intergovernmental organisations in anti-doping matters, while sensing that it was crucial to represent the interest of the doping laboratories in the discussions. Ultimately, it also enabled him to contribute to the *Explanatory Report on the Anti-Doping Convention*, adopted in 1989.[129] Therein, a specific section was attributed to the work and importance of the anti-doping laboratories. Whilst acknowledging the work of the IOC Medical Commission, the report reads that laboratories do not only conduct doping tests but also put considerable effort into research and the publication of it:

> The creation of doping control laboratories is an essential part of a coherent anti-doping strategy (see paragraphs 8, 10, 14, 16, 17 and 28 above). Their complexity is such that, in the vast majority of cases, such laboratories will be attached to an institution benefiting from public funds (hospital, university, etc.). A number of elements for the recognition of doping laboratories are relevant, in particular the criteria established by the International Olympic Committee. Their criteria are followed by virtually all sports organisations. It is their criteria, which the Monitoring Group will examine and approve. Research is an essential part of such laboratories' work (see paragraph 10) and should be incorporated in their assignment and taken into account in staff allocation. The rapid publication of research results is important: publication is a criterion for scientific consideration and for the divulgation of new techniques and/or discoveries, whether relating to analysis or to new doping methods. The development of new detection

---

[127] Letter, "Manfred Donike to August Kirsch, July 21, 1987," 6.

[128] Letter, "Manfred Donike to Hans Hansen, July 21, 1988," archive collection "Nachlass August Kirsch," File 088, "Doping (5)," CuLDA, Cologne.

[129] COUNCIL OF EUROPE, *Explanatory Report on the Anti-Doping Convention* (Strasbourg. Council of Europe, 1990).

methods should be made operational and applied in all laboratories as soon as possible.[130]

Manfred Donike also reiterated the significance of the doping laboratories and the need for governmental investment on the anti-doping seminar "Out-of-competition testing," that the Working Group on Effective Anti-Doping Measures organised in Borlänge (Sweden) at the end of 1988. At the seminar, he urged for the installation of out-of competition controls to detect the usage of anabolic steroid on a global scale.[131] Finally, the report of the Working Group on Effective Anti-Doping Measures to the European Sports Conference proposes an increase in the quality standards of the European anti-doping laboratories. It foresaw an annual update of laboratory staff members on technical and organisational matters in close cooperation with the members of the IOC MSD.[132] Hence, ensuring high-quality standards was an important outcome of these efforts as it confirmed the IOC MSD´s approach after the establishment of its anti-doping laboratory network.

Whilst all these activities concerned the a European framework, the IWG, including Manfred Donike and Don Catlin, continued its efforts to harmonise global anti-doping efforts and to implement the recommendations of the First Permanent Anti-Doping Conference. The IWG developed an organigram for a worldwide doping control system to coordinate the proposed global out-of competition tests, whilst trying to be consistent with the existing sport and anti-doping structures.[133] This proposal intended the installation of an International Olympic Anti-Doping Committee (IAODC) to determine the overall anti-doping policy, and to establish a strategy for its implementation. It therefore also reacted to the appeal of the "37th Meeting of Leaders of Sports Organisations in Socialist Countries," who requested the IOC to set up an international doping control

---

[130] Ibid., 22.
[131] EUROPEAN SPORTS CONFERENCE, WORKING GROUP ON EFFECTIVE ANTI-DOPING MEASURES, *Final report Anti-doping Seminar, 30 October - 2 November, Borlänge, Sweden* (Borlänge, 1988), 44.
[132] Report, "ESC, October 2-7, 1989," archive collection "Nachlass August Kirsch," File 089, "Doping (6)," CuLDA, Cologne, 8.
[133] Report, "Worldwide Doping Control System, by Manfred Donike, August 26, 1989," archive collection "Nachlass August Kirsch," File 089, "Doping (6)," CuLDA, Cologne, 5-7.

committee.[134] The IWG´s plans for the IAODC anticipated a constitution of representatives of the IOC Medical Commission, the IFs and a representative of the IOC Athletes´ Commission. The IOC-dominated structure reveals that Alexandre de Mérode led the meetings and attempted to retain control over the developments. He wanted to situate the IAODC very close to the IOC Medical Commission and proposed that it should become a subcommission, which would deal only with the execution of out-of competition controls.[135] Besides these important political and organisational considerations, the IOC accredited laboratories also occupied a central role within the suggested chains of command and report.[136] Whilst all three organisational levels – IOADC, IFs and NOCs or governments – could have their own sample collection teams at designated events, they had to send them to the IOC official laboratories. These laboratories would continue to undertake all global doping analysis but would report their analytical results to the corresponding authority *and* to the IOADC.[137] However, in opposition to the concrete proposals for the establishment of an international anti-doping body, only the seven annexes of the "International Olympic Charter Against Doping in Sport" were adopted at the "Second Permanent World Conference," held in Moscow in October 1989. The participants did not achieve a concrete implementation of the suggestions at this time.

Notwithstanding the dissatisfying results of the first attempts to harmonise international anti-doping rules – which were in fact only achieved through the foundation of WADA in 1999 – a very distinctive behaviour of the anti-doping laboratory experts in general and the IOC MSD in particular, can be identified. During the beginning of the phase of increasing multinational and intergovernmental involvement in international anti-doping politics, anti-doping laboratory experts were already contributing to the political processes in various working groups. Although their degree of participation was somewhat limited, it enabled them to emphasise the necessity for high-quality doping laboratories. The inclusion of the laboratories in almost all policy statements demonstrates that they were successful with this strategy. Their professional expertise was necessary for

---

[134] Press Release, "Appeal of the 37th Budapest Conference of Heads of Sports Organisations of Socialist Countries to set up an International Doping Control Committee, November 11, 1988," archive collection "Nachlass August Kirsch," File 088, "Doping (5)," CuLDA, Cologne.

[135] Minutes, "95th Session of the IOC in Puerto Rico, August 30 – September 1, 1989," archive collection "IOC Sessions 1894-2009," IOC Archive, Lausanne, 11 and Annex 9.

[136] Report, "Worldwide Doping Control System, by Manfred Donike, August 26, 1989," 5-7.

[137] Ibid., 4.

the execution of the doping control system in place. Unsurprisingly, the anti-doping laboratory experts welcomed the initiatives for more out-of competition controls as it strengthened their institutions´ raison d´être. Internally, the individuals made no secret of this strategy either, addressing the need to stress the importance of doping laboratories even more. This becomes most obvious in the remarks during a doping symposium ahead of the 1988 Seoul Olympic Games. The doping control laboratory in Seoul, in collaboration with Manfred Donike, had organised this symposium. Mainly members of the IOC Medical Commission attended the event. In their joint paper, Robert DUGAL and Manfred DONIKE welcomed the political processes as long as the laboratories could maintain high technical standards. For this, they demanded more financial support:

> These extremely positive developments in the political arena must however be accompanied by a parallel evolution of the scientific requirements for doping control analyses and by the definition of the highest scientific and technical standards that can be achieved by the use of currently available technology. (...) The strengthening of the criteria for IOC accreditation of laboratories in order to achieve greater analytical equivalence amongst laboratories constitutes a major improvement. It should not be forgotten that the competence of the doping control laboratories is at the very centre of an effective deterrence programme.[138]

One can amplify HUNT´s remarks that Alexandre de Mérode specifically envisaged and ensured that "the IOC would remain in command of the new anti-doping commission." as a result of the political processes at the end of the 1980s.[139] There is no doubt that the politically strategic intentions of Alexandre de Mérode provided for a centralisation of all anti-doping matters around the IOC. Significantly, for the anti-doping laboratory experts, the responsible body for the doping laboratories remained the IOC MSD. This investigation discloses that the leading anti-doping laboratory experts were also very active in their approach to remain relevant themselves. Thereby, they attempted to demonstrate that following the establishments of main procedures such as testing techniques, an

---

[138] Robert DUGAL and Manfred DONIKE, "International Olympic Committee Requirements for Laboratory Accreditation and Good Laboratory Practices," in: *Proceedings of the International Symposium on Drug Abuse in Sports (Doping)*, ed. Jong Sei PARK (Seoul: KAIST, 1988), 86.

[139] HUNT, *Drug Games*, 85.

anti-doping laboratory network, guidelines for laboratory work and educational initiatives, the focus had to be on an increase in scientific quality and reliability. As a result, individuals such as Manfred Donike as head of the IOC MSD became even more involved with administrative and political processes during this period. The IOC MSD was successful in its attempt to increase the number of doping controls drastically in this period. From 1986 until 1988, the number of analysed samples in IOC-accredited anti-doping laboratories increased from 32,982 samples to 47,069 samples.[140] Hence, the efforts of the IOC MSD resulted in the establishment of more doping controls overall.

THE ROLE AND PERCEPTION OF THE ANTI-DOPING LABORATORY EXPERTS AT THE 1988 OLYMPIC GAMES

It has been emphasised that in the period leading up to the 1988 Olympic Games, the phase of dominating institutional and individual positions of already established key figures continued. With the network of anti-doping laboratories progressively expanding, they pursued the strategy of increased quality control. Manfred Donike was the main advocate behind the installation of total quality management. Hence, he did not refrain from "controlling the controllers," as he argued in retrospect of the flaws in the doping analysis at the 1987 World Athletics Championships.[141] It is notable that the anti-doping laboratory experts occupied their leading roles prior to the positive doping test of Ben Johnson at the 1988 Seoul Olympic Games, which is today defined as the watershed of global anti-doping, because it alerted the public about the doping problem in sport and resulted in world-wide anti-doping measures.[142] It is important to investigate their role in the preparation, as well as during the doping controls for the 1988 Olympic Games, beginning with the 1988 Winter Olympic Games in Calgary.

---

[140] DUBIN, *Commission of Inquiry*, 398.

[141] Manfred Donike in "Anti-Doping Kampf: Kontrolle für Kontrolleure," *SID*, January 26, 1988, archive collection "Nachlass August Kirsch," File 088, "Doping (5)," CuLDA, Cologne.

[142] HOULIHAN, *Dying*, 150.

Troubled Preparation of Doping Controls at the 1988 Winter Olympic Games in Calgary

In August 1982, the Organising Committee of the 1988 Winter Olympic Games in Calgary (OCO `88) appointed Bruce Challis as chief medical officer,[143] and the IOC Medical Commission made him a temporary member in October 1982.[144] OCO `88 wanted to install the anti-doping laboratory for the Olympic Games at the Department of Laboratory Medicine at the Calgary Foothills Hospital under the leadership of scientific director Dr. Siu Chan and managing director Dr. Robert Baynton. The latter was the direct contact for the IOC MSD concerning for issues the doping analysis. However, in contrast to other laboratory representatives such as Don Catlin, he did not participate in official meetings. In December 1987, the IOC Medical Commission officially accredited the laboratory.[145]

In total, the laboratory staff used fourteen chromatographic systems during the Olympic Games.[146] There were technological advancements with the GC-MS methods. For example, whereas in 1984 in Los Angeles, most GC-MS analyses were still being performed with packed columns, all GC-MS analyses in Calgary were performed with capillary columns.[147] Moreover, the laboratory tested for beta-blockers, diuretics, probenecide, cannabinoids, corticosteroids and hCG for the very first time. One has to attribute these advancements to the efforts of the anti-doping laboratory experts following the 1984 Olympic Games. However, from the 424 samples taken, there was only one positive finding: the urine of the Polish ice-hockey player Jarosław Morawiecki displayed testosterone usage after

---

[143] "XV Olympic Winter Games. Inventory of the Records of the Operations Group, Part III,"   *City   of   Calgary*;   http://www.calgary.ca/CA/city-clerks/Documents/88olympics/operation_inventory_pt3.pdf?noredirect=1 [accessed July 13, 2014], 388.

[144] Fax, "Monique Berlioux to John Pickett, October 5, 1982," archive collection "Summer and Winter Olympic Games: Medical Files," folder "Medical matters (laboratory) at the 1988 Calgary Winter Olympic Games: correspondence and report," IOC Archive, Lausanne.

[145] Letter, "Claus Clausnitzer to Alexandre de Mérode, November 3, 1987," archive collection "Summer and Winter Olympic Games: Medical Files," folder "Medical matters (laboratory) at the 1988 Calgary Winter Olympic Games: correspondence and report," IOC Archive, Lausanne.

[146] Siu C. CHAN, George A. TOROK-BOTH, Debbie M. BILLAY, Peter S. PRZYBYISKI, Claire Y. GRADEEN, Kathleen M. PAP and Jitka PETRUZELKA, "Drug Analysis at the 1988 Olympic Winter Games in Calgary," *Clinical Chemistry* 37, no. 7 (1991), 1296.

[147] Ibid.

a match against France.[148] Clearly, only one positive doping test demonstrated that doping controls were not as efficient as the anti-doping laboratory experts had hoped.

A particularly precarious situation arose ahead of the Olympic Games because there was already an official anti-doping laboratory in Canada at the INRS. In fact, when accrediting the anti-doping laboratory in Calgary, the IOC MSD had recommended that it should request additional assistance of another IOC-accredited laboratory for the time of the Olympic Games, in order to ensure the necessary capacity for that period.[149] One has to consider this another attempt to raise the quality of the doping controls but also to involve an IOC MSD member more actively. Alexandre de Mérode made clear that according to him, it was logical that this support should come from the INRS and Robert Dugal.[150] Notwithstanding, it is evident from written exchanges between Bruce Challis, Robert Baynton and Robert Dugal that the latter had an interest not only to become involved in the laboratory work but also to take on considerably more responsibility. Once approached by Robert Baynton about possible assistance by four staff members from the INRS, Robert Dugal showed interest, but suggested the support of six staff members and more involvement of the personnel than was originally intended by OCO `88.[151] The Calgary laboratory perceived this reply as an intervention into its own plans, and assumed that exertion of influence through the INRS would leave the Calgary laboratory with little credibility after the Games.[152] Robert Baynton suspected that Robert Dugal wanted to prevent the long-term establishment of another official anti-doping laboratory in Canada,

[148] "The Best Organization," *Olympic Review* 45 (1988), 103.

[149] Fax, "Alexandre de Mérode to Sir Arthur Gold, January 17, 1988," archive collection "Summer and Winter Olympic Games: Medical Files," folder "Medical matters (laboratory) at the 1988 Calgary Winter Olympic Games: correspondence and report," IOC Archive, Lausanne.

[150] Ibid.

[151] Letter, "Robert Dugal to Bruce Challis, January 28, 1988," archive collection "Summer and Winter Olympic Games: Medical Files," folder "Medical matters (laboratory) at the 1988 Calgary Winter Olympic Games: correspondence and report," IOC Archive, Lausanne.

[152] "Olympic call for King's," *The Times*, January 15, 1988, archive collection "Summer and Winter Olympic Games: Medical Files," folder "Medical matters (laboratory) at the 1988 Calgary Winter Olympic Games: correspondence and report," IOC Archive, Lausanne.

thereby strengthening the position of his own institution.[153] Hence, OCO '88 looked elsewhere for the recommended support and approached the anti-doping laboratories in London and Los Angeles. Heavily interested in becoming involved in the doping tests of the Olympic Games themselves, both institutions agreed to provide four anti-doping laboratory technicians.[154] Don Catlin and David Cowan would act as senior consultants to Siu Chan, the head of the anti-doping laboratory, for one week each.[155] They reached this agreement without official consultation of the IOC MSD. Indeed, Raymond Baynton only informed Alexandre de Mérode and stated that both accredited laboratories were, "extremely compatible, not only with each other but with the staff of the Foothills Control Laboratory. They have actively collaborated in research as well as exchange of personnel during the past few years." [156] However, British sport officials were hesitant about a potential involvement of the KCL, because they were concerned that it would become inadvertently involved in the quarrel between Montreal and Calgary.[157] Significantly, whereas Alexandre de Mérode hoped the IOC Medical Commission could not be involved in such an internal problem, [158] Manfred Donike favoured Robert Dugal's proposal because it anticipated the involvement of Professor Dr. Robert Massé. He had been associate director of the INRS-led laboratories at the 1976 Montreal Olympic Games and at the 1980 Winter Olympic Games in Lake Placid, and had therefore experience in conducting doping analysis at Olympic Games. Ultimately, Manfred Donike's pressure – again displaying the necessity to arrange the best possible conditions for reliable analytical results – caused OCO '88 to back down, and it was agreed on a compromise to include five staff members from the

---

[153] Letter, "Robert Baynton to Alexandre de Mérode, January 18, 1988," archive collection "Summer and Winter Olympic Games: Medical Files," folder "Medical matters (laboratory) at the 1988 Calgary Winter Olympic Games: correspondence and report," IOC Archive, Lausanne

[154] Ibid.

[155] Ibid.

[156] Letter, "Robert Baynton to Alexandre de Mérode, January 28, 1988," archive collection "Summer and Winter Olympic Games: Medical Files," folder "Medical matters (laboratory) at the 1988 Calgary Winter Olympic Games: correspondence and report," IOC Archive, Lausanne.

[157] Letter, "Michele Verroken, on behalf of Sir Arthur Gold, to Alexandre de Mérode, January 15, 1988," archive collection "Summer and Winter Olympic Games: Medical Files," folder "Medical matters (laboratory) at the 1988 Calgary Winter Olympic Games: correspondence and report," IOC Archive, Lausanne.

[158] Fax, "Alexandre de Mérode to Sir Arthur Gold, January 17, 1988."

INRS laboratory.[159] As a result, OCO´88 annulled the agreements with the UCLA and the KCL.

The conflict of interest gives additional evidence to the dominant role of the anti-doping laboratory experts in 1988. It has already been addressed that the experts had undertaken several initiatives in order to maintain control over their expanding network, and Robert Dugal´s attempt to gain control over the anti-doping laboratory in Calgary is no exception. On the contrary, it proves that such dominant figures as Manfred Donike, Arnold Beckett and Robert Dugal did not refrain from pursuing individual interests whilst dealing with global anti-doping matters.

Doping Controls at the 1988 Seoul Olympic Games

Preparations

In 1982, the Organising Committee of the 1988 Seoul Olympic Games (SLOOC) appointed Dr. Ki Ho Kim as member to the IOC Medical Commission.[160] He had been the team doctor of the Korean Olympic team at the 1972 and 1976 Olympic Games and acted as head of the SLOOC Medical Advisory Commission.[161] In his role as co-opted member of the IOC Medical Commission, he had observed the health services and the work at the anti-doping laboratory during both 1984 Olympic Games. However, for the first time in the history of Olympic doping controls, there was a change in the representative of the OCOG on the IOC Medical Commission. From December 1986 onwards, Dr. Byung Ryun Cho

---

[159] Letter, "Robert Baynton to Alexandre de Mérode, January 31, 1988," archive collection "Summer and Winter Olympic Games: Medical Files," folder "Medical matters (laboratory) at the 1988 Calgary Winter Olympic Games: correspondence and report," IOC Archive, Lausanne.

[160] Fax, "Yong Shik Kim to Juan Antonio Samaranch, March 9, 1982," archive collection "Summer and Winter Olympic Games: Medical files," folder "Medical matters and doping controls at the 1988 Seoul Summer Olympic Games: correspondence," IOC Archive, Lausanne.

[161] Letter, "Sang Ho Cho to Juan Antonio Samaranch, January 17, 1984," archive collection "Summer and Winter Olympic Games: Medical files," folder "Medical matters and doping controls at the 1988 Seoul Summer Olympic Games: correspondence," IOC Archive, Lausanne.

replaced Ki Ho Kim because the latter one could not devote enough time to his work on the IOC Medical Commission.[162]

In terms of the anti-doping laboratory, the preparations appear to have been more straightforward than for the Winter Olympic Games in the same year. In particular, the arrangements for the establishment of the laboratory started considerably earlier, which one can contribute to the 1986 Asian Games, held in Seoul. In fact, it was the first time that the Olympic Council of Asia (OCA) undertook official doping controls at any Asian Games.[163] For that reason, the Korean authorities founded a doping control centre in the Korea Institute of Science and Technology (한국과학기술연구원, KIST),[164] a multi-disciplinary research institute in Seoul, in April 1984.[165] Dr. Moon Hi Han[166] headed the centre. The Korean Ministry of Science and Technology, SLOOC and KIST agreed that the government financed the basic costs for research, acquisition of all technical equipment and the training of the laboratory staff.[167] After the establishment, SLOOC was responsible for the payment of the analytical equipment from 1986 onwards. In contrast to most previous Olympic Games, the anti-doping laboratory was not based within a university setting, but the strong governmental support enabled the laboratory staff to undertake a lot of research prior to the Olympic Games, too. This resulted in the publication of numerous scientific articles on GC-MS methods in the *Journal of Analytical Toxicology* in 1990.[168]

---

[162] Letter, "Seh Jik Park to Alexandre de Mérode, December 2, 1986," archive collection "Summer and Winter Olympic Games: Medical files," folder "Medical matters and doping controls at the 1988 Seoul Summer Olympic Games: correspondence," IOC Archive, Lausanne.

[163] Jong Sei PARK, Song Ja PARK, Dong Suk LHO, HP CHOO, Bong Chull CHUNG, Chang No YOON, Hong Gi MIN and MJ CHOI, "Drug testing at the 10th Asian Games and 24th Seoul Olympic Games," *Journal of Analytical Toxicology* 14, no. 2 (1991), 66-72.

[164] KIST was founded in 1966 but between 1981 and 1989, the institution was known as Korea Advanced Institute of Science and Technology. Consequently, the official documents of the doping laboratory at the 1988 Seoul Olympic Games all use the abbreviation KAIST. For reasons of simplicity, only the abbreviation KIST is used in this book.

[165] ORGANISING COMMITTEE OF THE GAMES OF THE XXIII TH OLYMPIAD, *Official Report of the 1988 Olympic Games in Seoul,* Volume 1, Part 3 (Seoul: Organising Committee of the Games of the XXIII th Olympiad, 1988), 786.

[166] Dr. Moon Hi Han (born 1932) was Head of the Doping Control Centre from 1985 until 1988. Following the Olympic Games, he was replaced with Jong Sei Park.

[167] Ibid.

[168] A listing of the most relevant papers can be found in: HEMMERSBACH, "History," 843.

Furthermore, the KIST laboratory cooperated very closely with the Cologne anti-doping laboratory from the first approach onwards. In fact, staff members from Cologne had already supported the KIST laboratory during the 1986 Asian Games and Manfred Donike had reported positively about the laboratory work, arguing, "no major problem from the sight of the current status should be expected for the Olympics."[169] Nevertheless, the supervision and support through the Cologne laboratory did not take place by official appointment by the IOC MSD but rather as an appointment of Manfred Donike as advisor to the Organising Committee of the Asian Games on a personal basis.[170] The close link allowed Manfred Donike to control considerable parts of the laboratory preparations and clearly, his instructions made a big impact. In fact, SLOOC had already acquired all necessary analytical equipment before the Asian Games, so it had only supplementary purchases to make in order to deal with the greater number of samples.[171] Moreover, it is important to note that the head of the KIST laboratory, Dr. Jong Sei Park, was already in charge during the 1986 Asian Games and continued in his position for the Olympic Games. Similar to the other heads of anti-doping laboratories, he had a background in chemistry.[172] He had spent most of his professional career in the USA, but he returned to the Republic of Korea following his appointment as head of the KIST laboratory in 1986.[173] He was responsible for the extensive research on the GC-MS, and thus accepted by

---

[169] Minutes, "Meeting of the IOC Medical Commission's Subcommission Doping and Biochemistry of Sport, November 12 and 13, 1986," Annex 5.

[170] Letter, "Alexandre de Mérode to Young Jin Om, July 26, 1985," archive collection "Summer and Winter Olympic Games: Medical files," folder "Medical matters and doping controls at the 1988 Seoul Summer Olympic Games: correspondence," IOC Archive, Lausanne.

[171] 585 samples were collected at the 1986 Asian Games and it is reported that 3.2% contained a banned substance, offenders were sanctioned accordingly. Jong Sei PARK, "Doping test report of 10th Asian Games in Seoul," *Journal of Sports Medicine and Physical Fitness* 31, no. 2 (1991), 304. The exact numbers of analytical equipments used during the 1986 Asian Games and the 1988 Seoul Olympic Games can be found in Jong Sei Park's report on the doping controls. Report, "Review of the Seoul Laboratory Activities – Seoul Olympic Games 1988," by Jong Sei Park, May 18, 1988, archive collection "Summer and Winter Olympic Games: Medical files," folder "Medical matters and doping controls at the 1988 Seoul Summer Olympic Games: report on the medical facilities and services, services and list of the meetings of the medical commission and conference on the laboratory activities," IOC Archive, Lausanne.

[172] Jong Sei PARK, *A Study on Doping Control* (Gwacheon: Ministry of Science and Technology, 1992).

[173] Ibid.

the IOC MSD because he focused on traditional fields of doping analysis. Such research was necessary, because there was a rapid development of the mass spectrometers after the Los Angeles Olympic Games. Hence, despite no new major analytical procedures, this resulted in the installation of new types of mass-selective detectors.[174] Because of these processes, the KIST laboratory was in a very good position when it applied for official IOC accreditation in April 1987.[175] It underwent the accreditation procedure following the Asian Games in August 1987 under the supervision of Vitaly Semenov.[176] Remarkably, Manfred Donike appeared to be aware of possible accusations due to the close link of his own institution and the KIST laboratory. Hence, he sent 36 samples, instead of the required ten, to Seoul and left it to Vitaly Semenov to make the final choice.[177] This was an unusual procedure because usually Manfred Donike picked the ten samples and sent them directly to the laboratory. The KIST laboratory correctly detected and identified all of the samples. It received official accreditation in September 1987.[178] It made the institution only the third official doping control centre outside Europe and North America at that time.

In contrast to the unproblematic and uncharacteristic preparations of the anti-doping laboratory, considerable concerns arose regarding the general status of the medical services ahead of the Seoul Olympic Games. IOC Medical Commission member Ken Fitch, and Calgary medical representative Bruce Challis, reported these concerns following a visit to Seoul in spring 1988. The testified problems were mainly of organisational nature and included the communication system, the logistics of the transportation and the medical services supplied to training

---

[174] HEMMERSBACH, "History," 842.

[175] Letter, "Byung Ryun Cho to Alexandre de Mérode, April 16, 1987," archive collection "Summer and Winter Olympic Games: Medical files," folder "Medical matters and doping controls at the 1988 Seoul Summer Olympic Games: correspondence," IOC Archive, Lausanne.

[176] Letter, "Vitaly Semenov to Alexandre de Mérode, August 29, 1987," archive collection "Summer and Winter Olympic Games: Medical files," folder "Medical matters and doping controls at the 1988 Seoul Summer Olympic Games: correspondence," IOC Archive, Lausanne.

[177] Letter, "Manfred Donike to Vitaly Semenov, September 13, 1987," archive collection "Summer and Winter Olympic Games: Medical files," folder "Medical matters and doping controls at the 1988 Seoul Summer Olympic Games: correspondence," IOC Archive, Lausanne.

[178] Letter, "Alexandre de Mérode to Moon Hi Han, September 26, 1987," archive collection "Summer and Winter Olympic Games: Medical files," folder "Medical matters and doping controls at the 1988 Seoul Summer Olympic Games: correspondence," IOC Archive, Lausanne.

events. [179] Moreover, their treatment through Byung Ryun Cho dissatisfied them.[180] Whilst they acknowledged that the encountered problems were also a result of cultural differences, which they were not aware of, they suggested that most of the team doctors of the NOCs might be more critical. [181] Most importantly, in his recommendations to avoid such problems in the future, Ken Fitch concluded that there was a need to check the preparations of the medical services more vigorously ahead of Olympic Games. He voiced discontent with the high responsibility granted to the IOC MSD, and proposed that the entire IOC Medical Commission should deal with it accordingly:

> I know that I am fully supported by Bruce Challis when I suggest that visits such as we have just dertaken[sic] should be considered by IOC-MC to be mandatory for future Summer & Winter Games perhaps six months prior to the opening ceremony. Until now, only the anti-doping laboratory has been subject to such scrutiny. Perhaps it is time to rectify this imbalance, and in fact terminate the recent policy of having progress reports of all medical aspects of Games preparation submitted to the Doping & Biochemistry Subcommission. [182]

Ken Fitch regarded the emphasis on the work of the IOC MSD in comparison with the attention to general medical aspects a major imbalance within the IOC Medical Commission. As other medical experts before him, he acknowledged that such prominence led to a very detailed preparation of the anti-doping laboratory, which he purposefully excluded in his critique. However, he felt that the IOC MSD occupied a too dominant role and dealt with medical aspects, which went beyond its competencies.[183] Following the closing of the Olympic Games, Ken Fitch reiterated this stance, arguing that the IOC Medical Commission should

---

[179] Letter, "Bruce Challis to Alexandre de Mérode, July 15, 1988."

[180] Letter, "Ken Fitch to Alexandre de Mérode, April 12, 1988," archive collection "Summer and Winter Olympic Games: Medical files," folder "Medical matters and doping controls at the 1988 Seoul Summer Olympic Games: report on the medical facilities and services, services and list of the meetings of the medical commission and conference on the laboratory activities," IOC Archive, Lausanne.

[181] Ibid.

[182] Letter, "Ken Fitch to Alexandre de Mérode, April 12, 1988."

[183] Ibid.

increase its efforts in publishing work that does not relate to doping.[184] Moreover, he stressed his argument by recommending Bruce Challis as a permanent member of the IOC Medical Commission. He claimed that for more than 25 years, the IOC Medical Commission had not appointed a medical chief of an Olympic Games and that it could not allow a person of his expertise to leave its ranks.[185] His statement highlights the little emphasis on general medical issues in the IOC Medical Commission at that time, and with the increasing involvement of anti-doping laboratory experts in administrative issues, this development progressed constantly.

Finally, the preparations for the 1988 Seoul Olympic Games were the first in which Arnold Beckett did not play a central role. While he was still a member of the IOC MSD, contributing extensively to discussions, he did not travel to Seoul on his own initiative prior to the Olympic Games and did not communicate directly with the KIST laboratory. Certainly, the close link between KIST and Manfred Donike´s institution played an important role in this regard. However, one also has to attribute this to the slow retreating of Arnold Beckett from the international anti-doping scene. At the same time, other head of anti-doping laboratories besides the established figures became involved. This accounts especially for Jordi Segura, who acted as a doping control officer for the 1988 Seoul Olympic Games and observed the work in the laboratory.[186] He became the first head of laboratory for future Olympic Games who had been directly involved in the work of the doping control teams at the previous Games. This is evidence for the demonstrated process that more individuals began to contribute to the leading group of anti-doping laboratory experts, and this accounts particularly for those that headed an anti-doping laboratory at Olympic Games, such as Don Catlin and Jordi Segura, and to a lesser degree as Jong Sei Park.

Anti-doping Laboratory Experts´ Role in the Positive Doping Test of Ben Johnson

---

[184] Letter, "Ken Fitch to Alexandre de Mérode, October 20, 1988," archive collection "Summer and Winter Olympic Games: Medical files," folder "Medical matters and doping controls at the 1988 Seoul Summer Olympic Games: correspondence," IOC Archive, Lausanne.

[185] Letter, "Ken Fitch to Alexandre de Mérode, April 12, 1988."

[186] Letter, "Alexandre de Mérode to Jordi Serra, March 31, 1988," archive collection "Summer and Winter Olympic Games: Medical files," folder "Medical matters and doping controls at the 1988 Seoul Summer Olympic Games: correspondence," IOC Archive, Lausanne.

319 people worked during the execution of the doping controls at the 1988 Seoul Olympic Games in total. More than 70 people were involved in the work of the anti-doping laboratory.[187] The KIST laboratory analysed 1598 samples during the Olympic Games with ten athletes disqualified. These were the weightlifters Alidad (Afghanistan, furosemide), Kalman Csengeri (Hungary, stanozolol), Mitko Grablev (Bulgaria, furosemide), Angell Guenchev (Bulgaria, furosemide), Fernando Mariaca (Spain, pemoline) and Andor Szanyi (Hungary, stanozolol) along with 100m sprinter Ben Johnson (Canada, stanozolol), judoka Kerrith Brown (Great Britain, furosemide) and modern pentathletes Jorge Quesada (Spain, propanol) and Alexander Watson (Australia, caffeine).[188]

Similar to the unproblematic preparations, IOC Medical Commission members praised the quality of the anti-doping laboratory during the Olympic Games.[189] The IOC MSD considered this a result of their efforts in previous years. However, as anticipated by Ken Fitch and Bruce Challis, minor procedural and administrative errors occurred. Considerable concerns arose within the IOC Medical Commission when press reports appeared with rumours about positive doping cases. One press article quoted Moon Hi Han of the KIST laboratory, which Alexandre de Mérode regarded as a violation of the newly introduced Code of Ethics. Consequently, Moon Hi Han received a warning with a reminder about the regulations set out in the Code.[190] Another administrative problem concerned the official reports. Jong Sei Park and Byung Ryun Cho both submitted incorrect summaries to the IOC Medical Commission after the end of the Olympic Games. They mistakenly stated all IOC Medical Commission control samples and the additional analyses (which the IOC MSD demanded for future research) as positive doping tests, and included them in the total number of investigated samples.[191] Hence, Manfred Donike worked with them on their official reports to ensure that the final versions would be correct.[192] In SLOOC's *Official Report,*

---

[187] ORGANISING COMMITTEE OF THE GAMES OF THE XXIIITH OLYMPIAD, *Official Report,* 786.

[188] Individual Minutes, "Meetings of the IOC Medical Commission, September 14 to October 1, 1988."

[189] Ibid., 38.

[190] Letter, "Alexandre de Mérode to Moon Hi Han, September 28, 1988," archive collection "Summer and Winter Olympic Games: Medical files," folder "Medical matters and doping controls at the 1988 Seoul Summer Olympic Games: correspondence," IOC Archive, Lausanne.

[191] Report, "Review of the Seoul Laboratory Activities – Seoul Olympic Games 1988, by Jong Sei Park, May 18, 1988."

[192] Minutes, "Meeting of the IOC Medical Commission, April 15 and 16, 1989" 4.

the number (1598 samples) appears in the corrected version.[193] One can regard this as another example of Manfred Donike's responsibility as administrator for the entire anti-doping laboratory network.

It is important to address more details on the positive doping test of Ben Johnson because the role of the anti-doping laboratory experts confirms previously outlined processes. The incident stands symbolically for the significance of the technical developments of the doping analysis. Ben Johnson went for his doping control after his victory in the 100m sprint on September 24, 1988. On the next day, Jong Sei Park reported about the finding of stanozolol in the sample of Ben Johnson.[194] The IOC Medical Commission scheduled the analysis of the B-sample for September 26.[195] When this second investigation confirmed the original result, the Canadian delegation, led by Richard Pound, who was IOC vice-president at the time,[196] were ordered to attend the meeting of the IOC Medical Commission to discuss the case. Richard Pound attempted to defend Ben Johnson based on several arguments, including a likely involvement of other people that could have manipulated the sample, unfavourable pharmacological effects of stanozolol for a sprinter and negative doping tests at previous events.[197] He also commented, "[he] did not wish to challenge the scientific results." [198] Curiously, despite this awareness, Manfred Donike demonstrated that the allegations of the Canadian delegation were completely unsubstantiated based on the results of the doping analysis. In fact, according to the official minutes, he was the only IOC MSD member to speak about the conclusions of the analysis. He reasoned that the results were in contradiction to Richard Pound's argument, because it indicated a long-term application of

---

[193] ORGANISING COMMITTEE OF THE GAMES OF THE XXIIITH OLYMPIAD, *Official Report*, 787.

[194] Individual Minutes, "Meetings of the IOC Medical Commission, September 14 to October 1, 1988," 32.

[195] Ibid.

[196] REINOLD reports about the concerns of IOC Medical Commission members that in Richard Pound an IOC vice-president appeared to protect an athlete from his own country from a doping ban. As a result, it was decided that Alexandre de Mérode should speak with the IOC president to avoid such a situation in the future. REINOLD, "Arguing," 24.

[197] Individual Minutes, "Meetings of the IOC Medical Commission, September 14 to October 1, 1988," 33ff.

[198] Ibid.

stanozolol and was not consistent with a single-dose application.[199] Furthermore, he had a scientific explanation for the earlier negative doping tests:

> The traces of the steroid would disappear within 8 to 14 days depending on the amount. However, the steroid profile would remain depressed for a longer period. The steroid profile was less than 10 per cent of the normal value whereas the density of the urine was normal.[200]

Hence, as he had already done during the 1984 Los Angeles Olympic Games (see Chapter 6), Manfred Donike retraced the exact application of the drug. Therewith he discounted Richard Pound's argument by providing scientific evidence, which Richard Pound had not wanted to contest in the first place. In retrospect, Richard Pound noted that after the revelations of the exact findings of the doping analysis, he did not see a possibility to defend Ben Johnson any longer. He recalled the moment when Manfred Donike told him about the detailed results of the doping analysis:

> The end became all too apparent when Manfred Donike, the head of the doping subcommission, asked if I would be interested in the 'scientific results of the tests'. Any lawyer with experience in court knows that such a question means you are about to be dead in the water. I said that I was not sure I would understand them (since I could not say I had no interest) but that our team medical officer might. Donike read off a series of figures and expressions that I did not understand. I turned to the team doctor and whispered, 'What have we just heard?' He was as white as my shirt. He said that we had just heard that not only had Johnson tested positive for stanozolol, but that his results indicated that he was a longtime user.[201]

Due to the technical development of the doping analysis and the strict procedures of the IOC MSD, the Canadian delegation knew that there was no possibility of defence due to the given scientific evidence.

Whilst the consequences of Ben Johnson's positive doping test and the subsequent qualification for global anti-doping efforts are addressed later in this

---

[199] Individual Minutes, "Meetings of the IOC Medical Commission, September 14 to October 1, 1988," 35.
[200] Ibid.
[201] POUND, *Inside*, 52ff.

chapter, one has to bear in mind that the detailed analysis of Ben Johnson´s urine sample was not the first case of such kind. Furthermore, it was not the only one at the 1988 Seoul Olympic Games. In the cases of Jorge Quesada and Kerrith Brown, the members of the IOC MSD also proved that the athletes had not doped with the substances they claimed. [202] Even when the Hungarian delegation accepted the analysis of the positive A-sample by Kalman Csengeri, the IOC MSD ordered an analysis of the B-sample. [203] This was also a continuation of previously applied procedures, because the IOC MSD wanted to guarantee scientific validity of the doping analysis.

If one considers Manfred Donike´s behaviour during the meetings, a continuation of already addressed patterns becomes evident as well. As in previous cases, he wanted to have quick solutions once the B-analysis had confirmed the original analytical result. For example, Alexander Watson´s urine sample had shown a high amount of caffeine. Though the Australian delegation claimed it was the result of many cups of coffee and the consumption of energy tablets, Manfred Donike reasoned that there must have been an additional source. [204] He based his argument on the comparison of the caffeine ratio of Alexander Watson to that of other competitors in the modern pentathlon, who drank comparable amounts of coffee. Moreover, in the two unpunished cases of Linford Christie (Great Britain, pseudoephedrine) and Phillipe Battaglia (Monaco, norephedrine), Manfred Donike strongly favoured the declaration of a positive doping test on the basis of the analytical results. These clearly displayed the presence of the substances, but in both cases, the other IOC Medical Commission members outvoted him, giving both athletes the benefit of the doubt. In the case of Linford Christie, the IOC Medical Commission members were uncertain about the effects of ginseng, since the British delegation based its arguments on Linford Christie´s consumption of a couple of ginseng teas. [205] In the case of Philippe Battaglia, they accepted the excuse that the athlete had been ill prior to the Olympic Games, and recommended a general review of the regulations regarding ephedrine, which remained unclear. [206] Manfred Donike did generally not agree with such excuses.

---

[202] Individual Minutes, "Meetings of the IOC Medical Commission, September 14 to October 1, 1988," 23 and 42.

[203] Ibid., 28.

[204] Ibid., 19.

[205] Ibid., 44

[206] Ibid., 48.

Finally, it is important to mention the case of American basketballer Stacey Augmon, whose urine sample contained a T/E ratio over the allowed limit.[207] It appears that Manfred Donike specifically requested the participation of Don Catlin for this occasion, because he had analysed three urine samples of Stacey Augmon in the UCLA laboratory in the months leading to the Olympic Games. Don Catlin had detected T/E ratios close to six but had not reported the case and instead investigated into the luteinising hormone and testosterone ratio (LH/T).[208] This method provides additional details about the presence of exogenous testosterone. He demonstrated that the LH/T ratio was much lower than for people known to take exogenous testosterone.[209] Thus, Manfred Donike, confronted with the new method for the first time, undertook additional tests in the Seoul laboratory. He eventually regarded the sample as negative because of the additional evidence through Don Catlin's new method.[210] The other members of the IOC MSD followed Manfred Donike in his recommendation. Notwithstanding, the decision raised concerns by several IOC Medical Commission members on the treatment of previous positive doping cases on the T/E ratio. Moreover, Arnold Beckett, who confirmed the negative result, argued that any country without an eminent specialist in doping analysis such as Don Catlin would have had a positive doping case because the ratio of the original sample exceeded the upper limit.[211] Parallel with the case of Ben Johnson, this incident reveals that scientific evidence was prevailing in the IOC Medical Commission, even if the official regulations intended other procedures. This also accounts for Manfred Donike. Whereas in other cases he strongly pushed for punishment based on the analytical data, he appears to be convinced by the additional tests of Don Catlin and the supplementary scientific data. This provides further evidence to the fact that he placed scientific evidence the highest priority, even if it resulted in a different treatment.

Whilst these other incidents confirm the identified processes, it was because of the high profile of Ben Johnson that the uncovering of his positive doping test was the climax of the contribution of the anti-doping laboratory experts to the fight against doping. The combination of a high-quality laboratory, the development of the technical standards and the education of staff members of the KIST laboratory through Manfred Donike influenced Ben Johnson's doping test.

---

[207] Ibid., 30.

[208] Ibid.

[209] Ibid.

[210] Ibid., 31.

[211] Ibid.

Hence, all processes, which the IOC MSD had initiated since its establishment had a positive effect on the exposure of the most significant doping case in Olympic history. According to Ken Fitch, the case also influenced the entire IOC's fight against doping in the progress. He remarked, "the IOC Medical Commission had been placed in a much stronger position as far as testing on an international level was concerned."[212] Curiously, the fact that Ben Johnson had been tested eight times in the 17 months leading to the 1988 Seoul Olympic Games without any positive result,[213] demonstrates that at the same time, the anti-doping system as a whole was not as efficient as the anti-doping laboratory experts believed. On the contrary, the case caused a public uproar. Richard Pound confirmed this at the IOC Session in Puerto Rico in 1989, when he stated that the IOC had become "the focus of world attention regarding the doping problem."[214]

Commission of Inquiry and the "Monopoly of Laboratories"

The immediate effects for the anti-doping laboratory experts, due to the increased public attention concerning the issue of doping in sport are addressed later in this chapter. At first, it is important to highlight the results of the subsequent public investigations. Immediately after the 1988 Seoul Olympic Games, the Canadian federal government established the "Commission of Inquiry Into the Use of Drugs and Banned Practices Intended to Increase Athletic Performance" (Commission of Inquiry), led by Ontario appeal court chief justice Charles W. Dubin.[215] The inquiry was not only an investigation into the Ben Johnson case. Four positive doping cases by Canadian weightlifters prior to the Olympic Games had also contributed to its implementation. [216] It was instead, as Robert ARMSTRONG, counsel to the Commission of Inquiry, described it, a wide-ranging investigation into the usage of banned substances with a focus on Canadian athletes.[217] The inquiry officially started with its first public session in November 1988, and finished almost a year later. The Canadian government investigators questioned 119 witnesses from around the world, including steroid users, sport officials and the anti-doping laboratory experts Robert Dugal and Manfred

---

[212] Minutes, "Meeting of the IOC Medical Commission, April 15 and 16, 1989" 2.

[213] Daniel ROSEN, *A History of Performance Enhancement in Sports from the Nineteenth Century to Today* (Westport, CT: Praeger Publishers, 2008), 71.

[214] Minutes, "95th Session of the IOC in Puerto Rico, August 30 – September 1, 1989," 41.

[215] DUBIN, *Commission of Inquiry*, xxi.

[216] Ibid.

[217] Robert ARMSTRONG, "The Lessons Learned from Canada's Dubin Inquiry," *International Symposium on Sport and Law*, Monte Carlo, February 1, 1991, 3.

Donike.[218] Robert Dugal spoke on behalf of the Canadian INRS laboratory, whereas Manfred Donike appeared as a representative of the IOC Medical Commission. Due to its formulated intention, the outcome of the Commission of Inquiry was mainly a revelation of the network of relationships between the key actors in the doping system.[219] In terms of anti-doping policy, the report led to the general conclusion that the Olympic doping policy was limited in its approach, based on doping tests at Olympic Games only.[220] However, it also revealed a significant number of details about the behaviour and processes surrounding the anti-doping laboratory experts. Most of them confirm the illustrated findings.

First, the controlling attitudes of Alexandre de Mérode and Manfred Donike resurfaced during the investigations. When the Commission of Inquiry contacted Jong Sei Park, he wrote to Alexandre de Mérode about the way of proceeding, because he did not want to violate any regulations.[221] Alexandre de Mérode allowed him to compile the scientific data and the technical details, but he emphasised that such a process had to go through the IOC.[222] This is interesting since the Commission of Inquiry officially addressed Jong Sei Park on an individual basis. However, Alexandre de Mérode ordered Jong Sei Park to send his draft replies to Manfred Donike for correction, and the final version of the reply for review to an IOC legal advisor.[223] Furthermore, Alexandre de Mérode suggested that Manfred Donike should testify in front of the Commission instead of Jong Sei Park.[224] He justified this by arguing that Manfred Donike was head of the IOC MSD and had been responsible for the B-analysis of Ben Johnson's urine sample. Interestingly, Alexandre de Mérode did not speak at all in front of the

---

[218] A complete list of the witnesses, who testified in front of the Commission of Inquiry can be found in: DUBIN, *Commission of Inquiry*, Appendix B.

[219] Ivan WADDINGTON and Andy SMITH, *Sport, Health and Drugs: A Critical Sociological Perspective* (London: Taylor & Francis, 2000), 131.

[220] Ibid.

[221] In fact, Alexandre de Mérode had already sounded a note of caution to Jong Sei Park because a newspaper interview on the scientific details of the Ben Johnson test had appeared in the *New York Times*. It transpires from Jong Sei Park's reply that he intended to emphasise the good work of the IOC Medical Commission in an effort to keep the good relationship with the IOC body. Jong Sei Park appears intimidated by Alexandre de Mérode. Letter, "Jong Sei Park to Alexandre de Mérode, January 6, 1989," archive collection "Summer and Winter Olympic Games: Medical files," folder "Medical matters and doping controls at the 1988 Seoul Summer Olympic Games: correspondence." IOC Archive, Lausanne.

[222] Ibid.

[223] Ibid.

[224] Ibid.

investigators, so Manfred Donike was the only representative of the IOC Medical Commission to give testimony. In light of his, by then very privileged status, this seems understandable.

Second, in terms of the out-of competition controls, the Commission of Inquiry concluded that such measures had to be introduced in all countries and on a global scale.[225] The IOC should contribute to funding of programmes in countries whose resources were unable to afford the costs. Although these conclusions were not new and these initiatives had already begun before the 1988 Seoul Olympic Games, it stressed the need for more urgency. In this regard it confirmed the anti-doping laboratory experts' continuous calls for a worldwide introduction of out-of competition testing since the mid-1970s. In fact, Manfred Donike had also demanded out-of competition testing in front of the Commission of Inquiry, because of his own interests and a possible expansion of the doping control system for which he was partly responsible.[226] There was a significant increase in the budget estimate for doping analysis from 1989 onwards, linked to the introduction of the out-of competition controls.[227] As a result, there were more doping controls and therefore more work and research funds for the anti-doping laboratory experts. However, the enforcement of the introduction of global training tests was not the only concrete recommendation made. On another level, the Commission of Inquiry also suggested that national and international organisations increase their educational efforts, and apply a full range of public health education techniques to the problem of doping in sport.[228] Thereby, it repeated the IOC Athletes' Commission, which had already called for education of athletes, coaches and administrators to teach the dangers of doping in a statement during the Seoul Olympic Games.[229] This was reiterated by its chair Peter Tallberg[230] at the IOC Session in 1989, where he stated that increased work

---

[225] DUBIN, *Commission of Inquiry*, 544.

[226] "Untersuchungsausschuß in Toronto," *SID*, August 4, 1989, archive collection "Nachlass August Kirsch," File 090, "Doping (7)," CuLDA, Cologne.

[227] KRÜGER et al., *Doping und Anti-Doping*, 121.

[228] DUBIN, *Commission of Inquiry*, 547.

[229] Press Release, "Seoul Declaration, 1988," archive collection "Athletes' Commission," folder "Athletes' Commission: reports, statement, seminar, press releases, press cuttings and leaflets of the commission," IOC Archive, Lausanne.

[230] Peter Tallberg (born 1937) competed at five Olympic Games (1960-1980) and became an IOC member in 1976 when he was still an active athlete. He was the first chairman of the IOC Athletes' Commission and held this position until 2002. He was also part of several Coordination Commissions for Olympic Games. INTERNATIONAL OLYMPIC COMMITTEE, *Biographies*, 103.

in the educational field of doping prevention was required. [231] Consequently, whilst acknowledging the technical advancements and the reliability on scientific evidence, the investigators also called for a more holistic approach to solve the doping problem. This was a new tendency.

Third, concerning the network of the anti-doping laboratory experts and the role of the IOC MSD, the Commission of Inquiry came to the remarkable result that a "monopoly of international laboratories" existed. [232] A small group of individuals controlled this monopoly: the members of the IOC MSD. It categorically linked its result to the situation of the Calgary laboratory. Therefore, the conflict between Robert Dugal and the Calgary doping control centre at the Foothills Hospital emerged again. The Calgary laboratory had – as all other testing centres – to go through its reaccreditation procedure at the beginning of 1989. However, the laboratory was not successful in completing the test and was suspended from international testing afterwards. [233] Robert Baynton raised suspicions that the IOC MSD did not want to reaccredit his institution because they wanted to guarantee the INRS laboratory of IOC MSD member Robert Dugal the sole control over the Canadian doping system. After the attempt to gain influence in the laboratory process during the Olympic Games, Robert Baynton perceived the rejection of reaccreditation as a second serious intervention into the running of his institution. [234] Just as in the first incident, Manfred Donike supported Robert Dugal based on the presentation of the scientific results of the reaccreditation. However, Robert Baynton felt that such extensive quality controls, which the IOC MSD applied to the Calgary laboratory, were not demanded from other doping control centres. Amongst quoted written correspondence in the final report of the Dubin Inquiry, Robert Baynton wrote to Manfred Donike:

> If every I.O.C. laboratory was subjected to the same scrutiny and treated as unfairly as us, chances are the number of I.O.C. labs would only number five (5) – *exactly the number of members of the subcommission who are heads of I.O.C. laboratories.* We know of few other systems where vested interests control and adjudicate so directly.

---

[231] Minutes, "95th Session of the IOC in Puerto Rico, August 30 – September 1, 1989," 65.

[232] DUBIN, *Commission of Inquiry*, 402.

[233] Minutes, "Meeting of the IOC Medical Commission, April 15 and 16, 1989" 5.

[234] DUBIN, *Commission of Inquiry*, 408.

It is apparent that the subcommission wishes to have only one I.O.C. accredited laboratory per Country. Right or wrong, this should have been addressed before the Calgary Olympics. Our laboratory, its personnel, our Institution and its community have been put through great deal of anguish and financial stress, attempting to achieve what may be impossible. It is paradoxical that one of the purposes of doping control is to make competition fair (fairplay) and to keep the competition field 'level'. The subcommission seems to have lost sight of this in their own dealings [emphasis added].[235]

Unsurprisingly, Robert Baynton received support from the president of the Foothills Hospital Ralph Coombs, who reasoned that the double functions of the IOC MSD members were a severe contradiction in the laboratory accreditation process. He argued as follows:

The structure of the Subcommission, which permits your members to be the professionals who acts as consultants, then accreditors, subsequently adjudicators, and also the appeal group, while maintaining a monopoly commercial interest, defies common standards of public accountability. We expect that the Subcommission will eventually be persuaded to restructure and function in a more forthright and open manner. In the meantime, we are unable to commit sufficient finances to continue our program.[236]

Because the members of the IOC MSD, who controlled the accreditation process, were also heads of the leading accredited laboratories, it was believed that they could, and would downgrade rival institutions. As demonstrated, such inconsistencies had occurred before. Whilst Charles Dubin perceived the issue as "incongruous that IOC laboratory accreditation is determined by the heads of some of the very laboratories that receive accreditation,"[237] he did not solve the issue whether Robert Dugal or Manfred Donike had deliberately prevented the Calgary laboratory to gain reaccreditation. Notwithstanding, he made the recommendation concerning the laboratories and the accreditation procedure:

---

[235] Ibid.

[236] Ibid., 410.

[237] Ibid., 542.

RECOMMENDATION THAT to avoid conflicts of interest, the competence of laboratories, including laboratories accredited by the International Olympic Committee, be determined by persons at arm´s length from the laboratories under consideration, and in particular that the Canadian Olympic Association urge the IOC to take steps to remove the present conflict of interest that exists in the IOC laboratory-accreditation process.[238]

Without doubt, the recommendation highlights the arguments brought forward in this book. The initial IAAF accreditation procedure had already been developed by those anti-doping laboratory experts, who were in charge of the leading testing centres. They were the only individuals with the competencies to do so. Once the IOC took over the process and founded the IOC MSD, the power for these very few individuals became even more extensive. As the Commission of Inquiry explains, this did not only lead to a global doping policy, which focused almost entirely on doping testing and doping analysis, but it also resulted in a subjective evaluation of the state of the respective laboratories. In contrast to this, the anti-doping laboratory experts interpreted the new standards as a means for quality assurance, which secured their own institutions´ leading role within the network of accredited laboratories.

Thus, the conclusions of the Commission of Inquiry publicly uncovered for the first time the rise of the anti-doping laboratory experts on the back of the introduction of the laboratory accreditation system. At the same time, it emphasised its negative effects by the dominance of a few individuals. According to a press article, the FRG´s IOC member Willi Daume had made similar accusations and blamed Manfred Donike for its "monopolistic position" in 1989.[239] Although Willi Daume denied to have made such a statement,[240] it shows the general discontent about the dominating attitude of Manfred Donike in the FRG. In an undiplomatic way of proceeding, Manfred Donike complained about the statements in to Willi Daume directly.[241] However, as in the case of the

---

[238] Ibid., 543.

[239] Adolf SCHERER, "Analyse-Monopol von Donike stört Olympier," *SID*, May 1, 1989, archive collection "Nachlass August Kirsch," File 089, "Doping (6)," CuLDA, Cologne.

[240] Letter, "Willi Daume to Manfred Donike, April 25, 1989," archive collection "Nachlass August Kirsch," File 089, "Doping (6)," CuLDA, Cologne.

[241] Letter, "Manfred Donike to Willi Daume, April 24, 1989," archive collection "Nachlass August Kirsch," File 089, "Doping (6)," CuLDA, Cologne. Also see: Letter, Manfred Donike to Willi Daume, May 10, 1989, archive collection "Nachlass August Kirsch," File 089, "Doping (6)," CuLDA, Cologne.

Calgary laboratory, at which the main public attention remained over Ben Johnson's positive doping case and the exposure of extensive doping usage within elite sport, the accusations on the role of the anti-doping laboratory experts remained largely unnoticed and did not have any direct consequences. In light of the dependence of the global anti-doping policy on the anti-doping laboratories, this appears understandable.

EFFORTS TO DEAL WITH CONSEQUENCES THROUGH CONTINUATION OF ESTABLISHED INITIATIVES

With the positive doping test of Ben Johnson heralding a new phase of global anti-doping activities, characterised by more public attention and increased initiatives of external stakeholders,[242] it is necessary to investigate the dealings of the anti-doping laboratory experts from 1988 onwards. It is important to separate this examination from the results of the Commission of Inquiry, as the reaction of the anti-doping laboratory experts has not been investigated to date.

Tightened Reaccreditation Procedure and GLP

In order to guarantee more reliable tests, particularly outside the Olympic Games, the members of the IOC MSD increased their efforts to enhance the technical standards once more. Already in 1987, Manfred Donike had suggested a revised procedure for accreditation to control the laboratories more regularly.[243] The new procedure, which was implemented from 1989 onwards, regulated an annual reaccreditation, introduced proficiency tests with an analysis of four samples every four months and raised the amount of work for the laboratories to obtain reaccreditation.[244] The new rules required the screening of ten samples with five screening procedures. Therefore, the IOC MSD established a method to increase the scope of control on the laboratories. This can be seen at the example of the 1989 reaccreditation procedure, which saw the incorrect report of results by five laboratories: Calgary reported a false negative result for caffeine, Helsinki a false negative for clostebol, Indianapolis a false negative for testosterone, Prague a false negative for oxymesterone and Moscow a false positive for testosterone and

---

[242] HOULIHAN, *Dying*, 139.

[243] Minutes, "Meeting of the IOC Medical Commission, February 24-26, 1987," 3.

[244] Minutes, "Meeting of the IOC Medical Commission's Subcommission Doping and Biochemistry of Sport, February 6, 1989," archive collection "IOC Medical Commission," IOC Archive, Lausanne, Annex 1.

a false negative for caffeine.[245] The IOC MSD withdrew the official accreditation from the five laboratories but also gave them the possibility to redeem themselves for the incorrect results. It adopted a staggered approach for laboratories with wrongly reported results.[246] The new system classified the unsuccessful doping testing institutions in two phases and foresaw corrective measures to improve the performance of the laboratories. "Phase 1" anticipated a suspension of four months from all events with international participation and out-of competition controls. All positive samples from national tests were to be sent to an IOC accredited laboratory for confirmation. Moreover, the IOC MSD requested the laboratories to submit a plan to improve the laboratory standards and at the subsequent proficiency test, it had to analyse eight samples.[247] Once a laboratory fulfilled these conditions and once it had successfully performed the proficiency test, the IOC MSD upgraded it to "Phase 2." This second stage differed in a way that laboratories were allowed to analyse samples of international events, but also had to send positive samples for a re-check to an approved institution at which the B-sample was analysed again. Only once were there correct results reported within a four-month period, the IOC MSD granted the laboratory full IOC accredited status again.[248] The laboratory in Rome, which had reported all results correctly but submitted "unacceptable documentation," was classified into "Phase 2." All other laboratories, which failed the 1989 reaccreditation process, were integrated in "Phase 1."[249] With the exception of the Calgary laboratory, the IOC MSD eventually awarded all institutions full accreditation again during 1989.

Aware of the possibility of increasing juridical and public attention to the work of the anti-doping laboratories, Alexandre de Mérode continued to support the IOC MSD in its strict approach. He claimed that the data presented by the laboratories should be flawless since it might be used for scientific evidence.[250] The four laboratories, which achieved excellent results in the 1989 reaccreditation process were the ones based in Cologne, Los Angeles, Montreal and Kreischa.[251]

---

[245] Ibid.

[246] Note, "Requirements for Accreditation and Good Laboratory Practices," archive collection "Summer and Winter Olympic Games: Medical Files," folder "Medical matters (laboratory) at the 1988 Calgary Winter Olympic Games: correspondence and report," IOC Archive, Lausanne, Part A.

[247] Ibid.

[248] Ibid.

[249] Minutes, "Meeting of the IOC Medical Commission's Subcommission Doping and Biochemistry of Sport, February 6, 1989," 1.

[250] Ibid.

[251] Ibid., Annex 1.

This is an important finding because they were the institutions of the IOC MSD members Manfred Donike, Robert Dugal and Claus Clausnitzer as well as Don Catlin. It shows that they were in charge of the leading institutions, whilst it also gives evidence to the statements in the final report of the Commission of Inquiry, which stated that the IOC MSD gave preference to their own laboratories.

The reaccreditation procedure was in line with the IOC MSD´s policy to expand its quality control measures and one has to consider it in conjunction with the final adoption of the GLP. The document, which Robert Dugal and Manfred Donike had already started to develop in 1987 (see Chapter 6), was eventually enforced for doping control laboratories seeking accreditation as from November 1988. In January 1989, the IOC Medical Commission then officially adopted the GLP.[252] The 64-paged document consisted of three parts, two of them (Part A and Part C) dealing specifically with the analytical procedures and the accreditation process, including the already addressed renewed reaccreditation procedure.[253] Especially Part B on "Scientific and technical guidelines for laboratories engaged in doping controls" highlights how the IOC MSD tried to control the institutions. Besides guidelines on the analytical procedures and regulations on regular quality control, the IOC MSD made certain physical laboratory facilities, qualifications for laboratory personnel and recordkeeping compulsory requirements for all accreditation-seeking institutions.[254] In light of increasing multinational efforts to harmonise anti-doping efforts, the members of the IOC MSD thought such regulations to be an attempt to establish "comprehensive operational standards for all aspects of laboratory drug testing and laboratory procedures to be applied."[255] As the international initiatives regarded the IOC MSD as the responsible body for the doping laboratories, its members used its uncontested position to enforce stricter regulations. Overall, it was an obvious continuation of their policy to enhance the scientific standards based on their professional competencies in doping analysis, through which they already controlled large parts of the system.

Further Extension of the Laboratory Network and Growing Difficulties

Besides the reaccreditation of existing institutions, the IOC MSD continued to be active in the acquisition of new doping laboratories. However, the more detailed regulations within the GLP made it harder for laboratories to become accredited.

---

[252] Ibid., 1.

[253] Note, "Requirements for Accreditation and Good Laboratory Practices."

[254] Ibid., Part B.

[255] Ibid., Part B, B-1.

According to the GLP, the IOC MSD now requested a pre-accreditation procedure, where the laboratories had to analyse three sets of ten samples successfully over a period ranging between six and twelve months.[256] During official meetings, Manfred Donike even argued that the preparation of a laboratory for doping control could take up to four years. He made clear that the IOC MSD was not willing to accredit laboratories without the necessary qualities.[257] Nevertheless, in light of the increased national and multinational efforts to install anti-doping policies, more laboratories gradually applied for official approval. In 1989, a total of fourteen institutions were interested: Athens (Greece), Beijing (China), Breda (Netherlands), Christchurch (New Zealand), Ghent (Belgium), Havana (Cuba), New Jersey (USA), Sao Paulo (Brazil), Sydney (Australia), Sofia (Bulgaria), Vanderbilt (USA), Warsaw (Poland), and unknown institutions in Costa Rica and Puerto Rico.[258] Most of the applications were encouraged by governments and sports organisations, which, considering the increasing public interest, were making marked efforts to support institutions from their regions to set up anti-doping laboratories. For example, the Peruvian IAAF Council member Admiral Pedro Galvez raised concerns about global anti-doping efforts if there was no anti-doping laboratory in the South American area. He proposed an institution in Lima for instant accreditation.[259] Although Arne Ljungqvist made him, and other IAAF Council members, aware of the complicated procedures and the long preparations periods of two to three years, the IAAF eventually decided together with the International Volleyball Association (FIVB) and the IOC, to support the Lima laboratory financially.[260] However, whereas the acquisition of the equipment did not pose a difficulty, the preparation and training of personnel along with the correct submission of paper work proved a considerable obstacle.[261] Even after the IAAF increased its grant from \$50,000 to \$70,000, the Lima laboratory could not obtain accreditation, due

---

[256] Ibid., Part A.

[257] Individual Minutes, "Meetings of the IOC Medical Commission, September 14 to October 1, 1988," 7.

[258] Minutes, "Meeting of the IOC Medical Commission's Subcommission Doping and Biochemistry of Sport, February 6, 1989," Annex 2.

[259] Minutes, "IAAF Council Meeting, April 3, 1989," archive collection "Nachlass August Kirsch," File 123, "IAAF (2)," CuLDA, Cologne, 35.

[260] Minutes, "IAAF Council Meeting, September 3, 1989," archive collection "Nachlass August Kirsch," File 123, "IAAF (2)," CuLDA, Cologne, 4.

[261] Minutes, "IAAF Council Meeting, May 31, 1990," archive collection "Nachlass August Kirsch," File 123, "IAAF (2)," CuLDA, Cologne, 6.

to insufficient training of its staff.[262] The challenge to install more educational initiatives alongside the already existing workshops becomes evident with this example, but also reveals the successful attempt to raise the standards. This also applies for two more cases. The IAAF supported the establishment of an Egyptian Research Centre with $75,000 from 1990 onwards.[263] The institution was strongly supported by the Egyptian government and intended to set up the first anti-doping laboratory in Africa. A laboratory in Rio de Janeiro received a grant of $11,000.[264] However, in both cases, the IAAF had to realise that the institutions were not able to obtain official accreditation, due to the high technical standards, and withdrew its financial support at the end of 1992.[265]

In contrast to the problems with institutions in South America and Africa, the IOC MSD approved the anti-doping laboratory in Oslo and awarded it with official IOC accreditation in July 1988.[266] Its current director, Professor Dr. Peter Hemmersbach, headed the anti-doping laboratory (situated at the Aker University Hospital, which is today part of the Oslo University Hospital), already at the time of the accreditation.[267] He became an influential key figure within the network of anti-doping laboratory experts from the mid-1990s onwards. This illustrates that the larger institutional network naturally resulted in more involved individuals. With the increasing international governmental efforts in anti-doping issues, the situation in Asia and Oceania also improved. In 1989, the laboratory in Beijing at the National Research Institute of Sports Medicine gained official accreditation, as did the Australian Government Analytical Laboratories in Sydney.[268] Both laboratories were headed by later influential anti-doping laboratory experts in

---

[262] Minutes, "IAAF Council Meeting, August 11, 1992," archive collection "Nachlass August Kirsch," File 123, "IAAF (2)," CuLDA, Cologne, Appendix 1.

[263] Minutes, "IAAF Council Meeting, May 31, 1990," 6.

[264] Minutes, "IAAF Council Meeting, August 11, 1992," Appendix 1.

[265] Ibid.

[266] Minutes, "Meeting of the IOC Medical Commission's Subcommission on Doping and Biochemistry, September 14 and 15, 1988," archive collection "IOC Medical Commission," folder "IOC Medical Commission: sub-commission Doping and biochemistry of sport: meeting in Seoul on September-October 1988: working documents," IOC Archive, Lausanne, 103.

[267] Ibid.

[268] "Laboratoires de contrôle de dopage accrédités par le CIO," *Olympic Review* 275 (1990), 446ff.

Professor Dr. Zeyi Yang[269] and Professor Dr. Rymantas Kazlauskas. One has to consider the Australian and the Chinese efforts in relation to their intentions of applying to host the 2000 Olympic Games. For the same reason, Greek authorities invested into the establishment of an official anti-doping laboratory in Athens, and the IOC MSD approved the institution at the Olympic Athletic Centre in 1990. [270] However, following the first reaccreditation phase the IOC MSD downgraded it to "Phase 1",[271] because the head of the laboratory had resigned.[272] In 1992, the Doping Analysis Unit at the University Institute of Legal Medicine of the Vaud Cantonal Hospices in Lausanne received official accreditation.[273] It was in the interest of the IOC to have another laboratory in Switzerland after the closure of the only testing centre in Magglingen in 1989.[274]

In conjunction with the proposal to install an international anti-doping body, there was another model discussed at the end of the 1980s to deal with the doping controls in remote regions: the "flying" or "mobile" laboratory. Alexandre de Mérode had envisaged that the "mobile" laboratory was under the auspices of the new international anti-doping body, anticipated during the world conferences, but would be financed by the IOC and its sponsors.[275] Significantly, Alexandre de Mérode pushed the idea but there was little discussion amongst the technical experts. In 1989, Alexandre de Mérode presented the idea to the IOC Session and

---

[269] Professor Dr. Zeyi Yang (born 1943) became the first appointed head of the anti-doping laboratory in Bejing in 1991. He was vice-director of the National Research Institute of Sports Medicine in China and professor at the Bejing Sports University. INTERNATIONAL OLYMPIC COMMITTEE, *Commission Médicale*, 19.

[270] Minutes, "Meeting of the IAAF Doping Commission, January 11, 1991," archive collection "Nachlass August Kirsch," File 090, "Doping (7)," CuLDA, Cologne, 3.

[271] Minutes, "Meeting of the IAAF Doping Commission, January 10 and 11, 1992," archive collection "Nachlass August Kirsch," File 090, "Doping (7)," CuLDA, Cologne, 2.

[272] Minutes, "Meeting of the IOC Medical Commission's Subcommission on Doping and Biochemistry, October 25, 1991," Box 106 "Subcommission Doping & Lillehammer," Private Archive Jordi Segura, Barcelona, 1.

[273] Individual Minutes, "Meetings of the IOC Medical Commission in Albertville, February 9-22, 1992," archive collection "Summer and Winter Olympic Games: Medical files," IOC Archive, Lausanne, 11.

[274] No official source for the closure of the laboratory in Magglingen could be found. However, the institution is not listed in the official announcement on the IOC-accredited institutions for 1990 anymore.

[275] Minutes, "Meeting of the IOC Medical Commission's Subcommission Doping and Biochemistry of Sport, September 16 and 18, 1988," archive collection "IOC Medical Commission," folder "IOC Medical Commission: sub-commission Doping and biochemistry of sport: meeting in Seoul on September-October 1988: working documents," IOC Archive, Lausanne, 110.

approached Hewlett Packard in order to begin cooperation concerning the issue.[276] However, the anti-doping laboratory experts did not really support the idea, considering it impracticable to ensure a high technical quality in a "mobile" laboratory. They also raised concerns about the high costs.[277] It is possible that they feared a reduction in work for their own institutions. Hence, it also came into discussion whether a "mobile" laboratory would counteract the aim to install more testing centres worldwide.[278]

There were 23 IOC-accredited anti-doping laboratories by the beginning of 1992. Yet, for the leading anti-doping laboratory experts, the emphasis remained not on the quantity of the laboratories, but rather on high-quality standards. One can see this by the more sophisticated technical requirements and guidelines caused through the adoption of the GLP. At the same time, a growing institutional network led to the involvement of more heads of laboratories, such as Peter Hemmersbach, Zeyi Yang and Rymantas Kazlauskas.

More Initiatives of Educational Nature and Increased Knowledge Exchange

Although the number of laboratories did not increase dramatically between the 1988 Seoul Olympic Games and the 1992 Barcelona Olympic Games, considerable efforts were made to teach the laboratory staff of interested control centres about the new procedures of the GLP. The majority of the courses addressed potential doping control officers, who could supervise the sampling procedures. In particular, the IOC MSD and the IAAF Medical Committee continued to offer such initiatives under the supervision of Manfred Donike and in collaboration with Olympic Solidarity and the International Athletic Foundation (IAF) respectively, which financed the participation at the courses.[279] In light of the difficulties of establishing official laboratories in all regions of the world, they wanted to assure that the collection of the urine samples and the

---

[276] Minutes, "Meeting of the IOC Medical Commission´s Subcommission Doping and Biochemistry of Sport, February 6, 1989," 5. Also see: Minutes, "95th Session of the IOC in Puerto Rico, August 30 – September 1, 1989," archive collection "IOC Sessions 1894-2009," IOC Archive, Lausanne, 11.

[277] Minutes, "Meeting of the IOC Medical Commission´s Subcommission Doping and Biochemistry of Sport, September 16 and 18, 1988," 110.

[278] Ibid.

[279] INTERNATIONAL ATHLETIC FOUNDATION, *A Review of Projects 1989-1990 and Projects in Progress 1991* (Monte Carlo: IAF, 1991).

handling of them was done in an appropriate manner. This was the first step to ensure that a correct analytical result could be produced.

Moreover, there was an increasing need for an exchange between the staff of the official doping laboratories. The IOC MSD discussed such measures from 1988 onwards to enhance the communication between the accredited institutions. Certainly, the Cologne Workshop remained one of the main forums for this exchange and regularly attracted more biochemists from accredited and non-accredited institutions around the world. They presented papers on the improvement of analytical techniques so that Cologne Workshop differed considerably from the educational workshops to inform laboratory staff about doping controls. In fact, Manfred Donike admitted in 1992 that the annual meeting had "more elements of a symposium than of a real workshop where the participants work at bench."[280] Consequently, Alexandre de Mérode and Manfred Donike began to arrange more meetings with the heads of the IOC accredited laboratories from 1989 onwards.[281] Although it was originally intended to hold such meetings biannually, they organised them on a yearly basis. According to the official documents available, the first of the IOC's "Head of Anti-Doping Laboratories Meetings" took place in Moscow ahead of the "Second Permanent World Conference on Anti-Doping" in October 1989.[282] In contrast to the Cologne Workshop, which increasingly focused on scientific aspects, Manfred Donike used these meetings to discuss the challenges of running an official anti-doping laboratory.[283] Hence, it addressed the leadership.

The increased exchange between the institutions, which was also a result of the annual reaccreditation, resulted in an increased professionalisation of the communication and administration systems. From 1989 onwards, the IOC financed an assistant to support Manfred Donike in dealing with administrative tasks and the filing of the analytical results.[284] Moreover, the laboratories also began to feel the expanding commercialisation of the Olympic Movement through the TOP Programme, which provided free fax machines to all

[280] Manfred DONIKE, "Preface," in: *10th Cologne Workshop on Dope Analysis 7th to 12th June 1992 – Proceedings*, eds. Manfred DONIKE, Hans GEYER, Andrea GOTZMANN, Ute MARECK-ENGELKE and Susanne RAUTH (Cologne: Sportverlag Strauß, 1993), 12.

[281] Minutes, "Meeting of the IOC Medical Commission's Subcommission Doping and Biochemistry of Sport, February 6, 1989," 5.

[282] Minutes, "Meeting of the IOC Medical Commission, April 15 and 16, 1989," 6.

[283] Interview with Don H. Catlin, November 11, 2012.

[284] Minutes, "Meeting of the IOC Medical Commission's Subcommission Doping and Biochemistry of Sport, February 6, 1989," 5.

laboratories.[285] Finally, official and unofficial meetings were not the only ways to inform about newest scientific developments anymore. In view of the acceleration of the technical advancements, Manfred Donike proposed that each laboratory circulated a scientific paper every three months.[286] Thus, even though he played a significant political role, he was still heavily involved with advancing the technical standards of the doping control system. During a meeting of the IOC MSD in Moscow in October 1989, it was even suggested that all official laboratories should submit all of the scientific projects they performed in order to set up a data bank of publications and projects. As a first step, it introduced a biannual newsletter to increase "inter-laboratory communications."[287] This was another attempt to accelerate the scientific developments and to install new analytical techniques as fast as possible. Furthermore, Manfred Donike and his colleagues began to publish the proceedings of the Cologne Workshop in an edited collection from 1992 onwards.[288]

There was also cooperation between laboratories within the framework of national agreements to conducts tests amongst each other. VOY and DEETER have already addressed in detail an initiative to sign a USSR-USOC drug testing agreement, which involved the testing laboratories in Moscow and Los Angeles.[289] However, the initiative by the Americans and Soviets was not the only one. The laboratory in Barcelona, under the leadership of Jordi Segura, clearly pursued an outreach strategy to act as a consultancy and teaching institution for other laboratories. For example, it trained Heloisa Trinidade from the Institute of Chemistry of the Federal University of Rio de Janeiro for five weeks in Barcelona.[290] This IAF-sponsored initiative aimed towards the eventual accreditation of the anti-doping laboratory. Moreover, the laboratories in Seoul and Kreischa signed an agreement over joint research on doping analysis, which

---

[285] Ibid.

[286] Ibid.

[287] Minutes, "Meeting of the IOC Subcommittee on Doping and Biochemistry in Moscow, October 7, 1989," archive collection "IOC Medical Commission," IOC Archive, Lausanne, 4.

[288] DONIKE et al., *10th Cologne Workshop*. Since 1992, the organisers have published an edition of the proceedings for all subsequent workshops. These are accessible at the Central Library of the DSHS.

[289] VOY and DEETER , *Drugs*, 156ff.

[290] INTERNATIONAL ATHLETIC FOUNDATION, *A Review*, 37.

started at the beginning of 1989. This project also included the exchange of laboratory staff.[291]

Other than the IOC, the IAAF also provided the anti-doping laboratory experts with a platform to present the latest developments in doping controls and doping analysis. In June 1989 in Monte Carlo, it staged the "Second IAAF World Symposium on Doping in Sport," following its initiative from Florence in 1987. However, as had been the case already during the first symposium, the event was less of an exchange of information for those active with the actual doping controls, but instead a possibility to inform about general processes. Thus, the attendees presented advances in scientific research, new methods of detection and aspects of sample taking. Manfred Donike did not perceive such occasions as very successful, let alone productive, as he had previously remarked after the first symposium.[292]

The initiatives presented demonstrate an increased awareness for more educational initiatives, whilst also exchanging information on latest research projects in order to remain at the forefront of anti-doping strategies. In fact, this was a consequence of the network extension and the stricter regulations for anti-doping laboratories. Hence, the leading anti-doping laboratory experts accepted the challenge of their more administrative roles in this regard.

Challenges for the Anti-doping Laboratory Experts

Personal and Procedural Challenges

Whilst the leading figures within the network of the anti-doping laboratory networks continued to expand established processes, it is also necessary to outline the main challenges and changes for them. It has already been addressed that dealing with more substances resulted in the involvement of an increasing number of scientific experts to develop analytical procedures because the members of the IOC MSD had a specific research focus on the more traditional doping substances, such as anabolic steroids and stimulants. This process also continued after the 1988 Seoul Olympic Games.

---

[291] Contract, "Agreement concerning first year program for the joint research on doping control between Korea Advanced Institute of Science and Technology (KAIST) and Zentrales Doping Kontroll Labor Kreischa, October 2, 1988," archive collection "DR 510 Nationales Olympisches Komitee der DDR," folder "DR 510/968, Band 4, Medizinische Kommission des IOC, 1977-1987," Bundesarchiv, Berlin-Lichterfelde.
[292] Letter, "Manfred Donike to August Kirsch, June 16, 1989," archive collection "Nachlass August Kirsch," File 089, "Doping (6)," CuLDA, Cologne.

Don Catlin finally became an official member of the IOC MSD in 1989.[293] Remarkably, he did not replace any of the existing members, but rather added to the IOC body, which then consisted of six anti-doping laboratory experts. With the exception of the replacement of Victor Rogozkin by Vitaly Semenov, this was the first personnel change to the IOC MSD since its establishment in 1981. The addition of Don Catlin was an acknowledgement for the advisory role that he had occupied in previous years.

Another issue, which caused the expansion of the main network, was the growing evidence for usage of blood doping amongst high-performance athletes. Reports that athletes used erythropoietin (EPO) fuelled these assumptions.[294] Having already banned blood doping in 1985, there was still no reliable method to analyse blood samples by the beginning of the 1990s. As outlined above, part of the reason was the lack of expertise amongst the IOC MSD members. By 1991, there was an increased interest in the introduction of blood tests and Alexandre de Mérode reported to the Executive Board and the IFs that this type of testing had become a necessity.[295] Nevertheless, the IOC MSD members did still not have a solution. A definitive test for establishing the use of exogenous EPO or autologous blood transfusions was not available at the time.[296] Consequently, the IOC MSD decided to meet with representatives of the American biopharmaceutical company Amgen to discuss the possibility of conducting a trial study on the issue.[297] The discussion on blood doping revealed a well-known pattern: Arnold Beckett and Manfred Donike especially, were highly critical towards the introduction of an incomplete testing technique. In fact, the IOC MSD released a statement in 1992: "[a]definitive test for establishing use of exogenous EPO or autologous blood transfusion is not available at this time."[298] Whilst the IOC MSD members certainly began to realise the problem of blood doping, their main concern remained the reliability of analytical procedures. With none of the members dealing with blood doping in their research, they did not consider such a method becoming available in the near future. Notwithstanding, during IOC Medical Commission meetings at the 1992 Winter Olympic Games in

---

[293] INTERNATIONAL OLYMPIC COMMITTEE, *Commission Médicale*, 18.

[294] Minutes, "Meetings of the IOC Medical Commission, February 9-28, 1988," 41.

[295] HUNT, *Drug Games*, 94. For the original source, see: "The Executive Board and the Summer IFs in Barcelona," *Olympic Review* 283 (1991), 187.

[296] Minutes, "Meeting of the IOC Medical Commission's Subcommission on Doping and Biochemistry, October 25, 1991," 1.

[297] Ibid.

[298] Minutes, "Meeting of the IOC Medical Commission in Courchevel, February 7, 1992," archive collection "IOC Medical Commission," IOC Archive, Lausanne, 6.

Albertville, the Italian sports doctor Professor Dr. Francesco Conconi [299] – member of the IOC Medical Commission's Subcommission Biomechanics and Physiology of Sport – presented a study on the detection of EPO misuse in sport, which the members hotly debated.[300] This is further proof that blood doping was considered to go beyond the existing entire network of anti-doping laboratory experts. As a result of the discussion, the IOC Medical Commission demanded more research in order to obtain scientifically valid results, and Francesco Conconi appeared again before the IOC Medical Commission in 1993 to report about further experiments.[301] As in the previous case, the Commission was not yet satisfied with the results, and demanded more research.[302] However, it did approve blood sampling for the detection of foreign blood abuse in endurance events (cross-country skiing and biathlon) at the 1994 Winter Olympic Games in Lillehammer.[303]

The issue of blood doping is an example that by the beginning of the 1990s, the development of analytical procedures went beyond the traditional key figures within the network of the anti-doping laboratory experts. This resulted in slow progress over this issue, and also accounted for the issue of hGH, for which no test was available before the 1992 Olympic Games, although the Commission of Inquiry proved that athletes had made use of hGH.[304] Clearly, the blood doping issue reveals the increasing complexity of the anti-doping control system, and discloses the dilemma in which the experienced anti-doping laboratory experts

---

[299] Professor Dr. Francesco Conconi (born 1935) was Professor of Applied Biochemistry at the Faculty of Medicine at the University of Ferrara from 1965. In 1993, he became president of the UCI's Medical Commission. INTERNATIONAL OLYMPIC COMMITTEE, *Commission Médicale*, 21.

[300] Individual Minutes, "Meetings of the IOC Medical Commission in Albertville, February 9-22, 1992," 19ff.

[301] Minutes, "Meeting of the IOC Medical Commission in Lillehammer, February 28 to March 2, 1993," archive collection "IOC Medical Commission," IOC Archive, Lausanne, 6.

[302] Francesco Conconi described his research with 23 amateur triathletes as controlled experiments with EPO but reports that there was no testing method available. However, in reality, he had experimented with professional cyclists of the Carrera Jeans-Tassoni team. Furthermore, it has been revealed that Francesco Conconi has been involved in various doping activities that included providing EPO to numerous athletes. Alessandro DONATI, *Lo Sport Del Doping* (Torino: Edizioni Gruppo Abele, 2012).

[303] Minutes, "Meeting of the IOC Medical Commission in Lillehammer, February 28 to March 2, 1993," 7.

[304] Minutes, "Meeting of the IOC Medical Commission's Subcommission on Doping and Biochemistry, October 25, 1991," 4.

found themselves at the beginning of the 1990s. Whilst they had gained influence through their professional competencies in the domain of doping analysis, they now faced an issue that they could evidently not solve independently of other experts. This resulted in the dilemma to either include additional experts and cede influence/funding, or to leave the usage of blood doping unpunished. They opted for a compromise that included calling on other experts, but that was also a refusal of, in their view, unreliable methods.

The difficulties with the inability to detect blood doping in an athlete's urine along with the consultation of other experts was not the only challenge that the long-established anti-doping laboratory experts faced. After the proposal of the IWG to install an international anti-doping body, it became clear to the IOC Medical Commission that anti-doping initiatives had to become more differentiated. Evidence for this is the establishment of a temporary "Subcommission Out-Of Competition Testing" in December 1991. [305] Significantly, Alexandre de Mérode suggested that the new subcommission would consist of a maximum of fifteen people from various stakeholders of the Olympic Movement (NOCs, government authorities, sports confederations, IFs, IOC).[306] Technical specialists could be consulted if it was necessary.[307] Certainly, the suggestion to establish the body under the umbrella of the IOC enabled Alexandre de Mérode to keep control over the main decision-making processes. Moreover, two of the three IOC representatives were members of the IOC MSD: Manfred Donike and Don Catlin.[308] However, the fact that there was a second anti-doping body within the IOC Medical Commission also caused major concerns amongst the members of the IOC MSD. At the end of 1991, the growing anxiety amongst the anti-doping laboratory experts about losing control over their traditional fields of work becomes most evident. [309] Don Catlin suggested a revision of the GLP to maintain control over the accreditation process, arguing, "the accreditation system is seriously endangered if the deficiencies are not corrected."[310] Actually, Don Catlin faced the difficulty that the GLP was not consistent with the practice pertaining to testing urine in the USA anymore, and

---

[305] DIRIX and STURBOIS, *The First*, 43.

[306] Ibid.

[307] Ibid.

[308] Minutes, "Meeting of the IOC Medical Commission, February 28 to March 2, 1993," Box 106 "Subcommission Doping & Lillehammer," Private Archive Jordi Segura, Barcelona, Annex 1.

[309] Minutes, "Meeting of the IOC Medical Commission's Subcommission on Doping and Biochemistry, October 25, 1991."

[310] Ibid., 3.

he wanted to take into consideration other accreditation systems from outside sport, such as the ones by the National Institute of Drug Abuse in the USA and the Commission of the European Communities. Hence, he had to push for a change in the requirements, or face legal challenges. This demonstrates that general developments within scientific work had to be increasingly considered.[311] The minutes of the same meeting reveal that Manfred Donike was equally concerned about governmental intervention. In line with previous statements, he was of the opinion that the IOC MSD should leave no room for other organisations to step in, and should continue to apply strict and up to date regulations.[312] Hence, whereas the aim for inclusion of the accredited laboratories in the majority of the multinational policy agreements was a significant achievement, it also brought with it more responsibility in terms of strict observance by the GLP.

However, if one briefly considers the exact way of proceeding in the revision of the GLP, different approaches and previously described attitudes become apparent. Because the original suggestion for changes within the GLP came through Don Catlin, the IOC MSD assigned him to circulate a first draft. He complied with this request in December 1991, but he was aware that, "the enclosed document will generate considerable controversy."[313] His main amendments included a further differentiation of the accredited laboratories into various categories, the introduction of inspection visits to check the laboratory work and the participation in external blind quality control programmes. A response letter from Manfred Donike reveals that he did not agree with many of the suggested changes.[314] His main concern focused on the fact that doping analysis in sport differed significantly from other chemical control programmes, which Don Catlin used as the basis of his suggestions. In particular, due to the analysis of two samples, as opposed to urine sample in other areas, Manfred Donike reasoned that more substance-specific data was accumulated and the techniques, thus more informative. Consequently, Manfred Donike saw no need

[311] Letter, "Don Catlin to Alexandre de Mérode, Mary Glen Haig, Arnold Beckett, Manfred Donike, Robert Dugal and Vitaly Semenov, December 23, 1991," Box 106 "Subcommission Doping & Lillehammer," Private Archive Jordi Segura, Barcelona.
[312] Minutes, "Meeting of the IOC Medical Commission's Subcommission on Doping and Biochemistry, October 25, 1991," 3.
[313] Letter, "Don Catlin to Alexandre de Mérode, Mary Glen Haig, Arnold Beckett, Manfred Donike, Robert Dugal and Vitaly Semenov, December 23, 1991."
[314] Notes, "Comments in the draft of 'The IOC Laboratory Doping Control Program', Manfred Donike, June 6, 1992," Box 106 "Subcommission Doping & Lillehammer," Private Archive Jordi Segura, Barcelona.

for stricter regulations and did not agree with amending the GLP to meet regulations outside sport. Specifically, he objected to the classification of laboratories in different categories, outlining that it was:

> not acceptable for the work within the sport area as it was decided earlier by the IOC Medical Commission and its Subcommission either accredited or not accredited and maybe accreditation with some kind of restrictions.[315]

This is an interesting statement because he had previously always favoured a classification system, even introducing it in the original GLP. Hence, it is not surprising that Don Catlin showed considerable confusion in his response.[316] Manfred Donike also opposed an objective blind review of the reaccreditation process and thought that such measures were not applicable. Therefore, he entirely contradicted the intentions of Don Catlin, who even favoured the inclusion of external impartial experts to evaluate the reports from the laboratories.[317] Besides the fact that the disagreement between the two members of the IOC MSD led to a considerable delay in the revision of the GLP, the episode demonstrates that Manfred Donike would only support changes if they could be controlled by the IOC MSD. Implementations such as a blind review process, and the inclusion of external supervisors clearly objected to this attitude, although he generally supported a strict maintenance process. Whereas Don Catlin looked out to other scientific working areas, Manfred Donike opposed this and preferred to stick with the majority of the long-established processes that had been developed solely within the field of sports drug testing. One has to recall at this point that Arnold Beckett had already criticised Manfred Donike for such a narrow approach (see earlier in this chapter). Manfred Donike´s attitude slowed down the development of decisive processes, but due to prior negative experience with stakeholders outside the network of anti-doping laboratory experts, he had good reason to do so. He was not prepared to give away control to external partners.

Finally, with the fall of the Berlin Wall in November 1989, the preconditions for global anti-doping activities also changed for the leading anti-doping laboratory experts. Manfred Höppner was one of the first high-ranked officials to

---

[315] Ibid.

[316] Letter, "Don Catlin to Manfred Donike, June 29, 1992," Box 106 "Subcommission Doping & Lillehammer," Private Archive Jordi Segura, Barcelona.

[317] Ibid.

confess to his role within the GDR´s doping regime in an interview with the magazine *Stern* in November 1990.[318] The revelations were self-motivated and Manfred Höppner took documents to the interview that proved much speculation and caused huge public interest.[319] After the confession, he requested his resignation from all IAAF commissions.[320] However, the IAAF Council was of the opinion that they should not allow him to resign, but instead dismiss him accompanied by a public announcement. As a result, the IAAF Council issued the following statement:

> The Council had considered Dr. Manfred Hoeppner´s admission that he had coordinated a systematic programme of drug abuse. In the light of this, the Council believed that his continued membership in the Medical Committee and in the Doping Commission was entirely inappropriate and that he should be dismissed.[321]

Although the case of the Manfred Höppner did not have a direct effect on the community of the anti-doping laboratory experts, he had worked intensively with Arnold Beckett and Manfred Donike on the IAAF´s doping bodies since the 1970s. The minutes of the first meeting after the revelations read that Manfred Höppner´s occupation of a high position in the echelons of GDR sport and his direct involvement in the systematic doping of sports persons were noted with concern.[322] Interestingly, Manfred Donike remarked that this was not a big loss from a scientific point of view since Manfred Höppner, so Manfred Donike stated, "did not understand the first thing about analytical chemistry."[323] In the case of Claus Clausnitzer, the procedure of the IOC and particularly the IOC MSD was very similar. In November 1989, he had already admitted that there had been exit controls for GDR athletes going to international competitions in his

---

[318] "Doping – Der Beweis. Wie die DDR Sieger machte," *Stern*, November 28, 1990, archive collection "Nachlass August Kirsch," File 090, "Doping (7)," CuLDA, Cologne.
[319] Jutta BRAUN, "'Dopen für Deutschland' – Die Diskussion im vereinten Sport 1990-1992," in: *Hormone und Hochleistung. Doping in Ost und West*, eds. Klaus LATZEL and Lutz NIETHAMMER (Berlin: Böhlau, 2008), 152.
[320] Minutes, "IAAF Council Meeting, January 19, 1991," archive collection "Nachlass August Kirsch," File 123, "IAAF (2)," CuLDA, Cologne, 48.
[321] Ibid., 48.
[322] Minutes, "Meeting of the IAAF Doping Commission, January 11, 1991," 2.
[323] Manfred Donike in HOBERMAN, "How Drug," 251.

laboratory since 1979.[324] As a result, the IOC MSD saw itself not in the position to keep up the membership status for him any longer, and the IOC Medical Commission officially dismissed him in 1990. The IOC MSD replaced Claus Clausnitzer with Jordi Segura.[325]

In addition to personnel consequences, there were concerns about the IOC-accredited laboratory in Kreischa, which Claus Clausnitzer had led. In January 1991, Claus Clausnitzer had still proposed to become increasingly active in the cooperation with other countries and establish its profile as a service institution.[326] In his proposal he wrote that within Europe, the laboratory network was already very extensive but that Kreischa could cooperate with other countries and undertake their doping analyses.[327] By that time, the laboratory had been temporarily shut down, and the IOC MSD did not accredit the laboratory for 1992 because it was not able to carry out the reaccreditation test.[328] The IAAF also included the consequences on the institutional level in its public announcement:

> It should also pointed out that the accredited laboratory in Kreischa had reportedly been involved in these [doping] activities and would therefore not receive any samples for doping analysis from the IAAF until a thorough investigation had been conducted and the IAAF was satisfied that the laboratory could adequately discharge its proper functions.[329]

A process of rehabilitation for the anti-doping laboratory began, following the report of an independent inquiry panel. The so-called "Reiter-Kommission"[330] had been installed by the German Sport Association and the National Olympic

---

[324] Hans Joachim TEICHLER, "Doping in der Endphase der DDR und im Prozess der Wende 1898/90," in: *Hormone und Hochleistung. Doping in Ost und West*, eds. Klaus LATZEL and Lutz NIETHAMMER (Berlin: Böhlau, 2008), 147.

[325] Curiously, he was notified about his appointment in a very informal manner during a meeting of the IOC Medical Commission, when Alexandre de Mérode passed him a paper on which he was asked to join the IOC MSD. Interview with Jordi Segura, May 24, 2013.

[326] Letter, "Claus Clausnitzer to Wolfgang Gitter, January 15, 1990," archive collection "DR 510 Nationales Olympisches Komitee der DDR," folder "DR 510/969, Band 4, Medizinische Kommission des IOC, 1977-1987," Bundesarchiv, Berlin-Lichterfelde.

[327] Ibid

[328] Individual Minutes, "Meetings of the IOC Medical Commission in Albertville, February 9-22, 1992," 16.

[329] Minutes, "IAAF Council Meeting, January 19, 1991," archive collection "Nachlass August Kirsch," File 123, "IAAF (2)," CuLDA, Cologne, 48.

[330] The Commission was named after its Chairman Professor Dr. Heinrich Reiter.

Committee.[331] A specific paragraph of the final report dealt with the further proceedings of the laboratory in Kreischa. Therein, the "Reiter-Kommission" recommended in agreement with a doping working group by the BiSP (which also included Manfred Donike), the maintenance of the Kreischa laboratory.[332] It argued that the existing technical equipment and the well-educated staff members had to stay available for doping analysis in the future, particularly because the number of doping tests would increase significantly with the expansion of the out-of competition tests.[333] In contrast to the upholding of the institution, the main positions of the chemical staff were advertised again. Moreover, the "Reiter-Kommission" recommended that the new institution should have a very specific research focus, namely research into the detection of peptide hormones, which was non-existent in Germany at the time. Hence, it concluded:

> Die Kommission ist der Auffassung, daß das Labor in Kreischa trotz seiner Vergangenheit durch diese Maßnahmen ausreichend Glaubwürdigkeit und Anerkennung erreicht
>
> [The Commission is of the opinion that as result of these measures, the laboratory in Kreischa reaches sufficient credibility and recognition disregarding of its past].[334]

Eventually, the laboratory reopened in March 1992 under the new leadership of Professor Dr. Klaus Müller, and in 1994, the IOC MSD officially reaccredited it.[335]

In summary, there is no doubt that because of the GDR revelations, the credibility of the anti-doping laboratory experts became questioned. In fact, Claus Clausnitzer had contributed to the IOC MSD, the steering body of the anti-doping laboratory network, since its establishment in 1981. He appeared to be a rather

---

[331] In general terms, the "Reiter-Kommission" most importantly proposed a general amnesty for all avowing athletes but not of all parties. BRAUN, "'Dopen für Deutschland'," 153.

[332] "Bericht der Unabhängigen Dopingkommission," June 1991, *Gazetta*; http://www.cycling4fans.de/uploads/media/1991_Bericht_der_Reiter-Kommission_01.pdf [accessed August 28, 2014], 25.

[333] Ibid.

[334] Ibid.

[335] Minutes, "Meeting of the IOC Medical Commission´s Subcommission on Biochemistry and Doping, February 17, 1994," Box 106 "Subcommission Doping & Lillehammer," Private Archive Jordi Segura, Barcelona.

passive member, and did not actively oppose the introduction of new technical equipment, the extension of the laboratory network and the educational efforts. However, he indirectly undermined the work of the IOC MSD by making the information useful to the GDR´s doping regime. His exclusion was not taken as a big loss, but instead allowed the official integration of Jordi Segura, who had already been part of the inner circle of heads of anti-doping laboratories. This was important to the already prevalent key figures because reluctance towards giving away control can also be observed in this phase. This becomes most evident not only on research on blood doping testing techniques, but also Manfred Donike´s opposition to include external measures of quality control. Whereas Don Catlin showed awareness for laboratory guidelines from other areas, Manfred Donike considered his experience from within sports drug testing as more important. This discloses different attitudes on personal and institutional supremacy. In any case, the deceleration in this regard allowed the established anti-doping laboratory experts to maintain the control of the network and the development of testing techniques. This was enhanced through their inclusion in administrative and political roles.

Structural Changes

There is also evidence for structural changes in the global fight against doping, thus affecting the work of the anti-doping laboratory experts, particularly if one considers the processes within the IAAF. This allows a drawing of parallels with the installation of the accreditation procedure at the end of the 1970s, by which time the IAAF already occupied a leading role. Ultimately, it was the first decision, after a meeting of the IOC with all summer sports federations in 1989, that the IAAF officially introduced global out-of competition testing in athletics, while stressing that the most effective measure to combat doping was out-of competition testing.[336] Whereas this decision clearly served the heads of anti-doping laboratories, because it increased the number of doping analyses, the contents of the "IAAF Goteborg Manifesto on Doping," passed by the IAAF Council in April 1989, were more differentiated. [337] Therein, the IAAF summarised its intent to combat doping while emphasising that the aims could only be reached through initiatives on various levels. It intended doping controls as the main tool but also included investments in two main areas.

---

[336] Ibid.

[337] Brochure, "The IAAF Göteborg Manifesto on Doping," archive collection "Nachlass August Kirsch," File 089, "Doping (6)," CuLDA, Cologne.

First, the IAAF Medical Committee under the leadership of Arne Ljungqvist reacted to the growing interest of the media following the Ben Johnson scandal. Previously in 1989, it had begun with the regular execution of a media workshop on anti-doping.[338] At the same time, the IAAF produced a video on all aspects of doping controls that it distributed amongst all athletes, but also made it available to the media.[339] It realised the project by the end of 1990.[340] Moreover, discussions on a wide-ranging public relations campaign started within the IAAF Council at the beginning of the 1990s. This suggestion was made on the instigation of Arne Ljungqvist who revealed that he had been working together with an ex-colleague from the public relations and advertising field to refine the idea.[341] He reasoned that the main points of the campaign were the following:

- This would be the first initiative of its like to be conducted by an international sports authority

- The objectives would be to popularize athletics, to increase anti-doping knowledge, to initiate and develop worldwide national anti-doping programmes, to create a clear anti-doping opinion at all levels and to get new sponsors and organisers to participate actively.

- This would be achieved through a uniform marketing policy.[342]

One can learn from this statement that Arne Ljungqvist was clearly concerned about the bad reputation of athletics. IAAF President Primo Nebiolo perceived the proposal in a positive manner for the exact same reason, as stated in the minutes: "Dr. Nebiolo perceived that this campaign was necessary in order to improve the credibility of athletics."[343] The only argument which hindered an instant start of such a campaign was the proposed costs of around $1 million, and the IAAF Council decided that several sponsors should be approached in order to

---

[338] Minutes, "IAAF Council Meeting, September 3, 1989," archive collection "Nachlass August Kirsch," File 123, "IAAF (2)," CuLDA, Cologne, 5.
[339] Ibid., 6.
[340] Minutes, "IAAF Council Meeting, December 6, 1990," archive collection "Nachlass August Kirsch," File 123, "IAAF (2)," CuLDA, Cologne, 9.
[341] Minutes, "IAAF Council Meeting, January 20, 1990," archive collection "Nachlass August Kirsch," File 123, "IAAF (2)," CuLDA, Cologne, 26.
[342] Ibid.
[343] Ibid., 41.

realise the project.[344] Notwithstanding, it is of major significance that such initiatives were not driven by the anti-doping laboratory experts, but rather by the political level. In fact, the heads of anti-doping laboratories strongly opposed giving insights to the public and the media about all aspects of doping controls. The IOC MSD had actually rejected a proposal to stage a large workshop for the media including a visit to the KIST laboratory before the 1988 Seoul Olympic Games.[345]

Second, the IAAF was quick to integrate juridical experts into its anti-doping approach. Previously in 1989, discussions arose within the IAAF Council to organise a symposium on "sport and law," and planned to make legal procedures within the IAAF's anti-doping affairs a central theme.[346] Finally, the IAAF held an "International Symposium on Sport and the Law" in Monte Carlo in January 1991 and was attended by 177 participants from 27 countries.[347] One of the subjects was entitled "Anti-Doping Procedures and Legal Consequences – Medical and Ethical Factors and Conflicts of Interest." This illustrates that interest in anti-doping matters from the juridical field existed, and lawyers progressively began to challenge the role of anti-doping laboratory experts as the leading epistemic community in global anti-doping affairs. Direct consequences for the work of the anti-doping laboratory experts in anti-doping bodies of sport organisations resulted from this. Whereas their role on the scientific level could of course not be contested, it was in administrative tasks that juridical experts slowly gained influence. This becomes most evident at structural changes regarding the bodies that dealt with anti-doping matters. In 1990, the IAAF dissolved its IAAF Doping Subcommittee and established a new IAAF Doping Commission.[348] This change was provoked by the fact that the previous Subcommission did officially exist within IAAF rules because it only acted as

---

[344] Minutes, "IAAF Council Meeting, June 20, 1990," archive collection "Nachlass August Kirsch," File 123, "IAAF (2)," CuLDA, Cologne, 41.

[345] Originally, the Seoul laboratory planned to stage a five-day workshop plus a symposium on doping control prior to the Olympic Games. The proposal also foresaw the involvement of representatives from the media with detailed insights into the work of the doping laboratory. However, Manfred Donike rejected these. Letter, "Manfred Donike to Moon Hi Han and Jong Sei Park, March 1, 1988," archive collection "Summer and Winter Olympic Games: Medical files," folder "Medical matters and doping controls at the 1988 Seoul Summer Olympic Games: correspondence," IOC Archive, Lausanne.

[346] Minutes, "IAAF Council Meeting, September 3, 1989," archive collection "Nachlass August Kirsch," File 123, "IAAF (2)," CuLDA, Cologne, 7.

[347] INTERNATIONAL ATHLETIC FOUNDATION, *A Review*, 47.

[348] Minutes, "IAAF Council Meeting, January 20, 1990," 22.

working group of the IAAF Medical Committee. According to the IAAF Council, this represented a legal weakness in light of the growing global attention to the doping problem.[349] Importantly, the membership of the new IAAF Doping Commission differed from the previous body. Whereas Arne Ljungqvist, Arnold Beckett, Manfred Donike and Manfred Höppner (until the revelations of the GDR doping system) became members again, the IAAF increased the membership from four to five in order to include a person with knowledge of legal aspects of athletics and doping matters.[350] Hence, a new situation arose for the anti-doping laboratory experts, who now had to discuss all technical and organisational issues, which they had previously debated amongst each other, with a juridical expert. The IAAF Council appointed lawyer Frank Greenberg for this position.[351] The official minutes of the first meetings of the new IAAF Doping Commission reveal that traditional aspects such as the analytical procedures and the official laboratories were still subject to debate. However, discussion on positive doping cases and changes in the overall procedural guidelines of doping controls were increasingly regarded topics to be dealt with by Frank Greenberg. Significantly, the membership of the IAAF Doping Commission had changed again by the beginning of 1992. Neither Manfred Höppner nor Arnold Beckett, whose withdrawal from international anti-doping matters steadily continued, was a member. The IAAF replaced them with Professor Dr. Antonio Dal Monte (Italy) and Dr. Gabriel Dollé (France), both sport medicine specialists.[352] Consequently, by the time of the 1992 Barcelona Olympic Games, Manfred Donike remained the sole representative of the community of anti-doping laboratory experts within the IAAF. Thus, a break-up of the traditional structures becomes obvious.

The developments within the IAAF are exemplary for the processes on the global scale. In fact, the IAAF again occupied a forerunner role in the restructuring of its doping bodies, through the installation of the IAAF Doping Commission and the inclusion of a legal expert. It was only in 1993, when the IOC Medical Commission followed this example by installing a "Juridical Working Group."[353] This can be compared to the processes at the end of the 1970s when anti-doping laboratory experts had an important say within the IAAF.

---

[349] Minutes, "IAAF Council Meeting, April 4, 1989," archive collection "Nachlass August Kirsch," File 123, "IAAF (2)," CuLDA, Cologne, 29.

[350] Minutes, "Meeting of the IAAF Doping Commission, January 5, 1990," 1.

[351] Minutes, "IAAF Council Meeting, January 20, 1990," 22.

[352] Minutes, "IAAF Council Meeting, November 17 and 18, 1991," archive collection "Nachlass August Kirsch," File 123, "IAAF (2)," CuLDA, Cologne, 15.

[353] Minutes, "Meeting of the IOC Medical Commission, February 28 to March 2, 1993," 2.

Having established main testing procedures, an anti-doping laboratory network and educational initiatives for laboratory staff until the mid-1980s, the adoption of administrative roles for influential individuals such as Manfred Donike and Arnold Beckett gave them more power. This allowed them to continue developing the established initiatives. However, particularly with Manfred Donike´s rigorous stance to maintain control over the technical aspects solely within the inner circle of the anti-doping laboratory network, it decelerated certain aspects of the doping fight. Such concerns can be justified with his bad experiences in previous years. Nevertheless, whereas this strategy was partly successful for the technical level, their authority in administrative matters became increasingly challenged. Final decisions on doping offences and lengths of bans were assigned to juridical experts. The structural changes also disclose that the anti-doping laboratory experts became progressively victims of the growing complexity of the doping control system. The establishment of which, they had been instrumental in.

EFFECT ON DOPING CONTROLS AT THE TWO 1992 OLYMPIC GAMES

The processes also had an effect on the role of the anti-doping laboratory experts at the 1992 Olympic Games in Albertville and Barcelona. Thus, this sub-chapter investigates the operations of the anti-doping laboratory experts at the two events. Thereby, one has to acknowledge that the body of source material was not as extensive as it had been for the analysis at previous Olympic Games. In particular, the individual minutes of the meetings of the IOC Medical Commission during the 1992 Barcelona Olympic Games were not available. Despite this limitation, the available documents allow a focus on continuing personnel/structural changes.

Doping Controls at the 1992 Winter Olympic Games in Albertville

In November 1987, the Organising Committee of the 1992 Winter Olympic Games in Albertville assigned Dr. Patrick Schamasch as medial representative to the IOC Medical Commission.[354] The surgeon was the chief medical officer for the Organising Committee and had a professional background in the traumatology of sports. He was also the team doctor of the French ice hockey team.[355] The

---

[354] Letter, "Rémy Charmetant to Alexandre de Mérode, November 23, 1987," archive collection "Summer and Winter Olympic Games: Medical files," folder "Medical matters at the 1992 Albertville Olympic Winter Games: correspondence," IOC Archive, Lausanne.
[355] INTERNATIONAL OLYMPIC COMMITTEE, *Commission Médicale*, 12.

investigated documents leave no doubt that besides his important position in Albertville, Patrick Schamasch also stands exemplary for the ongoing changes. This can be justified with a brief perusal of his involvement after 1992. Due to the growing demands in the fight against doping, the IOC provided the IOC Medical Commission with a permanent secretariat at its headquarters in Lausanne from 1993 onwards.[356] This was an important step in the professionalisation and administration of its activities. Patrick Schamasch became the part-time medical director of the IOC.[357] Despite his professional background in traumatology, the IOC Executive Board considered his appointment a strengthening of "the IOC's activity in the field of medicine, and in particular in the fight against doping."[358] However, he was not only dealing with anti-doping in his new role. His main tasks entailed more generally the management of the secretariat and the support of the working processes of the IOC Medical Commission and its subcommissions. His job suitability was strengthened due to the administrative nature of the role, and the fact that he is bilingual in French and English. The creation of the position was a continuation of the ongoing processes, increasingly moving administrative tasks away from the heads of anti-doping laboratories by the beginning of the 1990s.

The IOC Medical Commission was confronted with two main challenges in the preparation of the doping controls for the 1992 Winter Olympic Games in Albertville. First, the collection of the urine samples posed a particular organisational challenge because the nine competition sites were up to 118 kilometres away from each other.[359] However, the medical teams on-site were very aware of this issue and installed doping control stations at all venues.[360] The challenge of the decentralised system and its adequate and efficient management is also noted in the *Official Report*.[361] Second, as had been the case in Canada, an

---

[356] DIRIX and STURBOIS, *The First*, 19.

[357] Minutes, "Meeting of the IOC Medical Commission, February 28 to March 2, 1993," 1.

[358] "The Executive Board met on 19th and 20th June," *Olympic Review* 309/310 (1993), 301.

[359] KLUGE, *Olympische Winterspiele*, 453. The 1992 Winter Olympic Games in Albertville are considered an environmental disaster due to the considerable intervention into the Alpine nature and irreparable damages on the biosphere.

[360] Letter, "Bruce Challis to Alexandre de Mérode, December 17, 1990," archive collection "Summer and Winter Olympic Games: Medical files," folder "Medical matters at the 1992 Albertville Olympic Winter Games: correspondence," IOC Archive, Lausanne.

[361] ORGANISING COMMITTEE OF THE XXVITH WINTER OLYMPIC GAMES, *Official Report of the 16th Winter Olympic Games in Albertville* (Albertville: Organising Committee of the XXVITH Winter Olympic Games, 1993), 219.

accredited anti-doping laboratory already existed in France (Paris) and hence it was feared that questions of authority would arise again. These concerns were underlined by the fact that in 1988, Patrick Schamasch reported that the Organising Committee deemed the laboratory in Paris too small and favoured the establishment of another doping testing centre in Lyon.[362] Nevertheless, although there was eventually an initiative in Lyon and its laboratory entered the pre-accreditation phase in 1990,[363] the French government strongly pushed the utilisation of the anti-doping laboratory in Paris. By no means did it want to create a political controversy such as the one before the previous Winter Olympic Games in Canada. In April 1990, the Secretariat for Youth and Sport (Sécretariat d´État à la Jeunesse et aux Sport, SEJS) officially nominated the anti-doping laboratory in Paris under the direction of Jean-Pierre Lafarge and IAAF Medical Committee member Gabriel Dollé to undertake the doping analysis at the 1992 Winter Olympic Games.[364] The IOC MSD accepted this proposal in February 1991.[365] Yet, the late date was, due to the already existing accreditation and the continuing success of Jean-Pierre Lafarge and his team in the reaccreditation procedure, not considered a big problem.[366] Nevertheless, some organisational problems remained. In order to undertake the doping analysis on site, the IOC MSD requested the laboratory to transport its equipment to the Alpine region. Eventually, in collaboration with Patrick Schamasch, a central location in an old hospital in Moûtiers was found.[367] Therefore, for the first time since the 1980 Winter Olympic Games in Lake Placid, the Organising Committee temporarily

---

[362] Minutes, "Meetings of the IOC Medical Commission, February 9-28, 1988," 19.

[363] Minutes, "Meeting of the IAAF Doping Commission, January 11, 1991," Annex 1.

[364] Letter, "Roger Bambuck to Juan Antonio Samaranch, April 27, 1990," archive collection "Summer and Winter Olympic Games: Medical files," folder "Medical matters at the 1992 Albertville Olympic Winter Games: correspondence," IOC Archive, Lausanne.

[365] Report, "Rapport d´Activites du Laboratoire Charge des Analyses Anti-Dopage by Jean-Pierre Lafarge, February 1992," "Summer and Winter Olympic Games: Medical files," folder "Medical matters at the 1992 Albertville Olympic Winter Games: activity reports (Medical Commission, anti-doping laboratory), reports on gender verification and on the World Congress on Sports Science," IOC Archive, Lausanne, 1.

[366] Minutes, "Meeting of the IOC Medical Commission´s Subcommission on Doping and Biochemistry, October 25, 1991."

[367] Report, Rapport d´Activites du Laboratoire Charge des Analyses Anti-Dopage" by Jean-Pierre Lafarge, February 1992." 1.

established an accredited laboratory at an Olympic site.[368] The finalisation of the laboratory in Moûtiers was only reached by the end of January 1992, and the late move of the equipment and instruments from Paris to Albertville caused complications with the reaccreditation process, which always took place at the beginning of the year. Eventually, the Paris laboratory and the facilities in Moûtiers received their reaccreditation at the end of January 1992.[369] The IOC MSD perceived the outcome favourably, as an accredited anti-doping laboratory undertook the doping analyses.

In total, the doping control officers took 523 urine samples.[370] The laboratory team analysed the samples with similar equipment to that in 1988. In this context, one has to remember, that despite the addition of EPO to the list of banned substances in 1989, no reliable detection method for blood doping was available yet. It used GC-MS as screening method with three types of screening: diuretics and masking agents, beta-blockers, anabolic steroids. It was the first time that a laboratory tested for diuretics as masking agents at Olympic Games because there was increased evidence for its usage.[371] Overall, the laboratory reported six positive findings to the IOC Medical Commission. However, these were the quality control samples of the IOC MSD, and therefore none of the urine samples of the 1992 Winter Olympic Games in Albertville were officially declared positive, whilst the IOC MSD praised the laboratory for its technical standards.[372]

Despite the apparently smooth conduction of the doping controls and the analytical procedures, the case of the Russian biathlete Sergei Tarasov demands closer investigation. A favourite in the biathlon competitions, he had to be hospitalised shortly before the start of his first event with what the Russian team

---

[368] Following the 1992 Winter Olympic Games in Albertville, this was to be the case in Atlanta (1996; laboratories in Indianapolis and Los Angeles in charge), Nagano (1998; laboratory in Tokyo in charge), Salt Lake City (2002; laboratory in Los Angeles in charge) and in Torino (2006; laboratory in Rome in charge).

[369] Fax, "Alexandre de Mérode to Manfred Donike, December 17, 1991," archive collection "Summer and Winter Olympic Games: Medical files," folder "Medical matters at the 1992 Albertville Olympic Winter Games: activity reports (Medical Commission, anti-doping laboratory), reports on gender verification and on the World Congress on Sports Science," IOC Archive, Lausanne.

[370] Report, "Rapport d'Activites du Laboratoire Charge des Analyses Anti-Dopage by Jean-Pierre Lafarge, February 1992," 10. The number differs from the 552 samples reported in CLASING, *Doping*, 170.

[371] Minutes, "Meeting of the IOC Medical Commission, February 28 to March 2, 1993," 2.

[372] Ibid.

doctors claimed to be a life-threatening food poisoning case.[373] The athlete had severe kidney failure and had to be treated with a kidney dialysis. However, several team doctors suspected that the complications did not arise from food poisoning, but were the result of blood doping instead.[374] Significantly, when the IOC Medical Commission members raised concerns, Patrick Schamasch and Alexandre de Mérode adopted a very reluctant stance concerning detailed investigations into the case. Whereas Alexandre de Mérode referred to problematic legal issues if the IOC Medical Commission were to investigate into the condition of a Russian athlete on French territory,[375] Patrick Schamasch claimed that the duty of the IOC Medical Commission, as well as the doctors, was, "to save the athlete´s life and not to analyse whether or not he had been blood doped."[376] He also appeared concerned about other members of the Olympic family, such as the IOC Athletes´ Commission, to deal with the issue.[377] This attitude is surprising because blood doping and possible methods of detection had been subject to intensive debate during the meetings of the IOC Medical Commission in Albertville. Although the mystery surrounding the case of Sergei Tarasov cannot be solved, it gives evidence to the complications regarding the detection of blood doping. In addition to this, Alexandre de Mérode´s reference to legal aspects proves that he increasingly sought juridical advice at the time.

Finally, it is important to emphasise that the continuing involvement of Patrick Schamasch was not the only personnel change to the IOC Medical Commission after the 1992 Winter Olympic Games in Albertville. Robert Dugal also left his position in the IOC MSD, so that after the dismissal of Claus Clausnitzer yet another of the five original members had to be replaced. The official reason for Robert Dugal´s resignation was his new position in the private pharmacological industry.[378] Thus, the withdrawal of the long established anti-doping laboratory experts from the official bodies continued.

In addition, a further aspect should be mentioned, which found continuation at the Albertville Games and gives evidence to a more multi-faceted approach to

---

[373] David WALLECHINSKY and Jaime LOUCKY, *The Complete Book of the Winter Olympics: The Vancouver 2010 Edition* (Vancouver: Greystone Books, 2009), 287.

[374] Individual Minutes, "Meetings of the IOC Medical Commission in Albertville, February 9-22, 1992," 15.

[375] Ibid., 25.

[376] Ibid., 15.

[377] Ibid., 25.

[378] Minutes, "Meeting of the IOC Medical Commission, November 30, 1992," archive collection "IOC Medical Commission," IOC Archive, Lausanne, 12.

combat doping: for the first time in Olympic history, the IOC Athletes'
Commission published a brochure with information on anti-doping.[379] Therein, it
also introduced its workshop on anti-doping, which it had organised for the first
time in Calgary in 1988.[380] This is proof for the continuation of increased
educational initiatives from the side of the athletes. Moreover, the IWG had
already made education the theme of its "Third Permanent World Conference on
Anti-Doping," previously staged in September 1991. The discussions during the
Conference revealed that athletes could play a vital role in the development of
educational anti-doping initiatives. The final declaration reflects this, identifying
various areas where educational initiatives could be implemented:

> - The need for more social research studies, particularly to determine
> those factors that influence an athlete to use drugs;
>
> - the need to collaborate with athletes when developing anti-doping
> strategies,
>
> - the need to work with experts in education;
>
> - the need to provide professional training for potential educators,
> particularly coaches
>
> - the need to start educating athletes at a young age;
>
> - the need to assess the effectiveness of anti-doping programmes;
>
> - the need to incorporate the ethical issue in anti-doping programmes.[381]

Although the Conference acknowledged additional "grey areas," where it
included a rapid reaction to possible new forms of abuse such as new substances

---

[379] Brochure, "Die Athletenkommission des IOC," archive collection "Summer and Winter
Olympic Games: Medical files," folder "Medical matters at the 1992 Albertville Olympic
Winter Games: correspondence and notifications," IOC Archive, Lausanne.

[380] Minutes, "Athletes' Seminar in Calgary, February 23, 1988," archive collection
"Athletes' Commission," folder "Athletes' Commission: reports, statement, seminar, press
releases, press cuttings and leaflets of the commission," IOC Archive, Lausanne.

[381] Minutes, "Meeting of the International Working Group on Anti-Doping in Sport (IWG),
September 21-23, 1991," archive collection "IOC Medical Commission," IOC Archive,
Lausanne, Annex 5.

and methods,[382] the declaration demonstrates the more wide-ranging approach to combat the doping problem. Because the discussions at the conference revealed that the athlete´s environment, in terms of coaches, sport administrators and media representatives contributed heavily to the problem of doping, it identified the demands on athletes by modern society as the topic for a planned fourth Conference in 1993.[383] Ultimately, the "Fourth Permanent World Conference on Anti-Doping" focused on "The Social Context of Doping."[384] This is not to say that the members of the IOC MSD did not participate in the conferences. They contributed to both conferences through Manfred Donike and Don Catlin,[385] but doping testing was clearly not the main emphasis.

In summary, one can therefore observe two continuing developments from the 1992 Winter Olympic Games in Albertville, which are both linked to the increasing differentiation within global anti-doping activities. First, educational initiatives became more important. Certainly, this posed a problem for the heads of the anti-doping laboratories, who had received the majority of the research funds for anti-doping matters until the beginning of the 1990s. The increasing recommendations to invest into social research projects such as "factors that led athletes to take drugs" and "social pressures," composed a threat to their monopoly.[386] Second, the structural and personnel changes also continued with the introduction of an IOC medical director and the turnover within the membership of the IOC MSD. The installation of Patrick Schamasch on a permanent basis also undermined the role of Alexandre de Mérode.

Doping Controls at the 1992 Barcelona Olympic Games: Arnold Beckett vs. the IOC MSD

Barcelona has the unique status of being the first host city of Summer Olympic Games since the introduction of the doping controls in 1968 to install an anti-doping laboratory years prior to staging the event (see earlier in this chapter). Due to Jordi Segura´s experience and involvement, no considerable quality concerns arose. Obviously, the IOC MSD regarded this favourably in light of the increasing public attention to the doping issue, and the resulting pressure to

---

[382] Ibid.

[383] Ibid., 2.

[384] THE SPORTS COUNCIL, *The Fourth Permanent World Conference on Anti-Doping in Sport* (London: The Sports Council with the International Olympic Committee, 1993).

[385] Ibid., 247.

[386] Minutes, "Meeting of the International Working Group on Anti-Doping in Sport (IWG), September 21-23, 1991," 4.

deliver correct analytical results. Hence, the extension of the leading circle of heads of anti-doping laboratories resulted in a more straightforward preparation of the doping controls at the Olympic Games for the first time.

Other than conducting regular doping controls, the Barcelona laboratory also positioned itself as a consulting institution on the international testing market. In this context, it is important to take into consideration that all official laboratories were in a competitive situation, and that there was another IOC-accredited laboratory in Spain (Madrid), which was mainly used by Spanish sports federations. Hence, the Barcelona anti-doping laboratory adopted an outreach approach for samples, while the ongoing developments of increased testing and the political desire to have a global distribution of doping laboratories favoured this strategy. Besides the training of a chemist from Rio de Janeiro, the preparation of the anti-doping laboratory for the 1991 Pan American Games in Havana (Cuba) was amongst its first major international tasks. Although there had already been strong interest from an institution in Havana to secure official accreditation in 1989, this initiative fell foul of the increasingly compelling technical regulations.[387] Actually, in February 1991, six months ahead of the event, the IOC MSD no longer had contact with the Organising Committee regarding the anti-doping laboratory facilities.[388] As a result, the IOC MSD decided that the Barcelona anti-doping laboratory should take the initiative and actively seek the cooperation.[389] One reason for this was that it was, together with the anti-doping laboratory in Madrid, the only official institution in a Spanish speaking country. According to Alexandre de Mérode, the doping controls at the 1991 Pan American Games were eventually successful, largely due to the efforts of the staff of the Barcelona anti-doping laboratory, which he praised for "the mobility and efficient work." [390] One has to consider this initiative a groundbreaking development. In previous cases, the IOC MSD would have raised major doubts if the laboratory staff of the upcoming Olympic Games became involved with other projects so shortly before the Games. This was not the case this time and it demonstrates how well-advanced the Barcelona laboratory was in

---

[387] Minutes, "Meeting of the IOC Medical Commission's Subcommission Doping and Biochemistry of Sport, February 6, 1989," Annex 2.
[388] Minutes, "Meeting of the IOC Medical Commission in Albertville, February 9-11, 1991," archive collection "IOC Medical Commission," IOC Archive, Lausanne, Annex 4.
[389] Minutes, "Meeting of the IOC Medical Commission in Barcelona, October 27-29, 1991," archive collection "IOC Medical Commission," IOC Archive, Lausanne, 11.
[390] Ibid.

1991.[391] The official report of Kenneth Fitch, who observed the medical facilities some months before the start of the competitions, confirms this finding.[392]

Despite the additional focus on the training of other laboratories, the doping analysis during the 1992 Barcelona Olympic Games ran smoothly. It received 1,871 samples, with athletics (248) and volleyball (144) undertaking the most doping controls.[393] Although this was not the highest total number of samples at Olympic Games, the more than 40,000 conducted analyses demonstrate that the analytical procedures rose considerably in quantity and set a new record for analyses.[394] The large laboratory team of 80 employees, plus 45 graduates in pharmacy and chemistry, who volunteered for three months,[395] is further evidence for this. In terms of the technical equipment, the laboratory staff used thirteen GC-MS instruments for the screening and the confirmation procedures of the anabolic steroids and non-volatile stimulants, beta-blockers and narcotics.[396] Due to the extensive research, which had taken place at the Barcelona laboratory since its accreditation and led to 18 published scientific papers and 47 presentations at international congresses and symposia ahead of the Olympic Games,[397] there were also minor technical advancements. HEMMERSBACH reports that for the first time, the staff used liquid chromatography-mass spectrometry (LC-MS) with a particle beam interface and a quadruple as the MS detector to confirm diuretics and labile compounds.[398]

---

[391] Significantly, following the Olympic Games, the laboratory continued to pursue the strategy of supporting laboratories all over the globe to become accredited. It was actively involved in the set-up of official testing centres in Rio de Janeiro, Istanbul, Bangkok, Mexico City and Doha. Interview with Jordi Segura, May 24, 2013.

[392] Report, "Report to the IOC Medical Commission on the Inspection of the Barcelona Medical Facilities," archive collection "Summer and Winter Olympic Games: Medical files," folder "JO/BARCELONE 1992/MEDICAL," IOC Archive, Lausanne.

[393] Report, "Antidoping Laboratory - Report of Activities. Games of the XXV Olympiad Barcelona '92," Private Archive Jordi Segura, Barcelona, 156f.

[394] Minutes, "Meeting of the IOC Medical Commission, February 28 to March 2, 1993," 4.

[395] Report, "Antidoping Laboratory - Report of Activities. Games of the XXV Olympiad Barcelona '92."

[396] Jordi SEGURA, Rafael DE LA TORRE, José Antonio PASCUAL, Rosa VENTURA, Magi FARRÉ, Robert EWIN and Jordi CAMI, "Antidoping control at the games of the XXV Olympiad Barcelona '92. Part II," in: *Recent Advances in Doping Analysis – Proceedings of the 12th Cologne Workshop*, eds. Manfred DONIKE, Hans GEYER, Andrea GOTZMANN and Ute MARECK-ENGELKE (Cologne: Sportverlag Strauß, 1995), 413.

[397] Minutes, "Meeting of the IOC Medical Commission, February 28 to March 2, 1993," 4.

[398] HEMMERSBACH, "History," 844.

According to the official report of Jordi Segura, the laboratory staff detected fifteen positive samples.[399] However, after the evaluation of the results and the hearings of the delegations, the members did not consider all cases positive. In particular, there were five cases of over-the-counter products, where the concentration in the urine only indicated a therapeutic use for the following substances: ephedrine derivatives, dihydrocodeine, caffeine and codeine (twice). [400] Such differentiated results were a consequence of the more sophisticated testing techniques. The laboratory also correctly detected and identified the five control samples of the IOC MSD. Consequently, the number of definite positive cases was five. These urine samples belonged to the following athletes: marathon runner Madina Biktagirova (Unified Team[401], norephedrine), volleyballer Wu Dan (China, strychnine), long jumper Nijole Medvedeva (Lithuania, mescocarb), shot putter Bonnie Dasse and hammer thrower Jud Logan (both USA, both clenbuterol).[402] There had also been three cases of a T/E ratio higher than six, but lower than ten, and the IOC Medical Commission decided not to disqualify these athletes.[403]

Despite the lack of documentation available, it is important to subject the doping cases of the two American athletes, who tested positive for clenbuterol, to critical scrutiny. This becomes necessary due to the resulting conflict between Arnold Beckett and the other members of the IOC MSD. In fact, the actual controversy surrounding clenbuterol had already begun ahead of the Olympic Games on July 11 and 12, when the British weightlifters Andrew Saxton and Andrew Davies were subject to out-of competition controls of the British Amateur Weightlifters Association (BAWLA). The analysis of the samples, undertaken by the laboratory at the KCL, showed that both of them contained clenbuterol. As a result, David Cowan, who had become the director of the KCL laboratory in 1990, reported the two cases to the Sports Council and stated that

---

[399] Report, "Antidoping Laboratory - Report of Activities. Games of the XXV Olympiad Barcelona '92," 156f.

[400] Ibid.

[401] Previously in Albertville, a Unified Team (Equipe Unifée) consisting of athletes of the former USSR, participated in the Olympic Games. For Barcelona, the Unified Team included athletes from ten Commonwealth of Independent States (CIS) and Georgia. KLUGE, *Olympische Sommerspiele. Die Chronik III*, 576n24.

[402] Bill MALLON and Ian BUCHANAN, *Historical Dictionary*, 371.

[403] Minutes, "Meeting of the IOC Medical Commission, February 28 to March 2, 1993," 4.

clenbuterol was both a stimulant and an anabolic agent.[404] However, at the time of the analysis, the two athletes were already at the Olympic village. Hence, a highly problematic issue arose because the BAWLA had to withdraw the athletes from Olympic competitions and ban them from the Olympic village. At this point, Arnold Beckett appeared as defender of the athletes. He thought that David Cowan should not have reported the appearance of clenbuterol in the samples. According to him, it did not belong to the class of anabolic androgenic steroids as stated in the IOC rules.[405] This was an important detail, because had it been regarded purely as a stimulant, IOC rules would have permitted its use in training. Arnold Beckett declared that he had objected to this rule before but backed down to the pressure of the other members. Whilst he accepted that clenbuterol was pharmacologically related to anabolic steroids, he thought that it was not related to androgenic anabolic steroids in tests conducted in men. The two British athletes in their proceedings against David Cowan later picked up this argument.[406] Importantly, the BOA appealed against the decision following Arnold Beckett's advice, and subsequently the IOC MSD debated the case. Manfred Donike and Don Catlin did not agree with Arnold Beckett and strongly pushed for a disqualification of the athletes. According to them, the performance-enhancing effect of clenbuterol for weightlifters was obvious. Eventually, they were successful and the IOC Medical Commission banned clenbuterol.[407] It reasoned that the list of banned substances was only a list of examples, and thus many unspecified substances were banned because of their chemical or pharmacological relationship to named banned substances. The majority of the IOC MSD believed Clenbuterol one such case because it was an anabolic agent and an extremely potent β_2-agonist with a stimulatory effect.[408] Arnold Beckett believed the transference of β_2-agonists into the class of androgenic anabolic steroids by the sports organisations to be a "big intellectual jump," with which he did not agree.[409] Importantly, the IAAF Doping Commission, of which Arnold Beckett was not a member anymore, supported the decision. These discussions

---

[404] Letter, "Herbert Smith to Don Catlin, August 20, 1997," archive collection "Summer and Winter Olympic Games: Medical files," folder "JO/BARCELONE 1992/MEDICAL," IOC Archive, Lausanne.

[405] Martin CHILDS, "Professor Arnold Beckett: Sports doping expert who later changed sides and supported those accused of drug use," *The Independent*, March 29, 2010.

[406] Letter, "Herbert Smith to Don Catlin, August 20, 1997."

[407] Ibid.

[408] Letter, "Bryan Wotton, September 3, 1992," archive collection "Nachlass August Kirsch," File 114 "Doping/Hochleistungssport (3)," CuLDA, Cologne.

[409] Arnold BECKETT, "Clenbuterol and sport," *Lancet* 340 (1992), 1165.

formed the basis for the declaration of the two American athletes Bonnie Dasse and Jud Logan at the Olympic Games.

Moreover, the reasoning by the majority of the IOC MSD caused Arnold Beckett also to advance the previously stated reason that Manfred Donike, who was for him the key figure behind the suspension of the athletes, was "only" a biochemist without broad and advanced pharmaceutical knowledge. [410] He received support from Joseph Keul, who also accused Manfred Donike and the IOC Medical Commission's Chairman Alexandre de Mérode of making uninformed decisions following the Barcelona Games. [411] A positive test of German athlete Katrin Krabbe for clenbuterol caused the involvement of German officials and sports medical experts. [412] This episode provides additional evidence for the fact that the expanded list of banned substances due to more sophisticated testing techniques resulted in more controversies. For clenbuterol, this was the case even amongst the leading anti-doping laboratory experts. Consequently, the aftermath of the much-debated and widely publicised clenbuterol case during the 1992 Barcelona Olympic Games encouraged the critics of Manfred Donike to combine efforts. In fact, there has been (unproven) speculation that Arnold Beckett's fallout was caused by his proximity and involvement with the pharmaceutical industry. [413] It remains unclear whether this really contributed to the final fallout with the IOC MSD. However, it is evident that in view of the difficult relationship between Arnold Beckett and Manfred Donike at the beginning of the 1990s, one can also attribute the controversy to their previous bitter altercations about authorities and expertise. Such was the extent of the dispute and growing personal animosities that it was Arnold Beckett's last involvement with the IOC Medical Commission, because he left the body following the 1992 Barcelona Olympic Games.

Although the limited body of source material only allows an incomplete picture of the anti-doping laboratory experts at the 1992 Barcelona Olympic Games to be drawn, it led to three significant findings. First, the clenbuterol cases

---

[410] Randy HARVEY, "Drug Dispute Might Alter Suspensions: Clenbuterol: Logan and Dasse could benefit from experts' differences on whether stimulant also has anabolic effects," *Los Angeles Times*, November 14, 1992.

[411] "Jeden Dreck, jeden Blödsinn reingehauen," *Der Spiegel*, September 14, 1992.

[412] KRÜGER et al., *Doping und Anti-Doping*, 152f.

[413] Following his retirement from his work on the medical bodies of sports organisations in general and the IOC Medical Commission in particular, Arnold Beckett started a successful business career. He linked up wth one of his former students and founder of Vitabiotics, Dr. Kartar Lalvani and become the company's a non-executive chairman for 18 years. CHILDS, "Professor Arnold Beckett."

before and during the Games marked the end of an era in the history of the anti-doping laboratory experts within the Olympic Movement. Arnold Beckett was involved from the establishment of the IOC Medical Commission in 1967, and represented the anti-doping laboratory experts from then onwards. Moreover, since Vitaly Semenov also retired from his position on the IOC MSD,[414] only Manfred Donike remained from its long lasting composition. Second, a consequence of the clenbuterol controversy was that the IOC MSD was unsuccessful in its attempt to regain its credibility in the public eye. On the contrary, the debate amongst themselves triggered even more mistrust in its work and consequently also the anti-doping laboratory experts. Third, it becomes evident that the general character of the Barcelona anti-doping laboratory, through its outreach approach and the involvement of Jordi Segura in the IOC MSD, reflects the ongoing developments of alteration and expansion within the community of the anti-doping laboratory.

INTERIM RESULTS FOR THE PERIOD 1985-1992: FROM CONTINUATION OF ESTABLISHED PROCESSES TO WITHDRAWAL OF KEY FIGURES

The implied challenges of the anti-doping laboratory experts′ initiatives, mainly within the framework of the IOC MSD, continued in the period between 1985 and 1992. Two main tasks can be identified in this regard: the attempts to regulate the extending anti-doping laboratory network through the introduction of administrative processes and more positive doping tests resulting in differences with leading sport administrators. However, the political agility of Alexandre de Mérode especially, but also the contribution of single anti-doping laboratory experts to decision-making processes supported the IOC MSD to maintain a highly significant position within Olympic anti-doping policy.

The anti-doping laboratory network benefited from this position, because the number of doping tests increased and public authorities allocated considerable amounts of research funding to the field of doping analysis. For example, in Germany, the budget estimate for doping analysis increased threefold.[415] On the international level, the effect is just as significant: from 1986 until 1992 the number of doping tests analysed by the IOC-accredited anti-doping laboratories

---

[414] Minutes, "Meeting of the IOC Medical Commission in Lillehammer, February 28 to March 2, 1993," 1.

[415] KRÜGER et al., *Doping und Anti-Doping*, 121.

increased from 32,982 to 87,808.[416] The most influential anti-doping laboratory experts, the members of the IOC MSD, sustained their administrative roles and continued to tighten measures within their specific sphere of activity through the introduction of stricter regulations for anti-doping laboratories, such as a regular reaccreditation procedure and the introduction of the "Code of Ethics," the development of more sophisticated analytical methods and the expansion of educational undertakings for laboratory staff. It also allowed them to support the increasing urgency for worldwide out-of competition testing to further improve the doping control system through their participation in political debates where even more external stakeholders participated. The anti-doping laboratory experts' professional expertise in doping analysis was required in these meetings because of its inevitable necessity for the doping control system. Thus, the processes they had created by convincing Alexandre de Mérode to install the IOC MSD, along with their subsequent work in the IOC MSD, became the prerequisite for even more relevance. Certainly, such inclusion also served their intention to obtain more research funds and financial resources for the execution of the doping analyses.

Whilst these necessary measures were a continuation of the established procedures, and mirrored the intentions of the anti-doping laboratory experts to expand and improve the doping control system, such commendable developments did not result in long-term success. For example, despite evidence for the wide-ranging usage of blood doping, efforts to develop a testing procedure appeared to be undertaken only with limited willingness. One explanation for this was a lack of expertise by the leading and long-standing experts such as Manfred Donike and Arnold Beckett in this scientific field. They appear to have been reluctant to actively engage with experts in detecting substances in blood.

However, the established procedures by the anti-doping laboratory experts, such as the high-quality anti-doping laboratory in Seoul, and sophisticated analytical methods for traditional substances such as anabolic steroids, also added to Ben Johnson's conviction. In this regard, one has to emphasise especially Manfred Donike's line of argument of reducing the Canadian delegation's defence to absurdity. Consequently, one has to consider the positive doping test of Ben Johnson as the peak of the anti-doping laboratory experts' work. However, Ben Johnson scandal had such a big impact that it also resulted in consequences for the anti-doping laboratory experts. It revealed to the public, and to governments, the extent of the doping problem in sport. The investigations of the

---

[416] Oliver DE HON, Harm KUIPERS and Maarten VAN BOOTENBURG, "Prevalance of Doping Use in Elite Sports: A Review of Numbers and Methods," *Sports Medicine* 45 (2015), 60.

Commission of Inquiry gave evidence for this assumption, while not refraining from unveiling the monopolistic role IOC MSD members. Those members continued with their administrative efforts nonetheless, since it perceived an increased standardisation necessary to deal with the rising demands on their field of work. This eventually led to the introduction of the GLP, who essentially summarised all important aspects defining high-quality anti-doping laboratory work and foresaw that accredited institutions increase the quality of their procedures. The instrument of control became the annual reaccreditation process for all official laboratories from 1989 onwards. However, the progressively greater involvement of governments and governmental organisations resulted in a more differentiated approach to the doping problem. It implicated in a growing awareness of the need for more educational and preventative measures, and the inclusion of juridical experts to deal with questions regarding bans. Within their own area of activities, the established key figures were increasingly forced to include other individuals too. This accounts in particular for the inclusion of more influential heads of anti-doping laboratories, such as Jordi Segura and Don Catlin, the latter attempting to include procedures from outside the world of sport to match up with standards from other scientific areas. In this period, Manfred Donike appeared to be reluctant to give away degrees of control, thus causing hesitations in implementation processes. Eventually, all of the developments contributed to structural changes within the anti-doping bodies of the leading sport organisations: the IAAF dissolved its Doping Subcommittee and the IOC installed medical director Patrick Schamasch. The withdrawal of influential and merited anti-doping laboratory experts, such as Robert Dugal and Arnold Beckett from the IOC MSD, also forced a change in power structure.

The phase between 1985 and 1992, where the long-standing anti-doping laboratory experts evidently had most political relevancy, also signifies another structural change. Their determining influence, beginning with the foundation of the IOC MSD, enabled them to advance the IOC's anti-doping activities, and they left a legacy from the investigated period. This accounts for the testing techniques, the GLP and the educational initiatives for laboratory staff, but most importantly for the institutional network of IOC-accredited anti-doping laboratories. However, it appears that by the beginning of the 1990s, they were unable to maintain a degree of control over all aspects of the doping control system any longer. Whilst their professional expertise was still needed to uphold the quality of doping analysis, the increasing complexity of anti-doping affairs caused structural changes.

CHAPTER 8

Conclusions

For the first time in sport historical research, this book has addressed the contribution of anti-doping laboratory experts to the IOC's fight against doping in a monograph with the support of multi-national and multi-lingual historical sources. The basis for the research were the documents on the IOC Medical Commission, obtained from the IOC archive in Lausanne but also the comprehensive material of August Kirsch's estate at the archive of the DSHS. With the aid of these documents, a large amount of these having been hitherto unknown to historical doping research, this books illustrates that sport organisations increasingly depended on a small group of anti-doping laboratory experts to pursue an anti-doping policy, based on reliable scientific evidence in doping testing from 1967 until 1992. Hence, it is not sufficient to only focus on political aspects if one aims to give a complete account of the IOC's fight against doping, so this publication is an expansion of previously undertaken research. This research points out that interpretations on the history of anti-doping are only possible in light of the significant role of the anti-doping laboratory experts and their efforts on the IOC MSD. Therefore, it is necessary to distinguish between the IOC Medical Commission and the IOC MSD in future research on global anti-doping history. In order to avoid monocausal conclusions in the context of the overall history of anti-doping, an examination of several levels was undertaken. For that reason, the study focused on the involved individuals, their institutions and their work on the relevant sport organisations. Most processes were centered on two key figures, namely Arnold Beckett and Manfred Donike, who were at the heart of the investigations.

The involvement and contribution of the anti-doping laboratory experts to the anti-doping bodies of sport organisations went through several phases. Whereas it has been demonstrated that sport medicine specialists already dealt with doping, its definition and its effects from the 1950s onwards, anti-doping laboratory experts did not take part in discussions on the issue until the mid-1960s. By that time, a shift in sport medicine had taken place, which went from considering sport solely as a source to gain data for human physiology research to supporting competitive sport. [1] Significantly however, parallel to the increased medical interest in doping in the 1950s and 1960s, extensive developments in pharmacy and biochemistry had been made to detect substances in bodily fluids. This allowed experts to develop competencies and methods in doping analysis, which made it considerably easier to install doping tests towards the end of the 1960s. However, only with the installation of the IOC Medical Commission in 1967 and the opening of the doping fight to *external* sport medicine specialists and Arnold Beckett, who had developed the analytical procedures for the doping controls at the 1966 FIFA World Cup, did the involvement of a then single anti-doping laboratory expert begin. Hence, this marks the beginning of the first phase of individual consultancy. Arnold Beckett benefited from the IOC Medical Commission's policy, geared towards a strict doping control system, for which reliable doping analysis was inevitable.

Because of the lack of personal medical and chemical understanding, the IOC Medical Commission's chairman Alexandre de Mérode relied heavily upon Arnold Beckett's consultancy in technical matters in the early years of the IOC Medical Commission's work. With his scientific competencies in the field of doping analysis, he contributed heavily to the establishment of the global doping control system. The investigation reveals that he adopted a pioneering role in this field. Sport historical research has ignored this significant aspect to date. One has to look beyond the person of Alexandre de Mérode in order to understand the personal motivations of the individuals involved in the global fight against doping. In fact, Arnold Beckett's scientific knowledge and experience from prior sporting events were essential for the installation of the first official Olympic doping controls in 1968. He had direct contact with the laboratory team in Mexico City, and was in charge of the preparation of the testing centre. Importantly, it was at the often-omitted 1968 Winter Olympic Games in Grenoble where official doping controls took place for the first time in an Olympic context. However, such as at the following 1968 Mexico City Olympic Games, the analytical aspects of the doping controls were not considered of major importance.

This changed entirely with the installation of the first standardised doping controls and anti-doping laboratory at the 1972 Munich Olympic Games. Manfred Donike activated this development in particular, who contributed immensely to intensive preparations of the doping controls, and especially doping analysis in a professional laboratory environment. Similar to Arnold Beckett,

---

[1] WADDINGTON, "The Development," 185.

Manfred Donike used his scientific expertise to advance doping analysis. The supervisor of the medical controls in Munich, Gottfried Schönholzer, who perceived the entire IOC Medical Commission counterproductively, also emphasised this. His detailed account on the problems within the Olympic anti-doping system is a decidedly early indication for the evolving significance of anti-doping laboratory expertise beyond the technical level. He distinguishes clearly between the role of anti-doping laboratory experts and the attitudes and competencies of sport medicine specialists and sport administrators. Such a distinction should be made in future research as one has to carefully consider the professional competencies of all doping controllers in order to avoid generalisations.

In fact, a network of laboratory experts and institutions did not exist at the beginning of the 1970s. There were attempts to standardise analytical procedures and to exchange information at the "Doping Technicians" meeting in 1969, the first of its kind, but regular meetings did not take place. Consequently, one can categorise the attempts of Manfred Donike and Arnold Beckett as individual efforts of a primarily technical nature that contributed immensely to the execution of 2,079 tests and 7 positive doping controls at the 1972 Munich Olympic Games.

Against the background of an increasingly apparent usage of performance-enhancing substances from 1972 onwards, the second phase of extended advisory by anti-doping laboratory experts began. This was a result of increasing dependence on their professional competencies. Initially, the installation of the tests for anabolic steroids in 1975 strengthened Arnold Beckett´s position in his extended advisory role. Arnold Beckett relied heavily on the support of Raymond Brooks and Manfred Donike, who were more sophisticated experts on the detection of steroids. It became evident at the time that Arnold Beckett needed support in his advisory position to keep pace with the analytical procedures. However, in the 1970s, Alexandre de Mérode appeared not to be concerned with such a need. Thus, Arnold Beckett remained the only expert in doping analysis on the IOC Medical Commission during this time.

Significantly, this was not the case in the IAAF Medical Committee, an important body in the global fight against doping, which has not been subject to prior research. Although it was not the focus to reveal organisational connections, the specific perspective and the rich body of source material allowed investigating the relationship between the IAAF and the IOC with highly valuable implications. The IAAF Medical Committee discussed scientific aspects in more detail and installed a working group, which developed strict and harmonised rules for the working procedures in an anti-doping laboratory from the mid-1970s onwards.

The working group also included Manfred Donike, and its efforts led to the recognition of official doping laboratories in 1975, and eventually the inaugural official accreditation procedure in 1979. Hence, the IAAF Medical Commission and the anti-doping laboratory experts involved played an extremely significant role for scientific aspects in general, and the accreditation of laboratories in particular. Decision-makers in the IAAF appeared to have quickly recognised the value of the experts in the field of doping analysis. As a result, whereas the IOC Medical Commission refrained from focusing extensively on analytical and chemical aspects, the IAAF Medical Committee proved to be the most powerful body for the anti-doping laboratory expert's attempts to make themselves more relevant before 1980. One can track the urgency of the IAAF back to the many regional and national events that were under the supervision of the IAAF, but also to the individual interests of the heads of laboratories, which anticipated more financial rewards and growing reputation for their institutions. Thus, one has to acknowledge the pioneering role of the IAAF Medical Committee. Manfred Donike also did, when he wrote in 1983:

> Specific work regarding the harmonization of the analytical procedures and the accreditation of laboratories has been done by the Medical Commission of the IOC and in *particular* by the Medical Committee of the IAAF [emphasis added].[2]

Following their more active involvement in the IAAF, Alexandre de Mérode slowly started to integrate more anti-doping laboratory experts towards the end of the 1970s. Hence, they slowly outstripped sport medical specialists, because they had other, more valuable competencies to maintain and advance the doping control system in place. Undoubtedly, this transition had major consequences for the anti-doping affairs in general. The number of doping controls increased steadily from the end of the 1970s onwards, the results became more reliable due to improved analytical methods, and slowly a network of anti-doping laboratory experts began to evolve. The latter point was also a consequence of more heads of anti-doping laboratories at Olympic Games, such as Robert Dugal and Viktor Rogozkin, becoming involved. All identified processes served the interests of the anti-doping laboratory experts because it gave their activities a firm basis to build upon. Hence, by the beginning of the 1980s, showing awareness for more reliable analytical procedures, but also striving for even more influence to generate more funding for anti-doping laboratory work, the scientists attempted to get more

---

[2] Letter, "Manfred Donike to German Ministry of the Interior, October 10, 1983."

influence in decision-making bodies. Arnold Beckett eventually proposed the installation of an IOC working group to deal solely with the accreditation of doping laboratories and analytical aspects of the doping control. Together with Manfred Donike, he intended to gain more influence for experts in doping analysis in order to strengthen their professional field. This discovery is essential for the understanding of the IOC's anti-doping strategy and the exertion of influence through anti-doping laboratory experts.

Following this proposal, Alexandre de Mérode seemed to become convinced about the necessity to include other anti-doping laboratory experts, and the most noteworthy transition in the history of the anti-doping laboratory experts took place through the foundation of the IOC MSD in 1980. This marked the beginning of the most influential period of the anti-doping laboratory experts within the Olympic Movement and where they began to obtain increasingly more responsibility as well as attempting to advance the technical aspects of doping controls. Through the "outsourcing" of all doping related aspects from the IOC Medical Commission to a body consisting only of anti-doping laboratory experts, they became highly decisive. Alexandre de Mérode allowed the IOC MSD members to have considerably more influence through the IOC MSD because they had proven in previous years that they could make highly valuable contributions to advance the IOC's fight against doping by their professional expertise in doping analysis. This becomes evident by a major increase in the number of doping controls, the introduction of more techniques (such as a method to detect testosterone), and educational initiatives for laboratory staff. Such developments were initiated and controlled by the leading anti-doping laboratory experts Manfred Donike and Arnold Beckett (and to a lesser extent by Robert Dugal, Claus Clausnitzer and Vitaly Semenov), who were all members of the IOC MSD and heads of anti-doping laboratories. From this point onwards, making a distinction between the IOC MSD and the IOC Medical Commission as a whole becomes inevitable.

Significantly, the increased influence by the IOC MSD also resulted in a changeover of the leading position within the network of the anti-doping laboratory experts. Manfred Donike's knowledge and experience with GC-MS meant he, and the laboratory in Cologne, occupied the leading position in doping analysis throughout the 1980s. By the mid-1980s, the laboratories did not use RI screening as extensively, so Arnold Beckett and colleagues' scientific competencies were needed less than the professional expertise of Manfred Donike. The Cologne Workshop, staged for the first time in 1983, is testimony for this leadership. It also highlights Manfred Donike's continuous efforts to exchange knowledge within the community of anti-doping laboratory experts. Jordi Segura also acknowledged this when he remarked, "Manfred was successful in trying to make this some kind of network and probably the key point was the Workshop, the annual Workshop."[3] Manfred Donike was the leading expert for anabolic steroid testing in particular, and the fact that in 1988, 216 of 254 positive doping tests in the FRG were anabolic steroids demonstrates that they were still the main problem.[4] Although he occasionally faced criticism from other experts concerning his controlling style of management, he was able to maintain this leadership until the mid-1990s. The implemented approach to consider the relationships within the scientific community helped to reveal such significant developments.

In addition to the personnel and technical developments because of the installation of the IOC MSD, this book also addresses the institutional perspective, and highlights that the steering role of the IOC MSD led to a considerable expansion of officially accredited doping laboratories, from six in 1981 to 23 in 1992. Whilst researchers have addressed the numeric increase before, they did not investigate in detail the relevance of a few individuals. Moreover, if one has a closer look at the structures and institutions that are involved in WADA on the scientific level today, one must say that WADA still relies on many laboratories that were set up and accredited during this period. In a recent publication on the consequences of the revision of the World Anti-Doping Code (WADC) for anti-doping laboratories, Sylvain GIRAUD et al. state that anti-doping laboratories today still play a "paramount role" in the fight against doping.[5] They explain that the entire WADC regime builds on the work of the laboratories, proving that the establishment of the anti-doping laboratory network had an effect on the global anti-doping system until today. This underlines the argument brought forward that the IOC MSD did much of the scientific groundwork from 1980 onwards with the majority of processes initiated until 1984, and it displays the degree to which WADA depended on the pre-existing institutional structures since its foundation. Therefore, this book contributes to an understanding of the present structures of the institutional anti-doping network.

In light of the established procedures in the first years of the IOC MSD, the role of the anti-doping laboratory experts became increasingly diverse after 1984. In particular, Manfred Donike occupied important administrative and political

---

[3] Interview with Jordi Segura, May 24, 2013.

[4] Report, "Jahresstatistik 1988 by Manfred Donike, January 26, 1989."

[5] Sylvain GIRAUD, Charles JOYE, Martial SAUGY and Marjolaine VIRET, "Role of Anti-Doping Laboratories in the Fight against Doping," *Causa Sport* 4 (2014), 344.

roles. In his role as head of the IOC MSD, he promoted the installation of stricter regulations for anti-doping laboratories in an attempt to make doping tests more reliable, and to build upon the existing procedures. Together with other stakeholders, the IOC MSD was also successful in its attempt to install out-of competition testing. This resulted in a significant increase in the number of conducted doping tests.

Starting with the Ben Johnson scandal at the 1988 Seoul Olympic Games, the final phase of the history of the anti-doping laboratory experts began. Whilst the IOC MSD still occupied a strong position at the end of the 1980s, the anti-doping laboratory experts also faced its growing expansion, which threatened their leadership role. In concrete terms, doping substances beyond the main expertise of the IOC MSD members, growing public attention to the doping issue and a withdrawal of long-established individuals began to confront them. The lack of urgency to support more research for a testing method for blood doping represents a specific dilemma, because it exceeded their traditional fields of research, but there was also reluctance to actively include other experts. Moreover, whilst the laboratories maintained an important role by the introduction of the out-of competition tests, public inquiries such as the Commission of Inquiry revealed the monopolistic character of the IOC MSD. The IOC MSD reacted to these accusations with the introduction of an extended quality control system, but at the same time, the internal differences grew, ending in a controversy at the 1992 Barcelona Olympic Games.

As a result, only Manfred Donike remained a key player after the incident. Tragically, he died only three years later of a heart attack on an aeroplane, travelling to Zimbabwe to prepare the doping controls of the All-Africa Games in 1995.[6] Hence, only fifteen years after the foundation of the IOC MSD, none of its original members contributed to its work anymore. In 1993, Alexandre de Mérode added endrocologist Professor Dr. Peter Sönksen[7] (Great Britain) to the IOC Medical Commission in order to develop a test for hGH, and the head of the IOC accredited laboratory in Beijing, Dr. Zeyi Yang, also joined. [8]

---

[6] "Obituaries," *Olympic Review* XXV, no. 5 (1995), 74.

[7] Professor Dr. Peter Sönksen (born 1936), after receiving his medical doctorate in 1967, became professor in Endocrinology 1979 St. Thomas Hospital Medical School in London. In 1989, he became clinical director in Endocrinology and Diabetes, and in 1996, chairman of the Division of Medicine. He dedicated much of his research to hGH, and founded the Growth Hormone Research Society in 1992. INTERNATIONAL OLYMPIC COMMITTEE, *Commission Médicale*, 20.

[8] Minutes, "Meeting of the IOC Medical Commission, February 28 – March 2, 1993," Box 107 "Lillehammer," Private Archive Jordi Segura, Barcelona, 1.

Simultaneously, the IOC Medical Commission also installed a new "Juridical Working Group" to deal with the growing legal issues. Against the background of the increasing influence of legal experts at the beginning of the 1990s, and the decreasing dominance of anti-doping laboratory experts, this installation appears to be the logical consequence. Clearly, once the first anti-doping laboratory experts, such as Manfred Donike and Arnold Beckett, had established main procedures to advance doping analysis, and once they occupied influential roles, international anti-doping efforts became increasingly more complex.

There is no doubt that besides the legacy on the institutional level with the numerous doping laboratories, the IOC acknowledged the contribution of its experts. Arnold Beckett received the Olympic Order in 1980,[9] and in June 1995, the 104th IOC Session awarded Manfred Donike with the same honour, presented posthumously to his family.[10] Consequently, discussing the scientific perspective of the anti-doping history does not merely contribute to understanding its multi-layered dimensions, but also illustrates the significance of personnel involvements and their consequences for the tendencies of anti-doping as a whole. Whilst this had been done for Alexandre de Mérode before,[11] this book is the first one that considers additional key agents to shape these processes. Hence, it extends HOULIHAN's study where he claims that doctors and scientists lack resources in order to influence policy debates.[12] Whereas this appears to be correct for the current situation, a small group of scientists were highly relevant to the IOC's anti-doping activities in the past, and by the 1980s, the had a lot of influence on the decision-making processes. Thus, they had a lasting effect on the doping control system.

Finally, in terms of the community of anti-doping laboratory experts as such, another body represents their interests today. This is the World Association of Anti-Doping Scientists (WAADS). Following the introduction of WADA, and the obvious loss of relevance for the anti-doping laboratory experts, due to the increased power for lawyers, the heads of the most influential accredited laboratories decided that a united organ to represent their interests was needed. Hence, Professor Dr. Larry Bowers (head of the Indianapolis laboratory), Professor Dr. Frans Delbecke (head of the Ghent laboratory), Professor Dr. Laurent Rivier (head of the Lausanne laboratory), Wilhelm Schänzer (head of the Cologne laboratory following Manfred Donike's death), Rymantas Kazlauskas

---

[9] "Olympic Awards," *Olympic Review* 154 (1980), 413.
[10] "Obituaries," *Olympic Review* XXV, no. 5 (1995), 74.
[11] DIMEO et al., "Saint or Sinner?"
[12] HOULIHAN, "Anti-Doping," 332.

(head of the Sydney laboratory) and David Cowan (head of the London laboratory) met in Frankfurt in 1998 to discuss a first set of regulations and a constitution. [13] Following amendments at the Cologne Workshop, which consequently continued to play a significant role for the network, the anti-doping laboratory experts founded WAADS, and David Cowan became the first president of the association in 2001. Its main objectives are:

- Maintain excellence in the science and practice of anti-doping programs in the interest of all athletes;

- Facilitate harmonization of modern scientific methodology for effective anti-doping control;

- Provide reliable information concerning the scientific aspects of anti-doping programs in the public interest;

- Foster good will and co-operation among members. [14]

It is interesting that such an association did not exist beforehand, but can be explained by the fact that the scientists had a powerful position through the IOC MSD, and as a result another association was not required. Moreover, in the Cologne Workshop, and later the heads of laboratories meetings, there had been enough exchange forums from the 1980s onwards. In comparison, WAADS is by no means as influential as the original anti-doping laboratory experts. However, according to Jordi Segura, WAADS president from 2012 until 2014, its foundation was more to maintain some "group perspective," but not to have a political influence. [15] Instead, WAADS focuses entirely on the technical and scientific reliability, whilst also keeping its own proficiency testing programme. In this way, WAADS keeps a degree of independence from WADA. A WADA "Laboratory Expert Group," which provides the accreditation and reaccreditation and maintains the International Standard for Laboratories also exists, [16] but it does not have decisive influence on the political level.

---

[13] WORLD ASSOCIATION OF ANTI-DOPING SCIENTISTS, "Who We Are," 2013; http://waads.org/about-us-welcome-message [accessed January 11, 2015].
[14] Ibid.
[15] Interview with Jordi Segura, May 24, 2013.
[16] WORLD ANTI-DOPING AGENCY, "Laboratory Expert Group," 2015; https://www.wada-ama.org/en/who-we-are/governance/ laboratory-expert-group [accessed January 19, 2015].

Despite the new numerous insights into the history of anti-doping through the attempt to address a gap in research, certain limitations remain. First, issues such as the dealing with blood doping after 1992, have to be investigated more thoroughly. Second, whereas the largely unknown sources from the estate of August Kirsch fill crucial gaps in research, it is important to take into consideration that these mainly contain the written exchanges of Manfred Donike. It follows on that this book deals in detail with his contribution to international anti-doping affairs and the network of anti-doping laboratory experts, for which he was a key player. However, it was not possible to gain access to other comprehensive sources – if they even still exist – which deal with individual anti-doping laboratory experts such as Arnold Beckett or Robert Dugal. Future research should attempt to undertake more investigations in this regard, in order to connect the personal accounts with each other. Third, for reasons of feasibility and accessibility to archival material, the investigations conclude with the doping controls at the 1992 Barcelona Olympic Games. In the future, research should focus on the period from 1992 onwards, in order to investigate the influence of anti-doping laboratory experts until today. It is clear that the first anti-doping laboratory experts involved left a wide-ranging legacy through the initial development and installation of doping tests, the network of IOC-accredited anti-doping laboratories, the guidelines for anti-doping laboratory work and educational initiatives to teach laboratory staff. However, the question remains how important these aspects are within today's doping control system. Therefore it is necessary to undertake these investigations on the individual and institutional level. Fourth, against the background of the nature of the body of source material, this book focuses on the IOC and the IAAF. However, there is evidence for the involvement of key anti-doping laboratory experts in other international sports federations. Manfred Donike was a member of the UCI's Medical Commission from 1991 onwards, and Arnold Beckett chaired the International Tennis Federation's (ITF) Medical Committee from 1985 until 1993. Although the IAAF Medical Committee had the most extensive influence on the IOC, it will be interesting to see whether Manfred Donike and Arnold Beckett showed the same behaviour and degree of influence on the smaller sports federation's medical bodies.

Archives and Bibliography

CONSULTED ARCHIVES

Carl and Liselott Diem-Archive, Cologne (Germany)

German Federal Archives, Berlin-Lichterfelde (Germany)

German Institute for Sports Science, Bonn (Germany)

International Olympic Committee Library and Archives, Lausanne (Switzerland)

King's College London – Archives and Special Collections, London (GB)

LA84 Foundation [online archive], Los Angeles (USA)

Private archive of Professor Dr. Don H. Catlin, Los Angeles (USA)

Private archive of Professor Dr. Jordi Segura, Barcelona (Spain)

BIBLIOGRAPHY

"A Brief History." *World Anti-Doping Agency*; http://www.wada-ama.org/en/about-wada/history/ [accessed July 13, 2014].

"After the Congress of the 'Association Internationale de Boxe Amateur'." *Bulletin du Comité International Olympique* 29 (1951): 16-17.

ALFES, Holger, and Dirk CLASING. "Identifizierung geringer Mengen Methamphetamins nach Körperpassage durch Kopplung von Dünnschichtchomatographie und Massenspektrometrie." *Deutsche Zeitschrift für die gesamte gerichtliche Medizin* 64 (1969): 235-240.

ANDERSSON, Carl-Ove. "Mass Spectrometric Studies on Amino Acid and Peptide Derivatives." *Acta Chemica Scandinavia* 12 (1958): 1353.

"Antidoping Laboratories." *Olympic Review* 213 (1985): 411.

ARMSTRONG, Robert. "The Lessons Learned from Canada's Dubin Inquiry." *International Symposium on Sport and Law*, Monte Carlo, February 1, 1991.

"Athletics mourns loss of Frederick Holder, IAAF Honorary Life Vice President." *International Association of Athletics Federations*; http://www.iaaf.org/news/news/athletics-mourns-loss-of-frederick-holder-iaa [accessed February 15, 2015].

"Athletics mourns loss of Frederick Holder, IAAF Honorary Life Vice President." *International Association of Athletics Federations*;

http://www.iaaf.org/news/news/athletics-mourns-loss-of-frederick-holder-iaa [accessed February 15, 2015].

BABA, S., Y. SHINOHARA and Y. KASUYA. "Differentiation Between Endogenous and Exogenous Testosterone in Human Plasma and Urine After Oral Administration of Deuterium-labelled Testosterone by Mass Fragmentography." *Journal of Clinical Endocrinology and Metabolism* 50, no. 5 (1980): 889-894.

BALE, John, and P. David HOWE, eds. *The Four-Minute Mile.* London: Routledge, 2008.

BARNES, Lan. "Olympic Drug Testing: Improvements Without Progress." *Physician and Sportsmedicine* 8 (1980): 21-24.

BARNEY, Robert K., Stephen R. WENN and Scott G. MARTIN. *Selling the Five Rings.* Salt Lake City: University of Utah Press, 2002.

BARTONíČEK, Jan. "K 80. narozeninám prof. MUDr. Miroslava Slavíka, CSc." *Ortopedie* 7, no. 5 (2013): 202.

BEAMISH, Rob, and Ian RITCHIE. *Fastest, Highest, Strongest: A Critique of High-Performance Sport.* London: Routledge, 2007.

BEAMISH, Rob. *Steroids. A New Look at Performance-Enhancing Drugs.* Santa Barbara: Praeger, 2011.

BECKETT, Arnold H. "Clenbuterol and Sport." *Lancet* 340 (1992): 1165.

BECKETT, Arnold H., and D.F. CASY. "The Testing and Development of Analgesic Drugs." In *Progress in Medicinal Chemistry*, edited by G.P. Ellis and G.B. West, 43-87. London: Butterworths, 1962.

BECKETT, Arnold H., and David A. COWAN. "Misuse of Drugs in Sport," *British Journal of Sports Medicine* 12 (1979): 185-194.

BECKETT, Arnold H., G.T. TUCKER and A.C. MOFFAT. "Routine Detection and Determination of Ephedrine and its Congeners in Urine by Gas Chromatography." *Journal of Pharmacy and Pharmacology* 19 (1967): 273-294.

BECKETT Arnold H., and M. ROWLAND. "Determination and Identification of Amphetamine in Urine." *Journal of Pharmacy and Pharmacology* 17, no. 1 (1965): 59-60.

BECKETT, Arnold H., M.A. BEAVAN and Anne E. ROBINSON. "Some Factors Involved in Multiple Spot Formation in the Paper Chromatography." *Journal of Pharmacy and Pharmacology* 12 (1960): 203-216.

BERENDONK, Brigitte. *Doping Dokumente. Von der Forschung zum Betrug.* Berlin: Springer Verlag, 1991.

BERENDONK, Brigitte. *Doping. Von der Forschung zum Betrug.* Reinbek: Rowohlt Taschenbuch Verlag, 1992.

BERG, Aloys, and Hans-Hermann DICKHUTH. "Nachruf auf Prof. Dr. Dr. h.c. Joseph Keul." *Deutsche Zeitschrift für Sportmedizin* 51, no. 7/8 (2000): 280.

"Bericht der Unabhängigen Dopingkommission." June 1991, *Gazetta*; http://www.cycling4fans.de/uploads/media/1991_Bericht_der_Reiter-Kommission_01.pdf [accessed August 28, 2014]

BERTRAND, Michel, Robert DUGAL, Cyrus VAZIRI, Gabriel SANCHEZ and S.F. COOPER. "A Special Dimension of the Nonmedical Use of Drugs. II. Systematic Approach to the Analytical Control of Doping]." *Union Med Can.* 104, no. 6 (1975): 952-960.

BEST, Mark, and Duncan NEUHAUSER. "Henry K. Beecher: Pain, Belief and Truth at the Bedside. The Powerful Placebo, Ethical Research and Anaesthesia Safety." *Quality Safety in Health Care* 19 (2010): 466-468.

BRAUN, Jutta. "'Dopen für Deutschland' – Die Diskussion im vereinten Sport 1990-1992." In *Hormone und Hochleistung. Doping in Ost und West*, edited by Klaus LATZEL and Lutz NIETHAMMER, 151-170. Berlin: Böhlau, 2008.

BROOKS, Raymond V., Richard G. FIRTH, and Nigel T. SUMNER. "Detection of Anabolic Steroids by Radioimmunoassay." *British Journal of Sports Medicine* 9, no. 2 (1975): 89-92.

BURSTIN, Stanislas. "Le dopage, ce 'mal' du Sport." *Vivre. Revue mensuelle d'information médicale, scientifique et de loisirs* 4 (1960): 10-14.

BURSTIN, Stanislas. "Le 'Dopage' Sportif." Paper presented at the Congress of the *Union Sportive Travailliste Du Nord et Du Pas-de-Calais*. Lens, March 20, 1960.

BURSTIN, Stanislas. "Problème medico-légal du dopage." *France Football* 749/750 (1960).

CALIFANO, Sergio. *Istituto di Medicina dello Sport di Firenze. Il "Centro delle Cascine": 1950-2005 Oltre Mezzo Secolo al Servizio dello Sport.* Florence: Commune di Firenze, 2005.

CANTELON, Hart. "Amateurism, High-Performance Sport, and the Olympics." In *Global Olympics. Historical and Sociological Studies of the Modern*

Games, edited by Kevin YOUNG and Kevin B. WAMSLEY, 83-101. Bingley: JAI Press, 2007.

CARL UND LISELOTT DIEM ARCHIV, ed. *Nachlaß August Kirsch.* Aachen: Verlag Mainz, 1998.

CARTER, Neil. *Medicine, Sport and the Body. A Historical Perspective.* London: Bloomsbury, 2012.

CATLIN, Don H., Craig KAMMERER, Caroline K. HATTON, Michael H. SEKERA and James L. MERDINK. "Analytical Chemistry at the Games of the XXIIIrd Olympiad in Los Angeles, 1984." *Clinical Chemistry* 33, no. 2 (1987): 319-327.

"Circular letter No. 5." *Official Bulletin of the Fédération Internationale de Médicine Sportive* 5, no. 4 (1965): 10.

CHAN, Siu C., George A. TOROK-BOTH, Debbie M. BILLAY, Peter S. PRZYBYISKI, Claire Y. GRADEEN, Kathleen M. PAP and Jitka PETRUZELKA. "Drug Analysis at the 1988 Olympic Winter Games in Calgary." *Clinical Chemistry* 37, no. 7 (1991): 1289-1296.

CHILDS, Martin. "Professor Arnold Beckett: Sports doping expert who later changed sides and supported those accused of drug use." *The Independent*, March 29, 2010.

CLARKE, E.G.C., and M. MOSS. "A Brief History of Dope Detection in Racehorses." *British Journal of Sports Medicine* 10, no. 3 (1976): 100-102.

CLASING, Dirk, Manfred DONIKE and Armin KLÜMPER. "Dopingkontrollen bei den Spielen der XX. Olympiade, München 1972 (III)." *Leistungssport* 4 (1975): 303-306.

CLIFFORD, Peter A., and John BUTFIELD. *The History of the Tour of Britain.* London: The International Cyclists Saddle Club, 1967.

COMMITTEE OF MINISTERS OF THE COUNCIL OF EUROPE. *Resolution on the Doping of Athletes (67/12), adopted by the Ministers' Deputies on 29th June 1967.* Strasbourg: Council of Europe, 1967.

CONSDEN, R., A.H. GORDON and A.J.P. MARTIN. "Qualitative analysis of proteins: a partition chromatographic method using paper." *Biochemical Journal* 38, no. 3 (1944): 224-232.

COUBERTIN, Pierre de. "Olympisme." In *Pierre de Coubertin: textes choisis. Vol. II*, edited by Norbert MÜLLER, 592-593. Zürich: Weidmann, 1986.

COUBERTIN, Pierre De. "Speech Given at the Opening of the Olympic Congress at the City Hall of Prague." In *Olympism. Selected Writings*, edited by Norbert MÜLLER, 555-556. Lausanne: International Olympic Committee, 2000.

COUNCIL OF EUROPE. *Explanatory Report on the Anti-Doping Convention.* Strasbourg. Council of Europe, 1990.

COURT, Jürgen, and Wildor HOLLMANN. "Doping." In *Lexikon der Ethik im Sport,* edited by Ommo GRUPE and Dietmar MIETH, 97-105. Schorndorf: Hofmann Verlag, 2001.

"Danish Oarsmen who took part at the European Championships in Milan were they drugged?" *Bulletin du Comité International Olympique* 28 (1951): 25-26.

DAVENPORT, Joanna. "Monique Berlioux: Her association with three IOC presidents," *Citius, Altius, Fortius* (became *Journal of Olympic History* in 1997) 4, no. 3 (1996): 10-18.

DE HON, Oliver, Harm KUIPERS and Maarten VAN BOOTENBURG. "Prevalance of Doping Use in Elite Sports: A Review of Numbers and Methods." *Sports Medicine* 45 (2015): 57-69.

DE MERODE, Alexandre. "Doping Tests at the Olympic Games in 1976." *Olympic Review* 135 (1979): 10-16.

DECKER, Wolfgang. *Sport in der griechischen Antike.* Hildesheim: Arete Verlag, 2012.

DIETZ, Werner, and Klaus SOEHRING. "Experimentelle Beiträge zum Nachweis von Thiobarbitursäuren aus dem Harn mit Hilfe der Papierchromatographie." *Archiv der Pharmazie und Berichte der Deutschen Pharamzeutischen Gesellschaft* 290, no. 2 (1957): 80-97.

DIMEO, Paul, Thomas M. HUNT and Matthew BOWERS. "Saint or Sinner?: A Reconsideration of the Career of Prince Alexandre de Merode, Chair of the International Olympic Committee's Medical Commission, 1967–2002." *The International Journal of the History of Sport* 28, no. 6 (2011): 925-940.

DIMEO, Paul. *A History of Drug Use in Sport 1876-1976.* London: Routledge, 2007.

DIRIX, Albert, and Xavier STURBOIS. *The First Thirty Years of the International Olympic Committee Medical Commission.* Lausanne: International Olympic Committee, 1998.

DIRIX, Albert. "The Doping Problem at the Tokyo and Mexico City Olympic Games." *Journal of Sports Medicine and Physical Fitness* 6 (1966): 183-186.

DONATI, Alessandro. *Lo Sport Del Doping.* Torino: Edizioni Gruppo Abele, 2012.

DONIKE, Manfred. "N-Methyl-N-trimethylsilyl-trifluoracetamide, ein neues Silylierungsmittel aus der Reihe der silylierten Amide." *Journal of Chromatography* 42 (1969): 103-104.

DONIKE, Manfred. "Acylierung mit Bis(Acylamiden): N-Methyl-bis-(trifluoracetamid) und Bis(trifluoracetamid), zwei neue Reagenzien zur Triflouracetylierung." *Journal of Chromatography* 78 (1973): 273-279.

DONIKE, Manfred. "N-Trifluoracetyl-O-trimethylsilyl-phenolalkylamine: Darstellung und massenspezifischer gaschromatographischer Nachweis." *Journal of Chromatography* 103 (1973): 91-112.

DONIKE, Manfred. "Der gas-chromatographische Nachweis von Catecholaminen im Femtomol-Bereich durch massenspezifische Detektion." *Chromatographia* 7 (1974): 651-654.

DONIKE, Manfred, Dirk CLASING and Armin KLÜMPER. "Dopingkontrollen bei den Spielen der XX. Olympiade München 1972 – Teil 2." *Leistungssport* 2 (1974): 192-199.

DONIKE, Manfred. "Zum Problem des Nachweises der anabolen Steroide: Gas-chromatographische und massenspezifische Möglichkeiten." *Sportarzt und Sportmedizin* 1 (1975): 1-6.

DONIKE, Manfred. "Preface." In *10th Cologne Workshop on Dope Analysis 7th to 12th June 1992 – Proceedings,* edited by Manfred DONIKE, Hans GEYER, Andrea GOTZMANN, Ute MARECK-ENGELKE and Susanne RAUTH, 11-14. Cologne: Sportverlag Strauß, 1993.

DONIKE, Manfred, Hans GEYER, Andrea GOTZMANN, Ute MARECK-ENGELKE and Susanne RAUTH, eds. *10th Cologne Workshop on Dope Analysis 7th to 12th June 1992 – Proceedings.* Cologne: Sportverlag Strauß, 1993.

DONIKE, Manfred, K.R. BÄRWALD, Karl KLOSTERMANN, Wilhelm SCHÄNZER and Johann ZIMMERMANN. "Nachweis von exogenem Testosteron." In *Sport: Leistung und Gesundheit,* edited by Hermann HECK, Wildor

HOLLMANN, Heinz LIESEN and Richard ROST, 293-300. Cologne: Deutscher Ärzte Verlag, 1983.

"Doping Control Laboratory." *Olympic Review* 215 (1985): 568.

"Doping." *Olympic Review* 90 (1965): 47-49.

DUBIN, Charles. *Commission of Inquiry into the Use of Drugs and Banned Practices Intended to Increase Athletic Performance.* Ottawa: Canadian Government Publishing Centre, 1990.

DUGAL, Robert, and Manfred DONIKE. "International Olympic Committee Requirements for Laboratory Accreditation and Good Laboratory Practices." In *Proceedings of the International Symposium on Drug Abuse in Sports (Doping)*, edited by Jong Sei PARK, 71-87. Seoul: KAIST, 1988.

DUGAL, Robert. "Doping Tests in Montreal." *Olympic Review* 116 (1977): 383-387.

DWYRE, Bill. "Doctor attended to sports stars," *Los Angeles Times*, July 7, 2008. http://articles.latimes.com/2008/sep/07/local/me-daly7.

DWYRE, Bill. "Doctor attended to sports stars." *Los Angeles Times*, July 7, 2008; http://articles.latimes.com/2008/sep/07/local/me-daly7   [accessed February 11, 2015].

EGGERS, Erik. "Geschichtliche Aspekte des Dopings in der präanabolen Phase." In *Doping in Deutschland: Geschichte, Recht, Ethik. 1950-1972*, edited by Giselher SPITZER, 47-70. Cologne: Sportverlag Strauß, 2013.

ERIKSSON, Bengt O., Tore MELLSTRAND, Lars PETERSON and Per RENSTRÖM. *Sports medicine.* Enfield: Guiness Publishing, 1990.

EUROPEAN SPORTS CONFERENCE, WORKING GROUP ON EFFECTIVE ANTI-DOPING MEASURES. *Final report Anti-doping Seminar, 30 October - 2 November, Borlänge, Sweden* (Borlänge: n.p., 1988.

EVANG, Karl. "Health Authorities and Sport." In *Sport and Health. International Conference on Sport and Health Oslo 1952*, edited by Otto JOHANSEN, 32-37. Oslo: The Royal Norwegian Ministry of Education State Office for Sport and Youth Work, 1952.

FAIR, John D. "Isometrics or Steroids? Exploring New Frontiers of Strength in the Early 1960s." *Journal of Sport History* 20, no. 1 (1993): 1-24.

FINISH CENTRAL SPORTS FEDERATION. *Nordic Anti-Doping Convention.* Helsinki: Finish Central Sports Federation, 1983.

FISHER, R.G., and H.E. ROBSON. " 'Doping' in the 1958 Empire and Commonwealth Games." *British Journal of Sports Medicine* 4, no. 2 (1969): 163-181.

FRANKE, Werner, and Brigitte BERENDONK. "Hormonal doping and androgenization of athletes: a secret program of the German Democratic Republic government." *Clinical Chemistry* 43, no. 7 (1997): 1262-1279.

GADAMER, Hans-Georg. *Truth and method* (2nd ed.). New York, NY: The Crossroad Publishing Corporation, 1989.

GEHRKE, Charles W., Robert L. WIXON and Ernst BAYER. "Prominent Chromatographers and their Research – Seminal Concepts in Chromatography/Separation Sciences." In *Chromatography. A Century of Discovery 1900-2000*, edited by Charles W. GEHRKE, Robert L. WIXON and Ernst BAYER, 107-598. Amsterdam: Elsevier Science, 2001.

GIRAUD, Sylvain, Charles JOYE, Martial SAUGY, and Marjolaine VIRET. "Role of Anti-Doping Laboratories in the Fight against Doping." *Causa Sport* 4 (2014): 331-344.

GLEAVES, John. "A Critique of Contemporary Sanctions For Anti-Doping Violations: Changing Directions." In *Doping and Anti-Doping Policy in Sport: Ethical, Legal and Social Perspectives,* edited by Mike MCNAMEE and Verner MØLLER, 233-245. New York, NY: Routledge, 2011.

GLEAVES, John. "Enhancing the Odds: Horse Racing, Gambling and the First Anti-Doping Movement in Sport, 1889-1911." *Sport in History* 32, no. 1 (2012): 26-52.

GLEAVES, John. "Manufactured Dope: How the 1984 US Olympic cycling team rewrote the rules on drugs in sport." *International Journal for the History of Sport* 32, no. 1 (2015): 89-107.

GLEAVES, John, and Matthew LLEWELLYN. "Sport, Drugs and Amateurism: Tracing the Real Cultural Origins of Anti-Doping Rules in Sport." *The International Journal of the History of Sport* 31, no. 8 (2014): 839-853.

GOHLKE, Roland S. "Time-of-flight mass spectrometry and gas-liquid partition chromatography." *Analytical Chemistry* 31 (1959): 535-541.

GOLDMAN, Bob, Ronald KLATZ and Patricia J. BUSH. *Death in the Locker Room.* South Bend: Indiana: Icarus Press, 1984.

GORDON, A.H., Archer J.P. MARTIN and Richard L.M. SYNGE. "Partition Chromatography in the Study of Protein Constituents." *Biochemical Journal* 37, no. 1 (1943): 79-86.

GORDON, A.H., Archer J.P. MARTIN and Richard L.M. SYNGE. "The Amino-Acid Composition of Gramicidin." *Biochemical Journal* 37, no. 1 (1943): 86-92.

GRAEVSKAJA, Nina. "The significance of the active motor regime for the preservation of health of the former leading sportsmen." In *Funktionsminderung und Funktionsertüchtigung im modernen Leben*, edited by Günter HANEKOPF, 454-458. Hamburg: Deutscher Sportärztebund, 1966.

GULLBRING, B., A. HOLMGREN, T. SJÖSTRAND and T. STRANDELL. "The Effect of Blood Volume Variations on the Pulse Rate in Supine and Upright Positions and During Exercise." *Acta Physiologica Scandinavica* 50, no. 1 (1960): 62-71.

HAAS, Peter. "Epistemic communities." In *International encyclopedia of political science*, edited by Bertrand BADIE, Dirk BERG-SCHLOSSER and Leonardo MORLINO, 787-791. Thousand Oaks, CA: SAGE Publications, 2011.

HARVEY, Randy. "Drug Dispute Might Alter Suspensions: Clenbuterol: Logan and Dasse could benefit from experts' differences on whether stimulant also has anabolic effects." *Los Angeles Times*, November 14, 1992.

HEGGIE, Vanessa. *A history of British sports medicine*. Manchester: Manchester University Press, 2011.

HEGGIE, Vanessa. "Volunteers for Science: Medicine, Health and the Modern Olympic Games." In *Perfect Bodies Sports Medicine and Immortality*, edited by Vivienne LO, 97-109. London: The British Museum, 2012.

HEIDEGGER, Martin. *Sein und Zeit* (16th ed.). Tübingen: Max Niemeyer, 1986.

HEMMERSBACH, Peter. "History of Mass Spectrometry at the Olympic Games." *Journal of Mass Spectrometry* 43 (2008): 839-853.

HENNE, Kathryn. "WADA, the Promises of Law and the Landscapes of Antidoping Regulation." *Political and Legal Anthropology Review* 33, no. 2 (2010): 306-325.

HENNE, Kathryn. "The Origins of the International Olympic Committee Medical Commission and its Technocratic Regime: An Historiographic Investigation of Anti-Doping Regulation and Enforcement in

International Sport." *Final Report to the IOC 2009 Postgraduate Research Grant Programme*, submitted December 31, 2009.

HENNE, Kathryn. "The Emergence of Moral Technopreneurialism in Sport: Techniques in Anti-Doping Regulation, 1966–1976." *International Journal for the History of Sport* 31, no. 8 (2014): 884-901.

HENRY, Ian, and Mansour AL TAUQI. "The Development of Olympic Solidarity: West and Non-West (Core and Periphery) Relations in the Olympic World." *The International Journal for the History of Sport* 25, no. 3 (2008): 355-369.

HOBERMAN, John M. *Mortal Engines: The Science of Performance and the Dehumanization of Sport*. New York, NY: The Free Press, 1992.

HOBERMAN, John M. "How Drug Testing Fails: The Politics of Doping Control." In *Doping in Elite Sport: The Politics of Drugs in the Olympic Movement*, edited by Wayne WILSON and Edward DERSE, 241-274. Champaign, IL: Human Kinetics, 2001.

HOBERMAN, John M. "Sports Physicians and the Doping Crisis in Elite Sport." *Clinical Journal of Sports Medicine* 12, no. 4 (2002): 203-208.

HOBERMAN, John M. *Testosterone Dreams: Rejuvenation, Aphrodisia, Doping*. Berkeley, California: University of California Press, 2005.

HOBERMAN, John M. " 'Athletes in handcuffs?' The criminalization of doping." In *Doping and Anti-Doping Policy in Sport: Ethical, Legal and Social Perspectives, edited by* Mike MCNAMEE and Verner MØLLER, 99-110. New York, NY: Routledge, 2011.

HOLLMANN, Wildor. "Sporthochschule – Heute und Morgen." In *Dokumente zur Gründung und zum Aufbau einer wissenschaftlichen Hochschule auf dem Gebiete des Sports*, edited by Dietrich R. QUANZ, 114-123. Cologne: Wienand, 1982.

HOLLMANN, Wildor. *Medizin – Sport – Neuland. 40 Jahre mit der Deutschen Sporthochschule Köln*. Sankt Augustin: Academia, 1993.

HOLLMANN, Wildor. *Ziel und Zufall - ein bewegtes Leben als Arzt, Universitätsprofessor, Forscher und Manager*. Cologne: Sportverlag Strauß, 2012.

HOLLMANN, Wildor and Heiko K. STRÜDER. *Sportmedizin. Grundlagen für körperliche Aktivität, Training und Präventivmedizin*. Stuttgart: Schattauer, 2009.

HOLLMANN, Wildor, and Kurt TITTEL. *Geschichte der deutschen Sportmedizin.* Gera: Druckhaus Gera, 2008.

HOLT, John. *Sport and the British. A Modern History.* Oxford: Oxford University Press, 1989.

HOULIHAN, Barrie. "Anti-Doping Policy in Sport: The Politics of International Policy Co-ordination." *Public Administration* 2 (1999): 311-334.

HOULIHAN, Barrie. *Dying to Win: Doping in Sport and the Development of Anti-doping Policy.* Strasbourg: Council of Europe Publishing, 1999.

HOULIHAN, Barrie. "Building an international regime to combat doping in sport." In *Sports and International Relations. An emerging relationship*, edited by Roger LEVERMORE and Adrian BUDD, 62-76. New York, NY: Routledge, 2004.

HOWALD, Hans. "Prof. Dr. med. Gottfried Schönholzer." *Schweizerische Zeitschrift für Sportmedizin* 27, no.4 (1979): 147-151.

HUNT, Thomas M. *Drug Games: The International Olympic Committee and the Politics of Doping, 1960-2008.* Austin, TX: University of Texas Press, 2011.

INTERNATIONAL ATHLETIC FOUNDATION. *A Review of Projects 1989-1990 and Projects in Progress 1991.* Monte Carlo: IAF, 1991.

"International Federations." *Olympic Review* 225(1986): 414.

"International Olympic Charter Against Doping in Sport." *Olympic Review* 253 (1988): 628-631.

INTERNATIONAL OLYMPIC COMMITTEE. *Proceedings of the XI Olympic Congress in Baden-Baden, 1980. Volume1.* Lausanne: International Olympic Committee, 1981.

INTERNATIONAL OLYMPIC COMMITTEE. *Répertoire. Directory. '84.* Lausanne: International Olympic Committee, 1984.

INTERNATIONAL OLYMPIC COMMITTEE. *Commission Médicale du C.I.O.* Lausanne: International Olympic Committee, 1994.

INTERNATIONAL OLYMPIC COMMITTEE. *Biographies of the Members of the International Olympic Committee.* Lausanne: International Olympic Committee, 1998.

INTERNATIONAL OLYMPIC COMMITTEE. *Biographies of the Members of the International Olympic Committee.* Lausanne: International Olympic Committee, 2009.

"Is the oxygenation of athletes a form of doping?" *Bulletin du Comité International Olympique* 45 (1954): 24-25.

"Jeden Dreck, jeden Blödsinn reingehauen." *Der Spiegel*, September 14, 1992.

JENNINGS, Andrew. *The New Lord of the Rings*. London: Simon & Schuster, 1996.

JOISTEN, Karen. *Philosophische Hermeneutik*. Berlin: Akademie Verlag, 2009.

JOYNER, Michael. "VO2MAX, blood doping, and erythropoietin." *British Jounral of Sports Medicine* 37, no. 3 (2003): 190-191.

JUNG, Matthias. *Hermeneutik zur Einführung*. Hamburg: Junius Verlag, 2001.

KAISER, Hans, and Heinz JORI. "Beiträge zum toxikologischen Nachweis von Dromoran 'Roche', Morphin, Dilaudid, Cardiazol Coramin und Atropin mit Hilfe der Papierchromatographie." *Archiv der Pharmazie und Berichte der Deutschen Pharamzeutischen Gesellschaft* 287, no. 4 (1954): 224-242.

KAMMERER, R. Craig. "What Is Doping and How Is It Detected?" In *Doping in Elite Sport. The Politics of Drugs in the Olympic Movement*, edited by Wayne WILSON and Edward DERSE, 3-28. Champaign, IL: Human Kinetics, 2001.

KAZLAUSKAS, Alanah, and Kathryn CRAWFORD. "Understanding International Scientific Expert Work." In *Recent Advances in Doping Analysis (11)*, edited by Wilhelm SCHÄNZER, Hans GEYER, Andrea GOTZMANN and Ute MARECK-ENGELKE, 247-256. Cologne: Sportverlag Strauß, 2003.

KAZLAUSKAS, Alanah, and Kathryn CRAWFORD. "The Contribution of a Community Event to Expert Work: an Activity Theoretical Perspective." *Outlines. Crtitical Pracice Studies* 6, no. 2 (2004): 63-74.

KETELAARS, H.J.C., and J.G.P. PETERS. "Determination of guaiphenesin and its metabolite, β-(2-methoxyphenoxy) lactic acid, in plasma by high-performance liquid chromatography." *Journal of Chromatography B: Biomedical Sciences and Applications* 224, no. 1 (1981): 144-148.

KICMAN Andrew T., and DB GOWER. "Anabolic steroids in sport: biochemical, clinical and analytical perspectives." *Annals of Clinical Biochemistry* 40 (2003): 321-356.

KINDERMANN, Wilfried. "Der Vater des Sportherzens – Herbert Reindell 100 Jahre." *Deutsche Zeitschrift für Sportmedizin* 59, no. 3 (2008): 73-75.

KLUGE, Volker. *Olympische Winterspiele – Die Chronik*. Berlin, Sportverlag, 1994.

KLUGE, Volker. *Olympische Sommerspiele. Die Chronik 1 – Athen 1896-Berlin 1936.* Berlin: Sportverlag Berlin, 1997.

KLUGE, Volker. *Olympische Sommerspiele. Die Chronik III: Mexiko-Stadt 1968 – Los Angeles 1984.* Berlin: Sportverlag Berlin, 2000.

KNORR CETINA, Karin. *Epistemic Cultures: How the sciences make knowledge.* Cambridge, Massachusetts: Harvard University Press, 1999.

KRIEGER, Jörg, and Stephan WASSONG. "Munich 1972: Turning Point in the Olympic Doping Control System." In *Problems, Possibilities, Promising Practices* (Proceedings of the 11th International Symposium for Olympic Research), edited by Janice FORSYTH and Michael HEINE, 62-67. London, Ontario: University of Western Ontario, 2012.

KRIEGER, Jörg and Stephan WASSONG. "Die institutionelle Formierungsphase und das frühe Wirken der Medizinischen Kommission des Internationalen Olympischen Komitees." In *Doping. Kulturwissenschaftlich betrachtet (Reihe Brennpunkte der Sportwissenschaft. Band 36),* edited by Eckhard MEINBERG and Swen KÖRNER, 101-116. St. Augustin: Academia Verlag, 2013.

KRÜGER, Arnd. "Viele Wege führen nach Olympia. Die Veränderungen in den Trainingssystemen für Mittel- und Langstreckenläufer (1850-1997)." In *Sportliche Leistung im Wandel* (Jahrestagung der DVS-Sektion Sportgeschichte), edited by Norbert GISSEL, 41-56. Hamburg: Czwalina Verlag, 1998.

KRÜGER, Michael. "Doping im Radsport – zivilisationstheoretische Anmerkungen zu einer langen Geschichte." *Sport und Gesellschaft – Sport and Society* 3 (2006): 324-352.

KRÜGER, Michael. "Doping in Cycling – Comments from the Theory of Civilization Point of View to a Long History." *Sport and Society* 3 (2006): 324-352.

KRÜGER, Michael, Christian BECKER, Stefan NIELSEN and Marcel REINOLD. *Doping und Anti-Doping in der Bundesrepublik Deutschland 1850 bis 2007.* Hildesheim: Arete, 2014.

KRÜGER, Michael, Stefan NIELSEN and Christian BECKER. "The Munich Olympics 1972: Its Impact on the Relationship Between State, Sports, and Anti-Doping Policy in West Germany." *Sport in History* 32, no. 4 (2012): 526-549.

LA CAVA, Giuseppe. "The Use of Drugs in Competitive Sport." *Olympic Review* 78 (1962): 52–53.

LAURIN, Carroll A., and Georges LÉTOURNEAU. "Medical Report of the Montreal Olympic Games." *The American Journal of Sports Medicine* 6, no. 2 (1978): 54-61.

LENNARTZ, Karl. "The 2nd International Olympic Games in Athens 1906." *Journal of Olympic History* 10 (2001/2002): 10-27.

LITSKY, Frank. "Dan Hanley, 85, U.S. Olympic Doctor, Dies." *New York Times*, May 10, 2001.

LJUNGQVIST, Arne. *Doping's Nemesis.* Cheltenham: Sportsbooks Limited, 2008.

LUCAS, John A. "The Great Gathering of Sport Scientists: The 1904 St. Louis Olympic Games Exposition Fair Physical Education Lecturers." *Journal of Olympic History* 12, no. 1 (2002): 6-12.

LYSOV, P.K., T.I. DOLMATOVA and G.A. GONCHAROVA. "Graevskaya Nina Danilovna - physician, scientist, educator." *Journal of Russian Association for Sports Medicine and Rehabilitation of Sick and Disabled People* 30, no. 3 (2009): 12-14.

MALLON, Bill. *The 1904 Olympic Games. Results for All Competitors in All Events, with Commentary.* Jefferson, Carolina: McFarland, 1999.

MALLON, Bill, and Ian BUCHANAN. *Historical Dictionary of the Olympic movement.* Oxford: Scarecrow Press, 2006.

MALLWITZ, Arthur. *Körperliche Höchstleistungen mit besonderer Berücksichtigung des Olympischen Sports,* Dissertation. Halle an der Saale, 1908.

MALLWITZ, Arthur, ed. *Sportmedizin und Olympische Spiele 1936. Festschrift der Sportärzteschaft.* Leipzig: Verlag Georg Thieme, 1936.

MALLWITZ, Arthur. "25 Jahre sportärztlicher Forschung." In *Sportmedizin und Olympische Spiele 1936. Festschrift der Sportärzteschaft,* edited by Arthur MALLWITZ, 15-17. Leipzig: Verlag Georg Thieme, 1936.

MANGAN, James A., and Patricia VERTINSKY, eds. *Gender, Sport, Science. Selected Writings of Roberta J. Park.* Abingdon: Routledge, 2009.

MARÓTI, Egon. "Gab es Doping im Altgriechischen Sportleben?" *Acta Classica universitatis scientiarum Debreceniensis* 40/41 (2004/2005): 65-71.

"Medical Commission." *Olympic Review* 145 (1979): 648.

MEDICAL COMMISSION OF THE INTERNATIONAL OLYMPIC COMMITTEE. *Doping.* Lausanne: International Olympic Committee, 1972.

MEIER, Henk E., and Marcel REINOLD. "Performance Enhancement and Politicisation of High Performance Sport: The West German 'air clyster' Affair of 1976." *The International Journal for the History of Sport* 30, no. 12 (2013): 1351-1373.

MEINBERG, Eckhard. "Hermeneutische Methodik." In *Zwischen Verstehen und Beschreiben. Forschungsmethodologische Ansätze in der Sportwissenschaft*, edited by Karl-Heinrich BETTE, Gerd HOFFMANN, Carsten KRUSE, Eckhard MEINBERG and Jörg THIELE, 21-77. Cologne: Bundesinstitut für Sportwissenschaft, 1993.

"Minutes of the Meeting of the Interfederal Medical Commission." *Official Bulletin of the Fédération Internationale de Médicine Sportive* 7, no. 2 (1967): 10.

MØLLER, Verner. "Knud Enemark Jensen's Death During the 1960 Rome Olympics: A Search for Truth?" *Sport in History* 25, no. 3 (2005): 452-471.

MOLZBERGER, Ansgar. *Die Olympischen Spiele in Stockholm. Zwischen Patriotismus und Internationalität*. Sankt Augustin: Academia Verlag, 2012.

MOLZBERGER, Ansgar, Caroline MEIER, Stephan WASSONG, Heike SCHIFFER and Ute GÖßNITZER. *Abgestaubt und Neu Erforschbar*. Cologne: Sportverlag Strauß, 2014.

MONDENARD, Jean-Pierre de. *Tour de France. Histoires extraordinaires des géants de la route*. Paris: Hugo Sport, 2012.

MOORE, Richard. *The Dirtiest Race in History. Ben Johnson, Carl Lewis and the 1988 Olympic 100m Final*. London: Bloomsbury, 2012.

MOROZOV, Vladimir I. "Professor Victor Alekseevich Rogozkin." *European Journal of Applied Physiology* 103 (2008): 379-380.

MOTTRAM, David R. "The evolution of doping and anti-doping in sport." In *Drugs in Sport*, edited by David R. MOTTRAM and Neil CHESTER, 21-36. London: Routledge, 2015.

MÜLLER, Norbert, ed. *Olympism. Selected Writings*. Lausanne: International Olympic Committee, 2000.

MÜLLER, Norbert. *One Hundred Years of Olympic Congresses 1894-1994*. Lausanne: International Olympic Committee, 1994.

MÜLLER, Rudhard K. "History of Doping and Doping Controls." In *Doping in Sports*, edited by Detlef THIEME and Peter HEMMERSBACH, 1-18. Berlin: Springer, 2010.

MÜLLER ENBERGS, Helmut, Jan WIEGOHLS, Dieter HOFFMANN, eds. *Wer war wer in der DDR. Ein biographisches Lexikon.* Berlin: Christoph Links Verlag, 2001.

NIKOLIN, Branko, Meliha LEKIC and Miroslav SOBER. "Introduction of the new analytical approaches to the doping control on the XIV Winter Olympic Games." *Bosnian Journal of Basic Medical Sciences* 3, no. 3 (2003): 45-49.

NOLTE, Martin. "Dopingbekämpfung anlässlich der FIFA Fußball-Weltmeisterschaft England 1966." In *Doping. Kulturwissenschaftlich betrachtet*, eds. Eckhard MEINBERG and Swen KÖRNER, 117-134. St. Augustin: Academia Verlag, 2013.

"Obituaries." *Olympic Review* XXV, no. 5 (1995): 74.

"Obituaries." *Olympic Review* XXVI, no. 27 (1999): 84-86.

"Obituary." *Olympic Review* 213 (1985): 400.

"Obituary." *Olympic Review* 213 (1985): 400.

"Olympic Awards." *Olympic Review* 154 (1980): 413.

"Olympic News." *Journal of Olympic History*, 2002, no. 10(3), 72f

"Olympic Order." *Olympic Review* 214 (1985): 472.

OLIARO, A. "Giuseppe La Cava (1908-1988)." *The Journal of Sports Medicine and Phyisical Fitness* 28, no. 3 (1988): 313-314.

ORGANISING COMMITTEE OF THE GAMES OF THE XXIITH OLYMPIAD. *Official Report of the 1980 Olympic Games in Moscow, Volume 1, Part 3.* Moscow: Organising Committee of the Games of the XXIIth Olympiad, 1981).

ORGANISING COMMITTEE OF THE GAMES OF THE XXIIITH OLYMPIAD. *Official Report of the 1988 Olympic Games in Seoul,* Volume 1, Part 3. Seoul: Organising Committee of the Games of the XXIIIth Olympiad, 1988.

ORGANISING COMMITTEE OF THE VIITH OLYMPIC WINTER GAMES. *Official Report of the VIIth Olympic Winter Games in Cortina d'Ampezzo 1956.* Cortina d'Ampezzo: Organising Committee of the Games of the VIIth Olympic Winter Games, 1956.

ORGANISING COMMITTEE OF THE X^TH WINTER OLYMPIC GAMES, *Official Report of the 1968 Winter Olympic Games in Grenoble*. Grenoble: Organising Committee of the Xth Winter Olympic Games, 1968.

ORGANISING COMMITTEE OF THE XITH OLYMPIC WINTER GAMES. *Official Report of the XIth Olympic Winter Games, Sapporo 1972, Part 1*. Sapporo: Organising Committee of the Games of the XIth Olympic Winter Games, 1972.

ORGANISING COMMITTEE OF THE XIITH OLYMPIC WINTER GAMES. *Official Report of the XIIth Olympic Winter Games, Innsbruck 1976*, Part 2. Innsbruck: Organising Committee of the Games of the XIIth Olympic Winter Games, 1976.

ORGANISING COMMITTEE OF THE XXIIITH OLYMPIC WINTER GAMES.*Official Report of the XIIIth Olympic Winter Games in Lake Placid 1980*. Lake Placid: Organising Committee of the XXIIIth Olympic Winter Games, 1980).

ORGANISING COMMITTEE OF THE XXVITH WINTER OLYMPIC GAMES. *Official Report of the 16th Winter Olympic Games in Albertville*. Albertville: Organising Committee of the XXVITH Winter Olympic Games, 1993.

OWEN, Raymond J. "The Organisation of the International Association of Olympic Medical Officers." *Olympic Review* 105 (1976): 372-374.

PARK, Jong Sei. "Doping test report of 10th Asian Games in Seoul." *Journal of Sports Medicine and Physical Fitness* 31, no. 2 (1991): 303-317.

PARK, Jong Sei. *A Study on Doping Control*. Gwacheon: Ministry of Science and Technology, 1992.

PARK, Jong Sei, Song Ja PARK, Dong Suk LHO, HP CHOO, Bong Chull CHUNG, Chang No YOON, Hong Gi MIN and MJ CHOI. "Drug testing at the 10th Asian Games and 24th Seoul Olympic Games." *Journal of Analytical Toxicology* 14, no. 2 (1991): 66-72.

PARK, Roberta J. "Physicians, Scientists, Exercise and Athletics in Britain and America from the 1867 Boat Race to the Four-Minute Mile." *Sport in History* 31, no. 1 (2011): 1-31.

PAYNE, Michael. *Olympic Turnaround*. Oxford: Infinite Ideas, 2005.

PEARSALL, Judy, ed. *The new Oxford Dictionary of English*. Oxford: Clarendon Press, 1999.

PIEPER, Lindsay Parks. "Sex Testing and the Maintenance of Western Femininity in International Sport." *International Journal of the History of Sport* 31, no. 13 (2014): 1557-1576.

POKRYWKA, Andrzej, Damian GORCZYCA, Anna JAREK and Dorota KWIATKOWSKA. "In memory of Alfons Bukowski on the centenary of anti-doping research." *Drug Testing Analysis* 2, no. 11/12 (2010): 540.

POUND, Richard W. *Inside the Olympics. A Behind-The-Scene Look at the Politics. The Scandals, and the Glory of the Games.* Toronto: Wiley, 2004.

PROKOP, Ludwig. "The struggle against doping and its history," *Journal of Sports Medicine and Medical Fitness* 10 (1970): 45-48.

PROKOP, Ludwig. "Zur Geschichte des Dopings und seiner Bekämpfung." *Sportarzt und Sportmedizin* 21, no. 6 (1970): 125-132.

REINOLD, Marcel. "Arguing against doping: a discourse analytical study on Olympic anti-doping between the 1960s and the late 1980s." *Final Report to the IOC 2011 Postgraduate Research Grant Programme*, submitted May 7, 2012.

REINOLD, Marcel, Christian BECKER and Stefan NIELSEN. "Die 1960er Jahre als Formationsphase von modernem Doping und Anti-Doping." *Sportwissenschaft* 42 (2012): 153-162.

RINGEN, Knut. "Karl Evang: A Giant in Public Health." *Journal of Public Health Policy* 11, no. 3 (1990): 360-367.

ROGGE, Jacques. "Foreword." *Olympic Review* 2003, no. 49: 7.

ROGOZKIN, Victor. *Metabolism of Anabolic Androgenic Steroids.* Boca Raton: CRC Press, 1991.

ROSEN, Daniel. *A History of Performance Enhancement in Sports from the Nineteenth Century to Today.* Westport, CT: Praeger Publishers, 2008.

ROUKHADZÉ, Marié-Hélène. "Artur Takac, the Stadium as Field of Experience." *Olympic Review* 233 (1987): 106-110.

"Royal Perth Hospital Emeritus Consultant Biographies." *Royal Perth Hospital*; http://www.rph.wa.gov.au/~/media/Files/Hospitals/RPH/PDFs/Emeritus %20Consultant%20Biographies%20vol%203.ashx [accessed February 17, 2015].

SANTOS, José Joaquim Ferreira. "Doping." *Olympic Review* 81 (1963): 56-57.

SCHANTZ, Otto. "The Olympic Ideal and the Winter Games: Attitudes Towards the Olympic Winter Games in Olympic Discourses – from Coubertin to

Samaranch." In *From Chamonix to Turin. The Winter Games in the Scope of Olympic Research*, edited by. Norbert MÜLLER, Manfred MESSING and Holger PREUß, 39-57. Kassel: Agon Sportverlag, 2006.

SCHÄNZER, Wilhelm. *Untersuchungen zum Nachweis und Metabolismus von Hormonen und Dopingmitteln, insbesondere mit Hilfe der Hochdruckflüssigkeitschromatographie.* Dissertation at the German Sport University Cologne (Cologne, 1984).

SEGURA, Jordi, Rafael DE LA TORRE, José Antonio PASCUAL, Rosa VENTURA, Magi FARRÉ, Robert EWIN and Jordi CAMI. "Antidoping control at the games of the XXV Olympiad Barcelona '92. Part II." In *Recent Advances in Doping Analysis – Proceedings of the 12th Cologne Workshop*, edited by Manfred DONIKE, Hans GEYER, Andrea GOTZMANN and Ute MARECK-ENGELKE, 413-430. Cologne: Sportverlag Strauß, 1995.

SEGURA, Jordi. "Antidoping Control, Cross Road Between Chemistry and Other Life Sciences." *Actualidad Analítica* 34 (2011): 16; http://www.seqa.es/ActualidadAnalitica/Ano2011Numero34.pdf.

SINGLER, Andreas, and Gerhard TREUTLEIN. *Doping im Spitzensport*, 6th edition. Aachen: Meyer & Meyer Verlag, 2012.

SPARKMAN, O. David, Zelda E. PETON and Fulton G. KITSON. *Gas Chromatography and Mass Spectrometry. A Practical Guide* Burlington, MA: Elsevier, 2011.

SPITZER, Giselher. *Doping in der DDR. Ein historischer Überblick zu einer konspirativen Praxis.* Cologne: Sportverlag Strauß, 1998.

SPITZER, Giselher, Erik EGGERS, Holger J. SCHNELL and Yasmin WISNIEWSKA. *Siegen um Jeden Preis. Doping in Deutschland: Geschichte, Recht, Ethik 1972-1990.* Cologne: Verlag Die Werkstatt, 2013.

STANLEY, Theodore H., Talmage D. EGAN and Hugo VAN AKEN. "A Tribute to Dr. Paul A.J. Janssen: Entrepreneur Extraordinaire, Innovative Scientist, and Significant Contributor to Anaesthesiology." *Anesthesia & Analgesia* 106, no. 2 (2008): 451-462.

STOKVIS, Ruud. "Moral Entrepreneurship and Doping Cultures in Sport." (ASSR Working Paper 03/04: 6); http://dare.uva.nl/document/2264 [accessed June 16, 2013].

TÄNNSJÖ, Torbjörn. "Commentary." *Journal of Medical Ethics* 3, no. 2 (2005): 113.

TAYLOR, Claire, and Gwyn WILLIAMS. eds. *King's College London. Contributions to biomedicine a continuing story.* King's College London: London, 2006.

TEICHLER, Hans Joachim. "Doping in der Endphase der DDR und im Prozess der Wende 1898/90." In *Hormone und Hochleistung. Doping in Ost und West*, edited by Klaus LATZEL and Lutz NIETHAMMER, 139-150. Berlin: Böhlau, 2008.

TITTEL, Kurt, and Howard G. KNUTTGEN. "The development, objectives and activities of the International Federation of Sports Medicine (FIMS)." In *The Olympic Book of Sports Medicine*, edited by. Albert DIRIX, Howard G. KNUTTGEN and Kurt TITTEL, 7-12. Oxford: Blackwell, 1988.

"The 80 years of Dr. Messerli. Ardent Disciple of Coubertin," *Olympic Review* 9 (1968): 225.

"The Best Organization." *Olympic Review* 45 (1988): 103-104.

"The Biographies of all IOC members, No. 99 Johannes Sigfrid Edström." *Journal of Olympic History* 18, no. 3 (2010): 43.

"The Biographies of all IOC members, No. 119 José Joaquim Ferreira Santos." *Journal of Olympic History* 18, no. 3 (2010): 54.

"The Biographies of all IOC members, No. 133 Comte Alberto Bonacossa." *Journal of Olympic History* 19, no. 1 (2011): 65.

"The Biographies of all IOC members, No. 149 Karl Ferdinand Ritter von Halt." *Journal of Olympic History* 19, no. 2 (2011): 45.

"The Biographies of all IOC members, No. 162 David George Lord Burghley." *Journal of Olympic History* 19, no. 2 (2011): 51.

"The Biographies of all IOC members, No. 168 Lord Arthur Espie Porritt." *Journal of Olympic History* 19, no. 3 (2011): 55.

"The Biographies of all IOC members, No. 172 Avery Brundage." *Journal of Olympic History* 19, no. 3 (2011): 57.

"The Biographies of all IOC members, No. 194 Josef Gruss." *Journal of Olympic History* 20, no. 1 (2012): 57.

"The Biographies of all IOC members, No. 221 Ryotaro Azuma." *Journal of Olympic History* 20, no. 2 (2012): 69.

"The Biographies of all IOC members. No. 223 Jean Bonnin de la Bonninière Count de Beaumont." *Journal of Olympic History* 20, no. 2 (2012): 70.

"The Biographies of all IOC members, No. 236 Agustin Arturo Sosa." *Journal of Olympic History* 20, no.3 (2012): 66.

"The Biographies of all IOC members, No. 262 Árpád Csánadi." *Journal of Olympic History* 2, no. 1 (2013): 63.

"The Biographies of all IOC members, No. 306 Dr. Eduardo Hay." *Journal of Olympic History* 22, no. 1 (2014): 60.

"The Executive Board met on 19th and 20th June." *Olympic Review* 309-310 (1993): 301-304.

THE PARLIAMENT OF THE COMMONWEALTH OF AUSTRALIA. *Drugs in Sport. An Interim Report of the Senate Standing Committee on Environment, Recreation and the Arts.* Canberra: Australian Government Publishing Service, 1989.

THE SPORTS COUNCIL. *The Fourth Permanent World Conference on Anti-Doping in Sport.* London: The Sports Council with the International Olympic Committee, 1993.

THEVIS, Mario. *Mass Spectrometry in Sports Drug Testing.* New Jersey: Wiley, 2010.

THYSSEN, Svenja. *Manfred Donike und das Institut für Biochemie der Deutschen Sporthochschule Köln - Geschichte und Leistung im Kampf gegen Doping.* Diploma thesis, Deutsche Sporthochschule Köln.

TODD, Jan, and Terry TODD. "Significant Events in the History of Drug Testing and the Olympic Movement: 1960-1999." In *Doping in Elite Sport: The Politics of Drugs in the Olympic Movement,* edited by Wayne WILSON and Edward DERSE, 65-128. Champaign, Illinois: Human Kinetics, 2001.

TODD, Terry. "Anabolic steroids: the Gremlins of Sport." *Journal of Sport History* 14 (1987): 87-107.

TODD, Terry. "A History of the Use of Anabolic Steroids in Sport." In *Sports and Exercise Science: Essays in the History of Sports Medicine,* edited by Jack W. BERRYMAN and Roberta J. PARK, 319-350. Urbana: University of Illinois Press, 1992.

TORRES, Cesar R., and Mark DYRESON. "The Cold War Games." In *Global Olympics. Historical and Sociological Studies of the Modern Games,* edited by Kevin YOUNG and Kevin B. WAMSLEY, 59-82. Bingley: JAI Press, 2007.

TOUCHSTONE, Joseph C. "History of Chromatography." *Journal of Liquid Chromatography* 16, no. 8 (1993): 1647-1665.

UNGERLEIDER, Steven. *Faust's Gold. Inside the East German Doping Machine.* New York, NY: St. Martin's Press, 2001.

VENERANDO, Antonio. "Italian Experiments on the Pathology of Doping and Ways to Control It." *Appendix to Council of Europe for Out-of-School Education, Doping of Athletes: Reports of the Special Working Parties*, 47-53. Strasbourg: Council of Europe, 1964.

VETTENNIEMI, Erkki. "Runners, Rumours, and Reaps of Representations: An Inquiry into Drug Use by Athletes in the 1920s." *Journal of Sport History* 37, no. 3 (2010): 415-430.

VOY, Robert, and Kirk D. DEETER. *Drugs, Sports and Politics.* Champaign, Ill: Leisure Press, 1991.

WADDINGTON, Ivan. "The Development of Sports Medicine." *Sociology of Sport Journal* 13 (1996): 176-196.

WADDINGTON, Ivan, and Andy SMITH. *Sport, Health and Drugs: A Critical Sociological Perspective.* London: Taylor & Francis, 2000.

WALLECHINSKY, David, and Jaime LOUCKY. *The Complete Book of the Winter Olympics: The Vancouver 2010 Edition.* Vancouver: Greystone Books, 2009.

WASSONG, Stephan. " 'Clean Sport:' A Twofold Challenge in the Contemporary History of the Modern Olympic Games." In *Pathways: Critiques and Discourse in Olympic Research. Ninth International Symposium for Olympic Research*, edited by Robert K. BARNEY, Michael K. HEINE, Kevin B. WAMSLEY and Gordon H. MACDONALD, 84-93. London, Ontario: International Centre for Olympic Studies, 2008.

"Wer war für die Doping-Kontrolle 1976 verantwortlich?" *Chemiereport* 8 (2010): 51.

WISE, Aaron N., and Bruce S. MEYER. *International Sports Law and Business.* The Hague: Kluwer Law International, 1997.

"What other People say." *Bulletin du Comité International Olympique* 53 (1956): 65-66.

WORLD ANTI-DOPING AGENCY. "Laboratory Expert Group," 2015; https://www.wada-ama.org/en/who-we-are/governance/ laboratory-expert-group [accessed January 19, 2015].

WORLD ASSOCIATION OF ANTI-DOPING SCIENTISTS. "Who We Are," 2013; http://waads.org/about-us-welcome-message [accessed January 11, 2015].

WRYNN, Alison. "The Human Factor: Science, Medicine and the International
    Olympic Committee, 1900–70." *Sport in Society: Cultures, Commerce,
    Media, Politics* 7, no. 2 (2004): 211-231.

"XV Olympic Winter Games. Inventory of the Records of the Operations Group,
    Part   III."   *City   of   Calgary*;   http://www.calgary.ca/CA/city-
    clerks/Documents/88olympics/operation_inventory_pt3.pdf?noredirect=
    1 [accessed July 13, 2014].

ZOJER,   Karl.   "Eindeutige   Aussagen   zu   komplexen   Fragestellungen."
    Chemiereport 5 (2010): 36-37.

TABLES

Table 1: Index of Selected Persons

Name	Country	Biographical Data
Beckett, Arnold	Great Britain	1920 - 2010
Catlin, Don	USA	1938
Challis, Bruce	Canada	1930
Daly, Anthony	USA	1933 - 2008
Danz, Max	FRG	1908 - 2000
Dirix, Albert	Belgium	1914 - 1999
Donike, Manfred	FRG	1933 - 1995
Dugal, Robert	Canada	1942 - 2003
Fitch, Kenneth	Australia	1932
Grashinskaya, Nina	USSR	1919 - 2008
Hanley, Daniel	USA	1916 - 2001
Hay, Eduardo	Mexico	1915 - 2005
Hollmann, Wildor	FRG	1925
Höppner, Manfred	GDR	1934
Howald, Hans	Switzerland	1937
La Cava, Giuseppe	Italy	1908 - 1988
Laurin, Carroll	Canada	1928
Ljungqvist, Arne	Sweden	1931
Keul, Joseph	FRG	1932 - 2000
Kuroda, Yoshio	Japan	1925
Mérode, Alexandre de	Belgium	1934 - 2002
Park, Jong Sei	Republic of Korea	1943
Porritt, Arthur	New Zealand	1900 - 1994
Prokop, Ludwig	Austria	1920
Rogozkin, Viktor	USSR	1928
Schamasch, Patrick	France	1947
Schänzer, Wilhelm	FRG	1951
Segura, Jordi	Spain	1949
Semenov, Vitaly	USSR	1937
Venerando, Antonio	Italy	1923 - 1990
Van Rossum, Jacques	Netherlands	1930
Vorobiev, Grigory	USSR	1929

Table 2: Index of IOC and IAAF Anti-Doping Bodies

Name	Year of Existence
IOC Doping Subcommittee	1961 - 1967
IOC Medical Commission	1967 -
IAAF Medical Advisory Panel	1970 - 1972
IAAF Doping Working Group	1970 - 1972
IAAF Medical Committee	1972 -
IAAF Working Group on Anabolic Steroids	1976
IAAF Anti-Doping Subcommittee	1976
Scientific Committee of the IOC Medical Commission	1976 - 1980
IAAF Doping Subcommittee	1977 - 1990
IOC "doping control sub-committee"	never in existence
IOC Subcommission on Doping and Biochemistry	1980 -
IAAF Doping Commission	1991 -

Table 3: Index of Accredited Anti-Doping Laboratories (1979-1992)

City	Country[1]	First accreditation	Head of Lab at time of accreditation
London	Great Britain	1979	Arnold Beckett
Cologne	FRG	1979	Manfred Donike
Montreal	Canada	1979	Robert Dugal
Leningrad	Soviet Union	1979	Viktor Rogozkin
Kreischa	GDR	1979	Claus Clausnitzer
Magglingen	Switzerland	1981	Hans Howald
Moscow	USSR	1982	Vitaly Semenov
Prague	Czechoslovakia	1983	Ruzena Slechtova
Tokyo	Japan	1985	Junichi Fukuda
Madrid	Spain	1983	Cecilia Rodriguez
Sarajevo	Yugoslavia	1984	Branko Nikolin
Los Angeles	USA	1983	Don Catlin
Rome	Italy	1983	Felice Rosati
Brisbane	Australia	1984	Les Johnson
Paris	France	1985	Jean-Pierre Lafarge
Huddinge/ Stockholm	Sweden	1985	Ingemar Bjorkhem
Helsinki	Finland	1983	Kimmo Kuoppasalmi
Nijmegen	Netherlands	1985	Jacques van Rossum
Barcelona	Spain	1986	Jordi Segura
Indianapolis	USA	1987	Carlton Nordschow
Zagreb	Yugoslavia	1987	Slobodan Rendic
Lisbon	Portugal	1987	Lesseps Lourenço Reys
Calgary	Canada	1987	Siu Chan
Seoul	Republic of Korea	1987	Moon Hi Han/ Jong Sei Park
Oslo	Norway	1988	Nils Norman/ Peter Hemmersbach
Sydney	Australia	1989	Rymantas Kazlauskas
Beijing	China	1989	Tong Hui Zhou/ Zeyi Yang

[1] Country name at the time of accreditation.

Athens	Greece	1990	John Kiburis
Ghent	Belgium	1991	Michiel Debackere
Lausanne	Switzerland	1992	Laurent Rivier
Copenhagen	Denmark	1992	Henrik Olsen

INDEX

CPSIA information can be obtained at www.ICGtesting.com
Printed in the USA
BVOW05s0613170216

437041BV00001B/3/P